# THE ATHLETE'S DILEMMA

# THE ATHLETE'S DILEMMA

## *Sacrificing Health for Wealth and Fame*

## John Weston Parry

ROWMAN & LITTLEFIELD
Lanham • Boulder • New York • London

Published by Rowman & Littlefield
A wholly owned subsidiary of The Rowman & Littlefield Publishing Group, Inc.
4501 Forbes Boulevard, Suite 200, Lanham, Maryland 20706
www.rowman.com

Unit A, Whitacre Mews, 26-34 Stannary Street, London SE11 4AB

Cover images (top, left to right) © iStock.com/KatarzynaBialasiewicz; iStock.com/Giorez; iStock.com/sofiaworld; iStock.com/lumelabidas; iStock.com/Poutnik; iStock.com/maska82. Pill © iStock.com/Just2shutter. Needle © iStock.com/Rtimages.

British Library Cataloguing in Publication Information Available

**Library of Congress Cataloging-in-Publication Data**

Names: Parry, John Weston, 1948– author.
Title: The athlete's dilemma : sacrificing health for wealth and fame / John Weston Parry.
Description: Lanham, Maryland : Rowman & Littlefield, 2017. | Includes bibliographical references and index.
Identifiers: LCCN 2016045936 (print) | LCCN 2017010641 (ebook) | ISBN 9781442275409 (hardback : alk. paper) | ISBN 9781442275416 (electronic)
Subjects: LCSH: Sports—Physiological aspects. | Sports injuries—Moral and ethical aspects. | Athletes—Health and hygiene—United States. | Athletes—Drug use—United States. | Doping in sports—United States. | Risk taking (Psychology)
Classification: LCC RC1235 .P37 2017 (print) | LCC RC1235 (ebook) | DDC 617.1/027—dc23
LC record available at https://lccn.loc.gov/2016045936

∞ ™ The paper used in this publication meets the minimum requirements of American National Standard for Information Sciences Permanence of Paper for Printed Library Materials, ANSI/NISO Z39.48-1992.

Printed in the United States of America

# CONTENTS

# PREFACE

**S**ports have provided me with a lifetime of enjoyment. My father, who grew up in the New York area, imprinted the pleasures of being a two-sport Giants fan, even after "our" baseball team moved to San Francisco in 1958. My baseball loyalty was cemented as a young child when the Giants swept the Cleveland Indians in the 1954 World Series. I still remember—spurred on by many replays—Willie Mays's famous over-the-shoulder catch and throw on Vic Wertz's blast to center field. I shared those precious moments with my dad, staring at shadowy images on a thirteen-inch black-and-white television set, listening to the eloquent play-by-play of Russ Hodges that only this languid game could engender. Little did I know that it would be fifty-six years until the Giants would win the World Series again, again, and again. Unpredictability is the magic of sports.

My first memorable experience with professional football was on December 28, 1958. My father and I listened to a transistor radio in Central Park, while playing catch, because the telecast had been blacked out in the New York area. Our Giants lost in "sudden death" to the Baltimore Colts in the championship that is considered by many to be the best ever played. Numerous football Hall of Famers participated, including Johnny Unitas, Frank Gifford, Sam Huff, Vince Lombardi, Tom Landry, Roosevelt Brown, and Emlen Tunnell. Pat Summerall was the Giants' "place-kicker." Yet, the first baseman's mitt my father wore on that chilly day is the far more precious memory. That glove sits on a shelf in our living room next to his ashes.

My professional basketball loyalty was not established until the early 1960s. Dad did not follow the sport, but he, my mother, and stepmother all supported equal opportunity and racial integration throughout my young life. Thus, as an adolescent, I was drawn to the team chemistry that allowed the pretty well-integrated Boston Celtics—led by Bill Russell, Red Auerbach, Sam and K. C. Jones, Bob Cousy, and John Havlicek—to win a multiplicity of championships over opponents with even better individual talent. Team defense, prodigious rebounding, exquisitely blocked shots, long release passes, "stop and pop," Auerbach's victory cigars, and the Celtics' parquet floor became forever etched in my psyche.

For me civil rights were best captured in sports by Paul Robeson, Arthur Ashe, Bill Russell and the Celtics, Willie Mays, and Shirley Povich. I did not fully appreciate Jackie Robinson until some years later, undoubtedly because he was a Dodger and Richard Nixon supporter. As a senior at Lake Forest College in Illinois I wrote my honors thesis on spectator sports in American society. I examined how those sports affected—and were affected by—law, politics, government, and perception. The social upheavals in our major sports, which were still percolating in 1970–1971, presented me with a grand opportunity, although it meant that my thesis became almost book length, if not book quality.

During my college years, I also became a Chicago Blackhawks fan. Hockey was the one major North American professional team sport that I had never followed more than casually. By close proximity and osmosis, however, I soon became captivated with the exploits of Bobby Hull, Stan Mikita, and Tony Esposito. My Blackhawks loyalty, however, did not endure, because in the early 1980s, a new and more engaging proximity made me a fan of Rod Langway and the defense-minded Washington Capitals.

Since law school, I have had a long career in Washington, D.C., focused on mental and physical disability law, disability and health rights, and diversity. My favorite pastimes have involved sports, particularly playing tennis and exploring the outdoors with close friends. Often, though, I have been a stationary spectator enthralled with the "thrill of victory and the agony of defeat."

Since the late 1990s, I have cheered for the Baltimore Orioles—except on the rare occasions when they have played the Giants—mainly because my daughter, Jennifer, became an O's fan as a child. My wife, Elissa, generally dislikes sports, although she will watch women's gymnastics and ice-skating in the Olympics, if it is scheduled conveniently. Elissa strenuously objects, however, when some "stupid" sporting event, particularly a football game, causes a delay or cancellation of a Sunday night television show she enjoys watching. For her, it is the infamous "Heidi" fiasco in reverse.

Elissa's sports animosity reflects an underlying love-hate dichotomy in America, which divides mostly along gender lines. That certainly has been true in my two households—both as a child and a married adult. It has been due not only to the natural inclinations and interests of those involved (Mars versus Venus), but also because, historically, organized sports—Title IX and other civil rights laws notwithstanding—too often have excluded or diminished the roles of girls and women. Fortunately, that type of gender bias has been receding, albeit too slowly.

Love-hate relationships were a part of several psychology courses that I took in college. In those days, psychology was influenced more by humanism and psychoanalysis than brain science, which predominates today. While Freud frequently mentioned the juxtaposition between love and hate, it was the Scottish psychiatrist Ian Dishart Suttie who elevated this fundamental human paradox to a psychological principle in *The Origins of Love and Hate.* [1]

Today, love-hate has both a common and a psychiatric meaning. In the vernacular, love-hate is part of the human chemistry, which—like the Western version of yin and yang—divides our perceptions about persons, objects, or aspects of society. The more familiar version encompasses the feelings and perceptions that many Americans have about organized sports. From a psychiatric perspective, though, love-hate can be viewed as a symptom of a mental condition, including what has been called "borderline personality disorder." [2]

In American society, this sports love-hate dynamic also encompasses what is known as cognitive dissonance. It is that dissonance that allows us to transform antisocial results into victories. Such dissonance is reflected in our reluctance to recognize, appreciate, and accept the destructive influences spectator sports have had on our society, including illicit drug use, concussions, mental illness, and other serious health-related problems. We much prefer to focus on the exhilarating entertainment that our athletic diversions provide us within a world of unsettling changes.

# INTRODUCTION

Health-related public controversies and scandals involving athletes in America's favorite spectator sports have not been limited to football. Similar—albeit often lesser—pathologies have infected baseball, basketball, hockey, soccer, Olympic competitions, tennis, and other popular sports, domestically and internationally. Athletes' health continues to be in jeopardy largely because powerful, revenue obsessed, and too often corrupt leagues and organizations run our most popular sports without any meaningful government oversight.

Whether it is the National Football League (NFL), Major League Baseball (MLB), the National Basketball Association (NBA), the National Hockey League (NHL), Major League Soccer (MLS), the National Collegiate Athletic Association (NCAA), the International Olympic Committee (IOC), the Fédération Internationale de Football Association (FIFA), the International Association of Athletics Federations (IAAF), the International Tennis Federation (ITF), the World Anti-Doping Agency (WADA), or one of their various affiliates, generally these sports cartels are beholden to no one but themselves. They are mostly exempt from federal antitrust and other laws that are supposed to govern corporate enterprises doing business in the United States. These sports entities are treated by governments and politicians as if they exist to serve the public interest, rather than to generate revenue and wealth for their owners, members, or organizers.

As a result, almost no one is protecting the health of elite American athletes who participate in these sports, often recklessly and irresponsibly for the promise or reality of wealth and fame. Instead, these sports cartels perpetuate environments in which such unhealthy risk taking thrives in order to better generate revenues. At the same time, due to myths and misleading perceptions that distort our views about spectator sports, the social impetus to intervene to protect these athletes' health has been greatly diminished, leaving these incubators of destructive behaviors and practices to flourish.

## THE MYTH OF THE OLYMPIC IDEAL AND OTHER SPORTS MISPERCEPTIONS

Myths and beliefs about sports being conduits of high moral values—including healthy competitions, fair play, and selfless amateurism—have established a sometimes impenetrable gap between perceptions and reality. Such shrouded perceptions help obscure the fact that our spectator sports heroes have been and remain a "Faustian bargain. . . . The[ir] . . . ruthless drive, narcissistic focus, [and] competitive obsession . . . are characteristics we'd find repulsive outside athletics."[1] Cognitive dissonance allows us to "keep faith in our games despite a century of evidence suggesting they [often] deserve our wrath."[2]

Beginning with the fragmented accounts of the ancient Olympics and the gladiatorial bread and circuses of Rome, the social and political roles spectator sports have played in supporting and influencing nation-states and community perceptions have been substantial and sometimes profound. Our favorite sports express American culture that millions of people share and revel in. The desire to make money, accumulate power, influence communities, and inculcate values largely explains how spectator sports evolved in the United States into complex and sophisticated commercial enterprises. Yet, that evolution is only part of the story because, in turn, our society has been shaped and influenced—both positively and negatively—by our favorite spectator sports. For much of our history we have uncritically glorified sports—much like religion and the military—as an institution that only promotes virtues and has no overwhelming blemishes.

The late chief justice Earl Warren reportedly embraced—and then went on to symbolize—this sports mythology with his pronouncement that he read the newspaper's sports pages first because they reflected our accomplishments, while the front page was a catalog of our failures.[3] Today, we keep that mythology alive by focusing on those atypical examples in which sports transcend selfish business concerns and practices to be special and morally uplifting—in addition to being extremely engaging and entertaining.

## SPORT: MIRROR OF AMERICAN LIFE

The American view of sports, which in large part was shaped by myths surrounding the modern Olympic ideal, began to change in the early 1960s when historian Robert H. Boyle wrote *Sport: Mirror of American Life.* Boyle revised our basic assumptions by demonstrating that sports, as reflections of what was happening in American society, were no better or worse than the developments in society itself. In his day, sports appeared in many different ways to mirror our society.

While Boyle illustrated with numerous rich examples how organized sports reflected our society in his time, and thus could no longer be viewed as a one-dimensional embodiment of the Olympic ideal, it soon became apparent to subsequent scholars that the nuanced interrelationships between sports and society were multidimensional and multifaceted. The reality was much more like two mirrors reflecting images off each other—the much smaller, yet expanding reflection representing sports and the larger one representing American society.

Due to profound societal and political changes after World War II and during the Cold War that followed, the influences of spectator sports on modern cultures steadily increased throughout the world. This is particularly true in the United States where it has been—and continues to be—the most dominant cultural presence for more than half our population. This fascination with sports encompasses mostly males, but increasingly females are joining the festivities, as well as the pathologies. But all of this may be changing because millennials have found and been given many other things that compete for their attention, especially electronically and virtually.

The America of the early 1960s was vastly different from what exists now, or even what existed during the late 1960s. Boyle's America appeared to be one of hope, economic prosperity, and incremental social progress, as well as relatively tepid social criticisms and insights. In those days, Americans were still in the process of ushering in the Kennedy era of human service, peace, space exploration, and good feelings toward humankind—in part to obscure the growing potential for nuclear catastrophe—so our views about sports were far more sanguine than not, even with their undeniable blemishes. Willie Mays, Mickey Mantle, Sandy Koufax, and Stan Musial were American heroes, and a less segregated, selectively integrated game of baseball was still the all-American sport and overwhelming fan favorite.

Soon after Boyle wrote his book, however, the United States entered a period of civil rights, a disputed war, changing values, expanded drug use, and protests against symbols of authority and inequity that often pitted children against their parents. These social upheavals had a profound impact on—and to a lesser extent were influenced by—spectator sports and athletics. The year 1968 turned out to be the pinnacle of such social unrest and turmoil. It made 2016 look like a walk in the park. Sports played a key role mostly as a dampener, but also on occasion as an instigator of tempestuous changes.

Once the nation had calmed down, many Americans overreacted in response to what had changed or had been threatened with change. The so-called me generation of values became dominant, which highlighted and accelerated for many Americans—whether or not they were direct participants—consumption, accumulation of assets, and corporate excesses. Like many other privileged segments of our society—bankers, stockbrokers, headline entertainers, and CEOs—American athletes, along with movie stars, reflected, represented, and perfected individual entitlements with their high salaries and spoiled affectations accompanied by moral corruption. "Many of our greatest athletic champions [came] from dark, needy places."[4] Spectator sports produced "weasels, scoundrels and lowlifes who would lift the pennies off their dead grandma's eyes."[5]

Moreover, our society was now incubating an obsession with violence and images of violence. Organized professional and major intercollegiate team sports, particularly the new fan favorite of football, often contributed to this unhealthy preoccupation with unbridled aggression. A number of sports, but especially football, became divining rods for those who wanted to exploit violence and greed for their own purposes. Recent times have been darker, less ethical, less principled, and more insecure than Boyle's post–World War II vision of an America that was populated by people who were later praised—and obviously overhyped—as "the greatest generation"[6] and "the best and the brightest."[7]

## THE POSTMODERN ERA AND THE EMERGENCE OF SPORTS CARTELS

Since the end of the twentieth century, the interactions between society and sports have continued to evolve, assimilating key characteristics of what has been aptly described as the postmodern era with the introduction, improvement, and expansion of personal computers; the Internet and instantaneous global communications; the metaphorical "cloud"; artificial intelligence; and virtual realities. Furthermore, in recent decades, psychology has repeatedly demonstrated that individual and group perceptions play a critical role in society, including spectator sports and athletics. Perceptions can be just as—and sometimes much more—influential in determining how human beings react or respond than reality.

That deception has been particularly true in spectator sports where hyperbole, self-promotion, and propaganda have become standard practices, even among many writers who deserve to be called journalists. Instead of Boyle's single mirror analogy, we now have multiple mirrors and a variety of influences, not always rational and almost always somewhat distorted. What is being perceived depends, among other things, on who is doing the viewing, where people stand, which direction they are gazing, what they believe in and are being taught, and what other social and environmental forces are present. In other words, deciphering reality can be a very complicated process.

The interplay of perceptions and beliefs has had a substantial effect on American sports, particularly since the end of the twentieth century, as professional, collegiate, and other elite organized sports have become an increasingly important force in our country's cultural development and identity, as well as meccas of economic opportunity. Spectator sports are both a key part of our other social institutions—particularly the media, television, entertainment, news, the military, and even religion—and a large, somewhat diffused institution in their own right, which can unite, segregate, and variously influence different groups and subcultures.

Under the broad umbrella of spectator sports that Americans follow, most encompass amateur, semiprofessional, and professional athletes; extreme sports; and global extravaganzas, such as the Olympics, Super Bowl, and World Cup. Yet, while the sports choices for American spectators have become far more varied and accessible, the accumulation of money, power, and influence has become concentrated in a few major spectator sports and global events. This has given rise to a number of powerful and influential, self-governing sports organizations, disparaged as cartels, which have been largely beyond the control of national and state governments. Among the most prominent sports cartels with a significant presence in America are the NFL, MLB, NBA, NHL, MLS, NCAA, IOC, FIFA, IAAF, ITF, and WADA.

## HEALTH-RELATED PATHOLOGIES IN OUR MOST POPULAR SPECTATOR SPORTS

These leagues, federations, committees, other organizations, and affiliates in somewhat different ways—both domestically and internationally—promote, change, profit from, control, and tend to corrupt the sports that Americans most like to watch and play. Thus, while generally there has been an extraordinary increase in the popularity and income-generating capacities of these favored sports, it has come with a steep price for those who play these sports, as well as American society. Given the mostly laissez-faire approach to legal regulation and enforcement combined with the unbridled commercialism, greed, and economic exploitation associated with how our most popular spectator sports are run, the fact that disturbing health-related pathologies have taken root and continue to grow worse should not be surprising.

Baseball, basketball, hockey, soccer, Olympic competitions, tennis, and other major sports have all had their well-publicized health-related transgressions and scandals, but our most popular sport of football has engendered the most notoriety. Football is exceptional because it, more than any other American sport, promotes—with essential assists from the NFL and NCAA—a culture of intentional harm and other antisocial attitudes and practices.

What befalls so many elite American male, and increasingly female, athletes—and many more elite athlete hopefuls—in our most popular spectator sports today has become a debilitating paradox. The overwhelming desire to attain the heightened fitness and training they believe is necessary to boost their performances leads athletes to: pain, injuries, and reliance on illicit and potentially harmful drugs while they are participating in their chosen sports; and poor physical and mental health, disability, addiction, and even premature death afterward. Too often these health-related pathologies become incorporated into their paths for success: playing with pain; using drugs to mask pain and speed recovery; relying on drugs and other risky medical interventions to enhance their athletic performances; and enduring repeated concussions and other physical or mental impairments that have long-term and sometimes catastrophic consequences. Making matters worse, the health care treatments and disability benefits that these athletes need to become whole again— or at least to improve—typically are inadequate or nonexistent once they leave or are jettisoned from their sports, unless they have the resources and insight to obtain those essential services themselves.

Many of the unconscionable stories originate in professional football, where careers tend to be shorter and debilitating injuries more prevalent, but these human tragedies befall American athletes in other favored spectator sports as well, both domestically and globally. Part of the problem for many former elite athletes is that they lack the financial acuity, knowledge, and temperament to thrive economically after their playing days end. This is especially problematic if they become addicted to painkillers, dementia sets in, or they become otherwise mentally or emotionally impaired.

Surprisingly, bankruptcy and impoverishment are no idle possibilities, even for the relatively few elite athletes who have successful professional careers. This has happened to athletes in America's favorite spectator sports, including those who played for years in the NFL, NBA, and MLB. Unfortunately, sports stories about financial mismanagement by professional athletes continue to occur on a regular basis. Furthermore, the financial situations for many elite athletes or wannabes, who never have professional careers or have ones that are cut short by injuries or waning or marginal talent, tend to be much worse. Being relatively poor and the long-term severity of a person's physical and mental impairments are closely linked. These two life challenges tend to feed off each other in extremely unhealthy ways.

The human toll can be enormous for athletes who play and fail, or play, fall, and never get back up again. Instead of shooting athletes to put them out of their misery, as happens with racehorses, teams and sports organizations typically push depleted athletes out the door, especially in pro football with the unilateral termination of their contracts and short professional playing careers. On the other side of fame, caveat emptor, free-market principles, good and bad fortune, and charity largely determine whether many former athletes will be able to live in relative comfort or suffer with extreme pain, disability, dementia, addictions, and/or poverty.

There usually is no safety net, and if there is one, it has many holes. Most of these negative health outcomes are pathogenic in the sense that they involve destructive practices and behaviors, which are spread like an infection among elite athletes, their teams, leagues, and sports organizations, and those who try to emulate elite athletes. Some of the worst sports problems are health related.

Those pathologies are allowed—and often encouraged—to breed, in large part, because the leagues, organizations, and federations—including the NFL, NCAA, MLB, NBA, NHL, MLS, IOC, FIFA, IAAF, ITF, WADA, and their affiliates—continue to be much more concerned with wealth and the wealth fame begets, than promoting healthy lifestyles for elite American athletes, or the millions of youngsters who aspire to become elite. These cartel-like entities, controlled or influenced by extremely wealthy corporate entrepreneurs, mostly look the other way or even help facilitate cover-ups, until their short- or long-term profits are jeopardized.

Moreover, increasingly youth sports are being run by people whose primary objective is to find ways, both legal and illegal, to line their pockets. The *New York Times* reported that embezzlement has become a common practice.[8] In addition, too often people connected with youth and high school sports receive money or gifts for unethically steering elite athletes to big-time college football and basketball programs.

At the same time, governments and politicians that should be protecting the health of their constituents allow—and are influenced to allow—these burgeoning sports enterprises to govern themselves with minimal or no regard to the laws that are supposed to apply to everyone else. The U.S. Department of Justice (DOJ) finally taking—or threatening to take—legal action against the widespread global corruption of FIFA and the Russian sports ministry should be viewed as remarkable political exceptions, not the general rule. It was not a coincidence that the DOJ focused on international sports cartels rather than the NFL, MLB, or NCAA.

# Part I

# Pain, Injuries, Drugs, and Team Doctors

# I

# REAL MEN PLAY HURT

## THE SPORTS LORE

Until recently there was near unanimity among male athletes in major professional and intercollegiate sports that to be real men they had to play through pain, even to the point of risking further injury, especially when championships, key rivalries, or other important games were on the line. That attitude still predominates, but with less gusto and universality than in the past. Nevertheless, the sports lore has defined the reality and immortalized certain modern-day athletes as being macho to the *n*th degree.

Former Oakland Raiders safety and football Hall of Fame member Ronnie Lott had part of his finger removed after the 1985 season, so he could avoid missing games while it healed. The lore was that Lott had it chopped off at halftime, so he could play the rest of a key game.

The iconic New York Knicks center Willis Reed appeared in uniform for the beginning of game seven of the 1970 championship, even though he had a badly torn muscle in his leg. That meant he was unable to do much more than bravely hobble around the court. The lore became that Reed had inspired the Knicks to their only NBA title.

Baltimore Orioles baseball legend Cal Ripken played in 2,632 consecutive games from 1982 until 1998, despite numerous nagging and painful injuries along the way. Ripken's bravado, which undoubtedly diluted his daily production, made him a hero to millions of fans and helped to lift baseball out of its work stoppage–inspired doldrums. With only a .276 career batting average, Ripken became a first ballot member of the Hall of Fame, with a higher voting percentage than much greater players, including Babe Ruth, Willie Mays, and Hank Aaron.

## FOOTBALL MENTALITY

Winners play when they are hurt; losers stand or sit on the sidelines. That remains the dominant ethos among elite athletes today, especially in football. As former Oakland Raiders defensive back George Atkinson explained after he retired, in old-school football—which many and perhaps most present-day players and coaches still practice or aspire to—if you held yourself out, you "wouldn't have a job. . . . You played every game and you played every down if you could, hurt or not."[1]

Until recently, the football nomenclature referred to brain concussions as dings in order to indicate that getting one's bell rung was something that most players experience on a regular basis, which should be viewed more as a temporary annoyance than a serious health risk. Former players, including ESPN commentator Mark Schlereth, brag that they had that type of loss of consciousness in almost every game they played in the NFL, sometimes for quarters at a time. Nonetheless, they played on, until their bodies would no longer let them. Schlereth in particular gained notoriety for having endured more than two dozen surgeries over his football lifetime. Playing with pain was a football constant for him and so many others like him.

That hardened—and arguably unenlightened—view still percolates throughout the NFL and collegiate football. In 2013, Washington linebacker London Fletcher acknowledged that he was apt to get his bell rung "a couple of times a game. . . . You see stars . . . and then you're back to normal. . . . It's just the way the game is."[2] Fletcher also admitted that in the 2012 preseason he had "suffered a concussion . . . and that lingering effects . . . bothered him until late in the year." He said nothing about his condition to the team, nor is it likely that anyone, except maybe a trainer, asked. He just continued to play on. In November 2016, Washington's Pro-Bowl tight end Jordan Reed, in light of repeated criticisms that he had become injury prone, claimed he would try to play with torn ligaments that reportedly had completely separated his left shoulder from his collarbone.

Even more irresponsibly, 2014 Super Bowl–winning quarterback Russell Wilson claimed that Reliant Recovery Water, a product that he had invested in, "helped him prevent a concussion" in the NFC Championship Game "after Clay Mathews leveled him." He insisted, even though he clearly had been stumbling around, his balance askew, that the recovery drink had saved him. As one sportswriter warned, Wilson's bravado might "lead to impressionable players misdiagnosing their own concussion."[3]

Ignoring, not diagnosing, minimizing, or self-diagnosing concussions is a continuing danger for athletes. According to Clint Trickett—a young assistant coach who decided to retire from football after receiving a string of concussions as West Virginia's starting quarterback—"It can be easy to hide a concussion. . . . Just keep your mouth shut."[4] In his family, apparently all the boys were expected to play football; quitting for any reason was unacceptable. This attitude still persists among too many fathers and mothers, even with all that is known about football's health risks.

Many of the manly football obsessions of playing hurt were vividly captured in a December 2015 *Sports Illustrated* article about Dallas Cowboy future Hall of Fame tight end Jason Witten. S. L. Price boasted on Witten's behalf that "concussions, sprained joints, a broken jaw—no amount of pain can keep [him] . . . from taking the field. It's just the way he was raised."[5] In this convoluted football world, the worst pain was not playing, rather than having to endure dozens of serious injuries during his football career. That is why he decided to suit up with "high ankle and deltoid sprains in his left leg; a lesser lateral sprain of his right ankle; [and] a Grade 2 sprain of his left MCL." For the Wittens, withstanding pain is a family ethic. His wife, Michelle, supposedly demonstrated her resolve by having two of their four children "without painkillers."[6]

## THE INSANITY OF PLAYOFF HOCKEY

Perhaps in no professional sport has playing hurt been more valued or expected than in the National Hockey League (NHL), particularly during the playoffs. In pursuit of the Stanley Cup, "players treat bruises, breaks, displacements and violent alterations to their facial features . . . as if they were . . . mosquito bites."[7] The movie classic *Slap Shot*, starring Paul

Newman, glorified this attitude, but even that comedy could not fully capture the body-shattering reality of NHL playoff hockey.

In the 2014 playoffs, Tampa Bay center Steven Stamkos returned to the ice a few minutes after being "knocked silly by a knee to the head." In those same playoffs, Patrick Kane played "wearing a brace" after missing the last twelve games of the regular season. In hockey players are celebrated for "skating through pain," and a great deal more, in quest of the Stanley Cup. [8]

The legion of honor goes back to at least 1952 when Montreal Canadiens Hall of Famer Maurice "the Rocket" Richard was "knocked cold . . . in the semifinals . . . but returned . . . to put the series winner past the goalie." In 1964, Toronto Maple Leafs defenseman Bob Baun reportedly broke his leg, but returned during that same game "shot up with Novocain." During the 1998 playoffs, St. Louis Blues defenseman Chris Pronger suffered a "cardiac arrhythmia after he was struck in the chest by a slap shot." Even though he had to be hospitalized and placed on a heart monitor, he was back in the lineup the next day. Ian Laperriere sustained a brain hemorrhage during the 2010 playoffs, but he returned to play a week later once the "bleeding in his brain had stopped and the blood was dry." [9]

Not surprisingly, given its culture, professional hockey has only disdain for those who appear to succumb to injury too easily. In game one of the 1989 finals, Montreal Canadien Claude Lemieux lay prone on the ice, not moving, after having been hit with a hockey stick. Reportedly, his coach, Pat Burns, irked at this unmanly display by one of his own players, told the trainer not to attend to Lemieux's injury. Burns also benched Lemieux for game two, even though the player had a deserved reputation for performing well in big games. [10]

## SLOWLY CHANGING ATTITUDES

Today, most professional athletes in team sports, if asked publicly whether they believe in the core value of playing hurt and with pain, probably would say they do, especially in football and hockey. The expectation or "overriding instinct . . . is to take care of the team, take care of teammates, do whatever it takes to win." [11] Yet, in private, away from the locker room, one might hear more equivocation than in the past. There is a growing awareness that players who put their team before their health are risking their careers and the rewards that accompany those careers. In addition, they may actually be hurting their teams.

As a result, many more professional players and athletes in contact sports, especially football, appear to be retiring early in order to protect themselves from chronic traumatic encephalopathy (CTE) and other crippling injuries, even though they could earn large salaries by continuing to play. Many others take much longer to recover from concussions than in the past. They also tend to be somewhat more open about describing their injuries to medical personnel.

Nevertheless, there remains a strong psychological imperative within the North American athlete culture, which believes overcoming pain and injury is what real men do. Research indicates "that when men's masculinity is challenged, they go to great lengths to be more 'manly' to compensate."[12] This bravado is greatly enhanced among elite athletes, in locker rooms and among fans. "We ask players to play hurt. . . . We make heroes out of those who do and vilify those who do not."[13]

# 2

# TEAMMATES, COACHES, FANS, AND OTHER UNHEALTHY INFLUENCES

## CLINGING TO THE MACHO ETHIC IN CONTACT SPORTS

### Football Players

Even if modern-day athletes try to be reasonable or cautious about injuries, teammates and coaches often try to step in to reestablish a more macho ethic, since those other team members are the ones depending on the athlete to play. In 2009, for instance, a public controversy erupted on the Pittsburgh Steelers when All-Pro and likely Hall of Fame quarterback Ben Roethlisberger was benched with a concussion. His key receiver, Hines Ward, questioned the team's decision,[1] but was criticizing his quarterback implicitly. Ward was not alone. Many athletes, coaches, and fans expressed the view that the quarterback should have manned up and played, even though the Steelers quarterback has long been regarded as one of the toughest players at his position, ever.

A few years earlier, Dallas Cowboys owner Jerry Jones told his future Hall of Fame quarterback Troy Aikman, who had experienced a number of concussions, not to be concerned "'since all the data . . . don't point to any lasting effects . . . from head trauma.'"[2] Aikman chose not to follow that dangerous advice and, perhaps not coincidentally, when he retired became mired in ugly and misleading rumors challenging his sexual manhood.

A similar type of macho nonsense was used to disparage Chicago Bears quarterback Jay Cutler during the 2011 NFC Championship Game. After he sprained his knee and could no longer continue to play effectively, either he or the coaching staff took him out of the game. As a result, Cutler was subjected to unrelenting criticism from many Bears fans and football observers. Even though Caleb Hanie performed extremely well as his replacement, it did not seem to matter much for Cutler's reputation.[3] Football priorities are so skewed in this regard that it seems as if many coaches, teammates, and fans would rather lose with an injured starter than improve their prospects by using a healthier substitute.

### Hockey Players

Not surprisingly, a similar ethos exists in hockey about playing hurt. Canadian studies have revealed that even when physicians diagnose a player with a concussion, hockey coaches will "defy" those doctors. One coach put it this way: "Unless something is broken, I want them out playing."[4] This ethic is so well ingrained in the hockey culture that when players on the two teams that were being studied had concussions they still remained on the ice. Similarly, there is an expectation in hockey that athletes will return to the ice almost immediately after their teeth have been knocked out or broken into stubs, or their head, face, or other body parts have been sewn up with stitches.

New concussion protocols are supposed to prevent these types of decisions from being made by the athletes themselves or by their teammates or coaches, but only with regard to head injuries. Furthermore, particularly in important games, players, assisted by their teams, still find ways to elude or evade medical common sense, while teammates and coaches push them to play hurt. Playing hurt is still what a loyal teammate is expected to do. And too often even the doctors and medical staff look the other way, defer to management, or hand out addictive pain medication as if it were aspirin.

### Coaches

Players are not the only ones to suffer from unhealthy practices. Coaches are subject to maladies as well due to the long hours and other stressful demands of their jobs. In college basketball, for example, "yelling is a way of life," which means many coaches do "permanent damage" to their vocal cords.[5] In addition, that constant yelling is extremely stressful, which takes a different toll on their health. Not surprisingly, those coaches tend to neglect their stress-infused health needs during the season, which increasingly is almost all year long. It is only when they physically collapse, like Golden State Warriors head coach Steve Kerr or Duke's Coach K have done in recent basketball seasons, that these coaches are apt to seek or receive medical assistance.

NFL coaches also are famous for placing their jobs before their health. Gary Kubiak and John Fox both experienced serious heart problems in the middle of the 2013 season. Fox returned to coach the Denver Broncos in the Super Bowl. Kubiak was fired at the end of the season but replaced Fox in Denver, becoming the winning coach in the 2016 Super Bowl.

Given the extreme pressure that coaches continue to place on themselves, it is not surprising that they expect their players to endure pain and discomfort and perform when they are hurt. This is part of the culture of professional and major collegiate sports teams. Those who are viewed as winners are given more slack; those branded as losers are more likely to be thrown to the proverbial wolves when they are absent during critical games. Furthermore, coaches are paid for winning now and thus have a vested interest in pushing their athletes to play hurt if it will—or appears likely to—improve their team's performance.

Perhaps the most glaring example of this type of obsessive behavior in coaching occurred in English professional soccer when the manager of Chelsea suspended the team doctor and her assistant in 2015 for racing onto the field to treat a hurt player at an inopportune moment. Chelsea's manager called the medical staff "'naïve' . . . saying they needed to 'understand the game [situation].' . . . He . . . was 'sure' [the player] had merely been tired, not hurt."[6] Somehow the manager had developed a unique ability to competently assess a player's condition from a relatively long distance without medical training. Similar coaching arrogance is on display in the NFL notwithstanding the new injury protocols.

## Changing Attitudes Slowly

Money, financial advisers, and lawyers may be changing that recklessness somewhat, but not quickly. Today, business and other outside influences help inform this issue of playing with pain and injury, especially in basketball and to a lesser extent baseball, which are not quite as invested in the macho culture, especially because they have so many star athletes who are moneymaking machines. Those celebrated athletes are more apt to protect their long-term financial security by shielding their bodies.

In addition, agents and loved ones, who have financial and emotional investments in those athletes, are more likely to warn them not to play injured. Even in football and hockey, superstar players, such as Roethlisberger and the Pittsburgh Penguins Sidney Crosby, respectively, tend to be more cautious than in the past. They realize that they have to look out for themselves, since others won't necessarily do so. For lesser players, though, who are competing to make or stay on their teams, playing injured becomes more a matter of career survival.

## CASE KEENUM AND THE NFL'S CONCUSSION AND SAFETY PROTOCOLS

In November 2015, Case Keenum, a backup quarterback—who due to an injury to the starter, Sam Bradford, played for the then St. Louis Rams— was rendered senseless when his head slammed into the turf. After trying to stand, his legs buckled.[7] In responding with what was supposed to represent the NFL's new concussion protocols, the trainer came onto the field and took a quick look at the player, but Keenum was not removed from the game. Clearly, this was inconsistent with the NFL's stated protocol. Almost everyone watching in person or on television thought— incorrectly as it turned out—that it was a blatant violation of the new policy, except for the Rams' coaching and medical staff, who had other priorities.

While this incident said a great deal about how the NFL continues to deal with concussions, it also was relevant to discussions about how the league and its teams practice health and safety. Sally Jenkins of the *Washington Post* blasted the league for forcing its players to make the decision whether to stay in the game, rather than stepping in to protect them when they are injured. This is all part of an unfortunate pattern in which the NFL "shift[s] liability . . . when it comes to player health and safety." Thus, one of the league's lawyers advised "woozy players not to 'hide their symptoms.'" In addition, the NFL employs a selfish double standard. It fines players for hitting their opponents in ways that are deemed inappropriate but "forgiv[es] coaches, trainers, and team doctors who turn a blind eye and leave players in the game to exacerbate their original injury."[8]

Ultimately, liability in the NFL—or its avoidance—tends to be defined by a player's contract, the collective bargaining agreement, and/or civil laws. Not surprisingly, when it comes to injuries and their treatment, all of these factors generally favor economic interests of the owners over the health of the players.

## IN BASKETBALL AND BASEBALL: A SOMEWHAT DIFFERENT VIBE

Due to this long-established ethic of playing hurt, there also have been publicly aired suspicions, and largely unsupported accusations, in the sports media that certain highly paid athletes have used phantom or exaggerated injuries to avoid playing when they are trying to leave a team or after they have signed large no-cut contracts. Derrick Rose, the once-beloved All-Star point guard for the Chicago Bulls, received constant criticism in 2013 for not returning to compete in the playoffs after going through an extended period of recovery and rehabilitation from surgery. Although "in the real world, playing hurt is stupid," many fans in Chicago thought Rose should have taken the risk and participated in the playoffs.[9] As it turned out, Rose's concerns were legitimate. Due to those very real injuries, Rose has not come close to regaining his basketball brilliance.

In baseball several years ago, the Washington Nationals Stephen Strasburg was roundly criticized, along with the team's general manager, for not objecting demonstratively enough when the player was directed to sit down in the playoffs. The GM had placed a strict limitation on the number of innings Strasburg would be allowed to pitch after returning from Tommy John arm surgery. John Feinstein, writing in the *Washington Post*, called "the decision to shut down . . . Strasburg . . . a debacle [and] disaster" that cost the team a "chance to win a World Series" both in 2012 and 2013.[10] That sentiment remains even today.

Yet, for Washington sports fans, Feinstein's well-received criticism turned out to be dripping in irony. That same year the city's professional football team chose to throw caution to the wind in dealing with its franchise player's health during the playoffs. In the process the presumed superstar quarterback-to-be, Robert Griffin, sustained a severe leg injury that significantly diminished his most prized football ability—to run extraordinarily fast—and contributed to his agonizing downfall in Washington.

# 3

# RG3'S PAINFUL STAY IN WASHINGTON

In 2012, football-related decisions that led to needless injuries to Washington's rookie phenom Robert Griffin III (RG3) created a chaotic and tempestuous relationship with his first professional head coach, two-time Super Bowl champion Mike Shanahan. Griffin's cautionary tale helped to incrementally change the ways in which the media, the public, teams, and athletes now speak about and react to the issue of playing with injuries. Intimate details about Griffin's medical situation were scrutinized in an often irrational media frenzy, much of it of the quarterback's own making.

## A GLORIOUS BEGINNING

RG3 began his football career in Washington under the tutelage of Shanahan and the head coach's son Kyle, who was the offensive coordinator. Many football commentators thought Griffin had the potential to become the type of football star and national celebrity who surfaces only once or twice in a generation. In order to get him, Washington had traded a handful of high draft picks to the (Los Angeles–bound) St. Louis Rams.

Despite the hype, Griffin proved to be a young quarterback with a good, but far from great, NFL arm in terms of touch and delivery, who appeared to be making many decent football decisions on the field. What he did possess was a unique ability to run faster and more elusively than anyone else in recent memory, and perhaps in football history at his position. He also was a marketing and promotional jewel: well spoken, intelligent, of color, and overtly Christian with military roots. Unfortunately, his two greatest strengths—the ability to run fast and to market himself—would become his greatest liabilities.

When he was drafted second out of the not yet highly regarded—nor scandalized—Baylor University football program, RG3 was viewed by most sports commentators as being just a smidgen behind Andrew Luck from Stanford, the other supposed once-in-a-generation quarterback, who had been drafted first. Yet, both by his own design and personal charisma, Griffin became the number one NFL media darling among the newly drafted players that year, easily surpassing Luck, who appeared to be resolute on learning how to play quarterback at an elite professional level. Almost immediately RG3 joined Peyton Manning and Tom Brady as one of the most visible and commercially valuable football commodities. He also endeared himself to the mercurial owner of Washington's football team, Dan Snyder, who seemed to be treating Griffin more like a special celebrity friend than a player.

Through training camp, the preseason, and the first four games, everything RG3 did appeared to be remarkable, both on and off the football field. Almost immediately he had become one of the most hyped players in the league. As a quarterback, who could run around linemen and linebackers as if they were standing still and was faster than almost every cornerback and safety, Griffin appeared to be an unstoppable force and threat to score each time he touched the football, which, at his position, was on almost every offensive play.

## TROUBLE IN PARADISE

The first troubling injury in his meteoric rise to fame occurred in a loss to the Atlanta Falcons early in October, when he was knocked unconscious while trying to elude defenders on one of his soon-to-be-famous cheetah-like sprints for large chunks of yardage. Although he had to be taken out of the game and did not return, the way his team described him as just being "shaken up,"[1] and not concussed, raised red flags. This parsing of words was significant because by then players who had suffered a diagnosed concussion were likely to be prohibited from returning for at least a game, whereas they could return almost immediately if no concussion was specifically identified.

The NFL felt that the presumed deception, which had become public, was serious enough to warrant fining Washington's team $20,000. By league standards this was a relatively paltry sum, but unusual because it had been levied against a team rather than a player. A couple of days later, however, despite Griffin's concussion symptoms, a league neurologist, as well as team officials, including Coach Shanahan, cleared Griffin to practice and to play the next game.[2]

Yet, there were lingering suspicions and concerns about Griffin because his symptoms had involved a brain injury, which, even in the non-journalistic sports media, was now being viewed as potentially serious, particularly if the player had been concussed previously. As one neurologist explained, even with a "'mild' concussion . . . the brain remains vulnerable."[3] By then everyone in the game of professional football, including the athletes and coaches, understood that those who revealed a loss of consciousness probably would be benched for at least another game after that type of injury had occurred. Multiple concussions were viewed as far more serious and could lead to several games out, which already had happened to no less a player than Ben Roethlisberger.

In the NFL, until fairly recent rule changes were made, quarterbacks were particularly vulnerable to these head injuries, many of which were never identified. In the past, huge defensive linemen or other blitzing behemoths could maul quarterbacks to their hearts' content as the crowds roared their approval. Nevertheless, even with modern quarterback protections, Griffin was particularly vulnerable in two respects.

First, as one former head coach remarked, RG3's running "skills are dazzling and effective, but . . . they're also dangerous."[4] Being elusive meant that every time he left the protected area known as the "pocket" and began to run, he became fair game for his opponents, as long as they did not obviously target his head. Second, even for a quarterback, Griffin's risk was magnified because by NFL standards he had a thin body frame, which appeared less able to absorb as much physical punishment as the bigger men he played against.

A few years earlier, former Washington quarterback Trent Green had to make a decision similar to Griffin's about placing his body and mental faculties in jeopardy, if he continued to play with reckless abandon. In 2007, even after sitting out half a season from a concussion, upon his return Green continued to marginalize the risks.[5] That was—and to a large extent continues to be—the culture of professional football and the one that Griffin grew up with as an athlete both in high school and college.

All-Pro Chicago Bears linebacker Brian Urlacher glibly acknowledged that "he would lie to cover up a concussion."[6] Good medicine, especially when concussions are involved, depends on patients being honest and feeling comfortable in reporting symptoms to their physicians, trainers, and coaches. This often is difficult, if not impossible, to do in the NFL, and in college and high school football as well.

## PLAYING INJURED

For a number of weeks, Griffin and his team employed an evasive strategy similar to what Green had used, and he continued to dazzle the NFL with his athletic gifts. RG3 had an opportunity to defy the odds and, for the first time in many years, lead Washington to a division title. The quarterback, however, had sustained what was publicly described as a grade 1 sprain of his lateral collateral ligaments.[7] Thus, the ongoing story for the rest of the season would be whether Griffin's health could be further jeopardized if he played, and even if it would, should he play anyway?

Washington was fortunate to have backup quarterback Kirk Cousins, another rookie, who played well when he had substituted for Griffin, helping the team beat the eventual Super Bowl champion Baltimore Ravens. Nevertheless, the media consensus was that as good as Cousins was on that particular occasion, making the playoffs would be unlikely if Griffin did not play. Griffin continually downplayed his leg injury, distinguishing it from the far more serious anterior collateral ligament (ACL) injury he had sustained in college.

Coach Shanahan shamelessly described it as a "mild sprain."[8] Against the less than mediocre Cleveland Browns, Griffin sat on the sidelines, while Cousins again led the team to victory. RG3 returned for the next two games and Washington won both contests and the division title. Griffin performed reasonably well, despite his obvious leg impairment, which was depriving him of the blazing sprinter's speed that had separated him from all the other quarterbacks in the league.

Despite his injury, the decision to use Griffin in the playoffs against Seattle was mostly viewed in Washington and elsewhere, among fans and the media, as worth the risk, at least before the game had been played. Unfortunately, as often seems to happen with injured players, the long-term risks were much worse than most fans understood or the team had disclosed. This type of secrecy and deception are typical of how old-school professional football is still handled in the NFL.

Bill Belichick has been the apparent puppet master of this strategic, but devious, ploy. His extreme lack of transparency as the head coach of the New England Patriots was—and continues to be—emulated because Belichick, a virtual lock for the football Hall of Fame, already had coached in five Super Bowls, winning three, and had been named NFL Coach of the Year three times. Perceived success typically breeds imitation, especially in professional sports.

Shanahan, Griffin, and the team—sometimes in different ways—tried to obscure what was actually wrong with the quarterback, using carefully worded descriptions of Griffin's status that appeared to be misleading at best. In hindsight, the decision to let the quarterback play in the playoffs was shortsighted, both as a football strategy and for the player's safety. Given what was revealed later about his injury, there should have been very little reason to think starting Griffin over Cousins would increase the chances for victory. In fact, the opposite appears to have been true. With respect to that one game, however, it really did not matter much which Washington quarterback played, because Seattle clearly was the superior team.

Making matters much worse, Washington's risk taking was soon transformed into a debacle when RG3 aggravated his leg injury during the game but still was allowed to play in a pretty much hopeless cause. Griffin's unnecessary bravado resulted in a severe ACL injury, which would have serious implications for his career and Washington's franchise. Because Griffin had suffered the same injury to the same leg in college, there were legitimate concerns that his leg impairment would become a long-term vulnerability and substantially diminish his talent.

## THE AFTERMATH

What actually happened, who was to blame, and what the likely impact would be on RG3's football career became murky as all the involved parties tried to shield themselves from criticism. Throughout his surgery and rehabilitation, the key decision makers—Shanahan, the team physician, and Griffin himself—changed their stories in different self-serving ways. The evolving popular consensus was that "the determination whether Griffin should keep playing . . . was made by Griffin himself, an overeager 22-year old rookie. And no one stopped him."[9] The only aspect of the story that all three of the principles could readily agree on was the one thing none of them could possibly have known: that there would be minimal impact on the quarterback's career, which, if it turned out to be true, meant there would be considerably less blame for them to share.

Part of the reason why the RG3 situation became so controversial and contentious was its juxtaposition with how the Washington Nationals had handled the reasonably comparable situation with their franchise pitcher. After Stephen Strasburg came back from Tommy John surgery on the elbow of his pitching arm, the team had acted cautiously—with little thought to any strategic playoff implications—by predetermining how many innings he would be allowed to pitch during the 2011 season. They were not anticipating a stellar regular season.

Thus, even though the team unexpectedly made the playoffs, the Nationals shut Strasburg down as promised, lost in the first round, and were roundly criticized. Later, Nationals manager Davey Johnson opined that "you do what's best . . . with an eye on tomorrow. Look at RGIII. They shouldn't have played him because they weren't looking at tomorrow."[10]

Two aspects about Griffin's ACL injury became readily apparent, even before any meaningful judgment could be reached about its ultimate impact on the quarterback and the franchise. First and perhaps foremost, no one involved in the decision-making process was willing to take responsibility for allowing Griffin to continue to play. This strongly supported the contention that new lines of responsibility should be drawn in the NFL, which would place the ultimate responsibility on the team and the league to protect the players. Griffin publicly proclaimed that the lack of clearly defined lines of authority resulted in the knee injury that required surgery.[11] Second, there was no indication that the team, particularly its head coach, had learned much from the experience, much less would assume responsibility. [12]

The 2013 season turned out to be a major disappointment for the Washington football team and Griffin, who clearly had less mobility. He lost the one attribute that had made him perform like an elite professional quarterback. After winning the division the year before, Washington finished last with a 3–13 record. The once-presumptive perennial All-Pro, who had been viewed as a consensus can't-miss superstar, became an uncertainty going forward. For a franchise that had given up so many draft choices, including two first-round picks to select him, the setback was stunning, but only a foreshadowing of what was to come.

Coach Shanahan was fired, a new coach was hired, and Griffin immediately promised that for the upcoming 2014 season he would take off the leg brace that had been protecting his knee. Griffin implied that he hoped to proceed on his road to superstardom, as if nothing had happened the past two years. By 2015, however, Griffin was benched; Kirk Cousins, his understudy, had become the starting quarterback; and Griffin, because of his rich contract, could not even be traded.

In addition, the former superstar-to-be somehow had evolved into one of the least liked players in the NFL among his peers. In part this was because he was perceived as being egotistical and the owner's favorite son. Also, he was viewed by some as being too "white" in his marriage, demeanor, and political preferences for a black man in a league dominated by African Americans.

Whatever the reasons, though, the Griffin brand had experienced a complete collapse after he, by playing injured, placed himself at heightened risk unnecessarily. In addition, for its cavalier and devious disregard for Griffin's health, Washington's football team had little to show for all those high draft picks it had sent to the Rams. Furthermore, the team would have to hire a new, inexperienced head coach. Making matters worse, there was the tantalizing possibility that Griffin might be signed, with no compensation to Washington, by those same Rams, who had just moved to Los Angeles. As it turned out, though, Griffin went to the lowly Cleveland Browns, who had recently cut ties with their emotionally troubled quarterback, Johnny Manziel.

# 4

# THE PITFALLS OF TEAM-DIRECTED MEDICAL CARE

**A**n overriding issue underlying the Griffin affair was how his situation related to the medical care NFL teams provide to their athletes. The accumulating evidence indicates that throughout the major professional leagues—especially in the NFL and NHL where deliberate bodily violence is an accepted component of the competition—health and safety issues have been dealt with poorly and often recklessly. Playing with pain and using drugs to mask pain and speed recovery appear to be rampant in all our major spectator sports. What is particularly distressing, however, is that the team doctors, other medical personnel, and trainers appear to be integral parts of these unhealthy practices. As a 2016 Harvard Law School study concluded, divided loyalty of team doctors "creates significant legal and ethical quandaries that can threaten player health."[1]

## THE NFL: THE WORST OF THE WORST

In the NFL, health care for the players has been substandard overall and negatively influenced by coaches and team management, who continue to push players to perform with injuries and pain. In RG3's case, even though it was readily apparent that the young quarterback was badly hampered by his knee injury, the team's medical personnel failed to interfere. He played injured, pushed along by his coaches, teammates, and management.

In professional football, health care is substandard. According to Sally Jenkins and Rick Maese, who conducted an in-depth investigation on the subject for the *Washington Post*, "There is medicine and National Football League Medicine, and the practice of the two isn't always the same." In order to satisfy the short-term interests of a team or head coach, "a central tenet of the Hippocratic oath—'Do No Harm'—[can be] turned on its head."[2]

A 2008 congressional report documented the discrepancies in the medical information that is given to professional football teams, compared to the more limited versions that are provided to the players, who are supposed to be the patients. Making matters worse, the team's confidential medical information and data about the athlete "are frequently leaked to the media," especially during the draft process or when trades appear to be imminent. Team doctors are beholden to their NFL employers, who pay them generous salaries and/or give them opportunities to promote and expand their medical practices. Reportedly "some health organizations pay seven figures for the right to call themselves official medical care providers for NFL teams."[3]

Combine this dependence on team management with the desire of everyone concerned to get players back on the field as quickly as possible, and there exists an environment that tends to override the traditional doctor-patient relationship and strains—and even breaches—medical ethics. According to a Georgetown law professor and health care expert who has studied the NFL, "To say there is no [medical] conflict of interest . . . is to have your head in the sand."[4]

Based on a NFL Players Association survey of all thirty-two league teams, 90 percent of the players surveyed did not trust their team's medical staff.[5] When asked how satisfied they were about the care they were receiving, nearly 80 percent responded that they were unsatisfied. By comparison, these same athletes indicated that they were much more confident in the care provided to them by their team trainers. In part this is because the trainers have been known to go beyond the rules—and the law—to provide the special pharmaceutical assistance that the athletes in their charge desire.

Some of the worst medical practices involve team doctors and members of training staffs who abuse what are supposed to be carefully prescribed and regulated pain medications that are highly addictive. The Obama administration launched a national campaign to curb the overuse of these drugs in the general population. Yet, their abuse appears to be rampant in all professional and major collegiate sports, particularly the NFL and NHL, which have been sued by former players because of such illicit drug practices.[6] Playing with pain appears to be synonymous with masking pain, medicinally, for the benefit of the team and to enhance the status of the players as perceived by their coaches, teammates, management, and fans.

A 2010 study at the Washington University School of Medicine of NFL players revealed more than half admitted "using narcotic painkillers during their career, with 71 percent of those misusing them."[7] In addition, based on court documents gathered as part of a Drug Enforcement Agency prosecution of the San Diego Chargers' team doctor, at least fifty-two other team doctors throughout the country had violated federal laws by writing "prescriptions . . . to themselves." In all likelihood many more sports doctors than that have been engaged in these illegal practices. According to one NFL player, the availability of pain-relieving narcotics is so commonplace that it is "like popping aspirin."[8]

Misusing drugs to control pain has become routine in the NFL, despite all the known dangerous side effects. When surveyed, more than half acknowledged taking them frequently.[9] Widespread drug abuse combined with the ethic to play hurt has contributed to permanent impairments and disabilities, chronic pain, dementia, and lifelong addictions for many of these former athletes.

## THE NORTH AMERICAN HOCKEY CULTURE

Problems with inappropriate and often illegal drug use to deal with pain, along with other questionable health practices associated with football, exist in other popular North American team sports as well, most notably hockey. Studies reveal that in Canada teams and coaches often ignore physicians when they offer opinions that conflict with the mantra that the athletes should play hurt, unless it is apparent that their injuries make it practically impossible for them to do so.[10] Injuries that are not apparent, especially concussions and mental impairments, tend to be dismissed, marginalized, and/or stigmatized. If significant pain or distress is involved, strong medications are dispensed by team doctors and other members of the medical and training staffs.

In 2012 the family of professional hockey player Derek Boogaard, who at age twenty-eight had died from a drug overdose while he was in the NHL's substance abuse program, sued the last two teams he had played for. His family contended that those teams "repeatedly prescribed painkillers and other drugs to Boogaard, even after his addiction to those types of drugs was well known."[11] After that initial suit was dismissed for a procedural violation, Boogaard's family brought a new claim against the NHL for wrongful death. They alleged the league had been "responsible for the physical trauma and brain damage Boogaard sustained during six seasons as one of the league's top enforcers, and for the addiction to prescription painkillers."[12] (See chapter 17.)

## BASEBALL, TORADOL, AND ALEX RODRIGUEZ

In baseball, which has been badly tarnished because of the widespread use of performance-enhancing drugs, multiple concerns have been raised about painkillers as well. One of the favorite pain-reducing substances in that sport is "the go-to elixir . . . Toradol, an injectable anti-inflammatory drug."[13] Toradol is legal when properly prescribed to treat an injury. Nevertheless, its medical benefits and negative side effects, including reinjury "because the warning signs of pain are muted," remain controversial. Moreover, much of the drug's use in baseball has been illicit, if not illegal. Too often Toradol is not properly prescribed or it is given to players without a doctor being directly involved. As a result, physicians of at least two Major League Baseball teams decided to stop prescribing it, even though it continues to be widely dispensed on other teams.[14]

The temptation to misuse painkillers to deal with nagging injuries over a very long 162-game baseball season, not including the playoffs, would seem to be compelling. Cal Ripken Jr. was the ultimate embodiment of this "try to play every game whether injured or not" philosophy. Yet, what may be much admired by teammates, coaches, management, and fans can be very unhealthy in the long run.

One of the countercharges that Alex Rodriguez—superstar turned media villain—made during MLB's investigation of him for using performance-enhancing substances was that the Yankees had played him while injured in hopes of shortening his career. His lawyer contended that team management put him on the field knowing he "had a torn labrum to his hip,"[15] which had been revealed by a magnetic resonance imaging test (MRI). Instead they supposedly said nothing and continued to use him in the American League playoffs.

Whether or not Rodriguez's accusations were accurate reflections of what actually happened to him—and there are good reasons to be skeptical—his lawyers took advantage of a perception—supported by considerable anecdotal evidence—that in baseball, like other major team sports, there is an ethical gap in medical treatments provided to the athletes. What is supposed to be prescribed in the best interests of the individual player is often eclipsed by what is viewed as being the best interests of the team and/or the coaches.

A medical conflict of interest exists when physicians are retained by teams, rather than by the players themselves or the unions representing those players. According to the Harvard Law School Study, these conflicts of interest exist whenever medical providers have obligations to both the team that pays them and the athletes who are the patients. Unfortunately, similar conflicts arise in all major professional and collegiate sports. Typically, the star and superstar players like Rodriguez can afford to obtain private doctors who treat them like patients. Most players, however, use the physicians paid for by management, in part because that is what management expects "team" players to do.

## BASKETBALL PLAYERS

Professional baseball, football, and hockey are not alone in failing to provide healthy environments for their players. A *Sports Illustrated* article chronicled the downfall of Rex Chapman. Twenty-five years earlier he had been a star at Kentucky and then the NBA. Toward the end of his basketball career the multimillionaire became addicted to painkillers. His life spiraled out of control until finally he lost all his money and was "arrested for theft and trafficking in stolen property."[16]

Chapman sought help from John Lucas, a former NBA basketball star, coach, and fellow substance abuser. In recent years many athletes, especially former basketball players, have visited the John Lucas Aftercare Program in order to overcome their addictions to painkillers. Lucas was never able to conquer his own drug problems as a player or a coach, but he was able to build a meaningful post-basketball career helping other athletes.

## CONCLUSION

In all our major professional team sports, addictions and other substance abuse problems tend to be magnified by the bravado of the athletes themselves and competitive pressures from teammates. Elite athletes continue to believe that playing hurt by managing pain with potentially harmful drugs is what real men are supposed to do. Teams reinforce this ethic by making it clear that a commitment to play injured and in pain will be rewarded during contract negotiations.

Conversely, players who cannot perform due to their injuries become known as injury prone. When that happens, the player's value and status are greatly diminished. In this unhealthy environment many athletes resort to using illegal or prohibited drugs. Team doctors, other health providers, and trainers often provide those drugs or look the other way when they are being used and abused. Ultimately, the patient–health provider relationships, which should help protect athletes from substance abuse, are undermined by the financial arrangements that these health providers have with their teams. These conflicts of interest work against providing competent medical and related services to the professional athletes under their care. They can only be resolved if team medical staff members are paid by player unions out of league or intercollegiate conference revenues. In addition, the ethical obligations of these team health providers should be to the athletes exclusively.

# Part II

# Performance-Enhancing Substances: The Perilous Search for the Holy Grail

# 5

# PERFORMANCE-ENHANCING MEASURES

## The Good, the Bad, and the Ugly

While our most popular spectator sports are primarily about entertainment and money, their essence is supposed to be about competition and being the best, or at least better than those one competes against. From this perspective everything that elite athletes do to improve—skills, endurance, recovery times, pain management, equipment, diet, nutrition, and mental acuity—in order to perform better than before may be deemed performance enhancing. What are deemed improper has become sport specific, often arbitrary and unfair, sometimes irrational, and almost always determined with profits in mind.

The modern Olympic sporting ideal of a level playing field for all competitors—which never really existed—has been frayed and distorted by many commercial if, ands, and buts. The greatest performance enhancements tend to favor the athletes who can most afford them. In that way our popular spectator sports today incorporate basic American economic values, much like the Olympics used to strongly favor well-to-do amateurs over those who had to work for a living. The propriety of performance-enhancing measures should be evaluated in the context of this free-market bias.

# WHAT MAKES A PERFORMANCE ENHANCEMENT IMPROPER IS LARGELY SUBJECTIVE

One area in which the free market intrudes in perplexing ways is performance-enhancing supplements. Sometimes banned substances have been known to be accidentally or purposefully introduced into what are marketed as nutritional supplements for athletes. This creates a grey area—as well as an escape from responsibility—for the athletes involved and the various anti-doping authorities that are supposed to be policing these substances. Athletes hope to get an edge on their competition, or at least keep up with the rest of their competitors and the rest of society by using various additives. Testosterone-like supplements, for example, are now heavily marketed to older men, as well as male athletes, online and in bodybuilding stores. If females use these supplements to gain an edge, however, they are liable to be accused of being males. [1]

In addition, sometimes retailers sell "supplements containing banned substances or prescription drug ingredients not listed on their labels." These illicit additives are advertised by word of mouth, or implications embedded in advertisements. A relatively small percentage of athletes have tested positive as a result of taking such substances, and almost all of them have been punished, regardless of their actual intent. Unfortunately, "the only way to avoid this risk is to avoid dietary supplements altogether." [2]

This all-or-nothing advice makes sense from an anti-doping perspective. Unfortunately, it goes against the primary motivation of athletes to improve, until they approach what for them is competitive perfection. For many or most elite athletes, the lure of seemingly enhancing their performance within the rules is what motivated them to take these over-the-counter substances in the first place.

Other controversies have surfaced over the use of drugs that were legal for many years and then, for political or other reasons, were made illegal, such as the Eastern European drug meldonium. That drug was first widely used by Russian soldiers to improve endurance and heart function. Later it was used by athletes in Russia, Eastern Europe, and elsewhere, but appears to have become a casualty of the state-sponsored drug cheating scandal involving the Russian government. On the other hand, platelet-rich plasma therapy, which is more costly and appears to be more performance enhancing than meldonium, was taken off the banned list.

Making matters worse, there is minimal uniformity or transparency with regard to how lab results are obtained or processed. Each sport, each country, and each lab tests somewhat differently—or at times not at all—even when they supposedly follow the overvalued, overhyped, and subjectively enforced World Anti-Doping Agency (WADA) protocols. Baseball is different from football, which is different from hockey, basketball, track and field, soccer, tennis, and the biathlon. For Olympic sports, each country has a different testing agency, except for the brief period when the Olympic competitions are actually being held. Thus suspicions abound.[3]

Moreover, the most popular excuses of athletes under suspicion tend to embrace plausible deniability over truth, much like the rest of today's lawyer-advised business world. To combat both reasonable and unreasonable suspicions, one would think there would be a greater push for transparency. Yet, transparency is an elusive, value-laden, and politically determined conceit that is difficult to define and implement, even in the best of circumstances.

Weeks before the Sochi Olympics, major problems were revealed with the Russian lab that had been designated to conduct drug screenings at those Winter Games.[4] The Russian protocols produced too many false positives and far too many false negatives, meaning that some athletes who were not using substances tested positive, while many more who were using escaped detection. This is a problem that all labs seem to share, but it appears to have been much more pronounced with those in Russia, whose results apparently were controlled—and arguably determined—by the government's Ministry of Sport with guidance from government security officials. Even when conducted properly those tests often are no better than screening tools that lack a high degree of reliability when compared to standards that are expected in scientific, medical, or social science research protocols, or even in most American courts of law. In Russia, apparently positive results for high-profile athletes were simply hidden away by replacing those samples as if they never had happened (see chapter 10).

# UNFAIR COMPETITIVE ADVANTAGES, REAL AND IMAGINED

Another complexity and challenge is that the notion that many of these banned substances substantially aid athletic performance can be anecdotal and presumptive. Oftentimes there is meager and/or inconsistent empirical and other scientific evidence that a particular banned substance is performance enhancing. Rumors and suspicions abound. To quote Peter Keating of *ESPN the Magazine*, the sports "world has essentially zero understanding of how much performance-enhancing drugs actually enhance performance."[5] At the same time, there are considerable financial incentives for those who provide these questionable substances to athletes to make misleading claims about their presumed effectiveness. This has led Keating to ask the question: "Who's Cheating Who?"

For many practical reasons and ethically based restrictions on trials involving human subjects, it is extremely difficult for researchers to do tests on questionable or disputed drugs. In one of the few quantitative analyses that has been done, two American researchers found that baseball pitchers who had been "suspended for flunking a drug test" only "increased their average fastball velocity by 1.07 mph."[6] Based on what American baseball fans presumed they saw with respect to Barry Bonds, Sammy Sosa, and Mark McGwire increasing their home run outputs, one would have thought the performance improvements of those pitchers would have been much more remarkable.

Unfortunately, when put to the test, science often proves common-sense assumptions and presumptions, like those about observations regarding performance-enhancing drugs, to be misleading, exaggerated, or incorrect. Another explanation for why home runs increased so dramatically is that it was due, at least in part, to changes that were made to baseballs,[7] which created more pop, making the balls go greater distances. Certain other physicists have disputed that theory,[8] but no one has offered conclusive proof one way or the other. Former MLB commissioner Bud Selig and his closest cronies may be the only ones who know for certain.

Despite the consensus about what presumably happened in baseball with regard to home runs, there still appears to be substantial doubt whether performance-enhancing drugs could account for most of that phenomenal increase. Weighing against the presumed conclusive explanation in the media are at least two compelling factors: the enhanced physical skills necessary to hit that many more home runs, unless the physics had changed; and the much smaller incremental increases in performance empirically measured for pitchers, and observed for athletes presumed to be using such drugs in other sports.

Given all those complexities and ambiguities, it is not surprising that there remains considerable debate about (1) what is or is not a performance-enhancing substance; (2) how much these various substances actually aid athletes, assuming they are performance enhancing; and (3) what protocols and due process protections drug enforcement authorities in sports should be required to use in making decisions about what drugs to ban or permit and how to fairly implement those rules. Yet, American courts are so reluctant to become involved in the flawed administrative decision making of the various sports authorities in the United States that NFL commissioner Roger Goodell was allowed to punish Tom Brady, even though the best scientific evidence indicated that he was innocent of improperly deflating footballs.

In international doping circles—largely governed by WADA—insulin-like growth factor 1 (IGF-1) has been a prohibited substance because it has been used to help certain animals heal more quickly when they have muscle damage.[9] Nevertheless, as with the recently banned drug meldonium, "there are no scientific studies with humans to show the expected effects actually occur." Making matters more confusing, in sports in which IGF-1 is not totally banned—including baseball, football, and golf—a number of athletes have been allowed to regularly ingest deer-antler velvet, which naturally contains small quantities of that substance, in order to give them the slight possibility of a competitive edge.

Scientists and doctors may be highly skeptical of the value of these products, "but that matters little if the right athlete becomes a believer, or, better yet, a proselytizer." Athletes are "desperate to enhance their performances."[10] The possibility of performance enhancement, even if it is remote, may appear to be better than no possibility at all, particularly if there is a strong suspicion one's competitors may be taking that substance.

At one time not so long ago being a professional athlete was viewed as an unfair competitive advantage. This was true even though amateurism clearly favored gentlemen athletes who had the independent financial means necessary to compete, while it severely handicapped those without such resources. Now our most popular spectator sports are dominated by performance-enhancing measures, some allowed, others prohibited. Every athlete and every team is trying to find an edge that will propel them to more victories, faster times, higher scores, and other improved outputs, especially more money and wealth. For instance, the Seattle Seahawks football team has been giving its players electronic wristbands to facilitate better sleep habits to encourage peak athletic performances. [11]

Even though blood doping remains improper and testing for that type of doping has been substantially increased, various athletes and teams—including the Washington Capitals—are using blood analysis techniques with the hopes of improving nutrition and athletic performances of their players. [12] Similarly, Quest Diagnostics has been working with the New York Giants football team to create "a program to help players get faster and stronger by measuring nutrition, hydration, and food allergies using detailed blood tests." [13] That company also is marketing its diagnostic information to professional and other serious athletes directly.

Today, if we were to regulate athletic competitions using the postmodern, so-called laissez-faire, big-business model—meaning few substantial restrictions, a great deal of paperwork, and meager enforcement—we undoubtedly would have fewer cheating violations. Much of what was once viewed as unfair competitive advantages would become common practice. That already has happened—albeit illicitly—in many sports, including football, baseball, cycling, weight lifting, and the biathlon. Perhaps, the most workable solution to this big mess is to allow any medically prescribed performance-enhancing substances, as long as they are in amounts that are not scientifically or medically known to jeopardize athletes' short-term or long-term health.

## WHY ATHLETES CHEAT

It should not be surprising, given the economic incentives involved, that our major spectator sports appear to embrace an ethos in which performance-enhancing measures are only a problem if the authorities actually catch an athlete violating the rules. Otherwise, that type of offense is like the proverbial tree falling in a forest without people being present: it never happened. Obviously, such pretenses rankle anti-doping organizations, health care providers, and commentators that view performance-enhancing measures in sports very differently from the athletes and teams.

Yet, these outsiders embrace highly divergent views about enforcement. Some views are somewhat compelling, others more self-serving. Only a few of them have consensus support, and none of them have proven to be consistently effective.

There are several prominent rationales that have been put forward to justify the banning of performance-enhancing substances, generally.[14] They include whether the substances (1) are physically and/or mentally harmful to the athletes who use them; (2) provide unfair competitive advantages to athletes or teams, undermining the traditional nature of the sport; (3) harm others in the sports community, including younger athletes who look up to these elite athletes as role models; and (4) harm our society.

In addition, major concerns have been raised about how performance-enhancing substances may affect the popularity of the sports involved, corporate sponsors, and the generation of revenue. When the bottom line is jeopardized, targeted actions protecting the sport are not far away. This type of self-protection happens in almost every major modern business enterprise.

In recent years, scandals regarding performance-enhancing substances have been frequent, involving many different professional, intercollegiate, and Olympic sports. Even though the mere accusation of being drug cheaters can be devastating to athletes' careers, particularly if they are deemed to be guilty of such offenses, our most popular sports continue to be riddled with this type of substance abuse. As former senator and MLB consultant George Mitchell explained, athletes are willing to take greater risks in using these substances because the monetary rewards continue to increase for doing so. He described anti-doping detection and enforcement as "an ongoing cat-and-mouse game between the cheaters, their enablers and those who use science to prevent cheating."[15] Practically speaking, however, it is not that simple, or that black and white.

Three important incentives appear to influence such illicit behavior in sports, beyond wanting to be known as the best or to make the most money by being the best. First, the rules governing which substances are permitted and in what amounts appear to be arbitrary and subjective, particularly since the world of elite sports "seems entirely dependent on technology"[16] and advances in training and nutrition. In that environment athletes tend to view these rules with skepticism and often contempt and ridicule.

What is the moral difference, for example, between professional athletes who take prescribed pain relievers to allow them to compete and a doctor prescribing human growth hormone to improve an athlete's recovery from an injury? Even if, as alleged, Peyton Manning did take medicine(s) to help him maximize his arduous rehabilitation so he could recover more quickly, why should that be improper, particularly if each substance he took was prescribed and monitored by a physician?

Second, because of the money involved, which depends on the interest of the fans and sponsors, those who are responsible for running revenue-generating sports tend to be considerably less than diligent in uncovering these drug abuses. There is a fear that more testing would reveal more doping, which is bad for business. Thus, a relatively low percentage of athletes who take these prohibited substances are discovered, much less effectively sanctioned. At the same time, too many athletes are found guilty by mistake.

It is not particularly difficult to avoid detection, especially for those athletes who can afford to pay for the camouflage and protection that hired experts can provide. There is little doubt that many athletes continue to cheat because they are convinced almost everyone else in their sport is cheating.

Most elite athletes are wired to have every edge on their side. For many of them, winning is much more important than living a long, healthy life, or even avoiding dementia, addiction, or other debilitating conditions. Assuming a relatively small risk of being caught, cheating seems almost trivial in comparison to the health-related consequences that can impair their lives.

Third, athletes have a relatively short time horizon when it comes to balancing risk and reward. Being in the moment is especially important in sports where most professional careers are measured in a few years and short-term goals and objectives become paramount. The strong tendency of Americans to overvalue what is likely to happen in the near future, and undervalue what is likely to happen later, is greatly magnified for serious athletes of any age. The longer athletes perform at an elite level and interact with others who are similarly talented and inclined, the more likely they will succumb to the temptation to cheat. This is especially true when it becomes apparent to the athlete that his or her career may be coming to an end or is in jeopardy.

## HOW PROHIBITIONS ARE ENFORCED

While there are a number of incentives that appear to be present in all of our most popular sports, which encourage this type of cheating, there are specific differences as to how such illicit behavior has manifested itself and been addressed in each of our major spectator sports. In addition, there are distinct differences as to how these issues have been dealt with domestically—most notably in baseball and football—and how they have been dealt with internationally—such as in Olympic sports, cycling, and tennis. Generally, these enforcement differences can be explained by cultural, economic, or organizational realities, and other practical factors and incentives, which distinguish these sports and the countries where they are played, more than by strong adherence to any overriding moral or scientific principles.

Plausible deniability and grudging integrity, followed by righteous outrage and arbitrary sanctions seem to be a large part of how all major spectator sports deal with these anti-doping issues when controversies and scandals emerge. The differences tend to focus on the nature of the denials and cover-ups, as well as the points at which enforcement is deemed necessary to protect the sport's revenue streams. Incremental and situation-based successes define even the most effective responses. Also, the burden is almost always placed on the athletes themselves, with few if any sanctions being directed at the individuals who own and manage the teams or sports enterprises. Virtually all of these approaches have been recipes for failure, frustration, hypocrisy, and under- and overreactions.

Widespread cheating by professional, collegiate, and Olympic athletes, combined with the difficulties in fair and reasonable enforcement, are important reasons why *Economist* has long doubted the justification for banning performance-enhancing drugs in sports. One approach to the cheating problem would be to allow athletes to use such substances, but require them to disclose what they have been taking to stay ahead of their competition.[17]

Unfortunately, the basic problem with that course of action would become apparent if corporate sponsors cut or eliminated paydays for athletes who were using these substances and/or the public condemned them for doping. The closeted cheating wars would likely resume. In addition, that free-market approach probably would encourage many athletes who might otherwise be resistant to breaking the rules to engage in unhealthy practices. The approaches that seem to make more sense and do more good would be focused on protecting the health of the athletes involved (see chapter 11).

# 6

# BASEBALL'S TARNISHED LEGACY

## WHY DOPING MATTERED SO MUCH IN BASEBALL

**B**aseball's reputation continues to be severely damaged by the use of performance-enhancing substances. It has seen more scandals and critical stories about the misuse of these substances than any other American sport. In part, that is because baseball is still viewed by many as the national pastime. Furthermore, it continues to be embraced by scholars and intellectuals, who appear—at least on the surface—to have higher ethical thresholds than the average sports fan, certainly as compared to those who closely follow football.

Of greater significance, though, is the fact that in baseball—more so than any other sport—records are important to fans wanting to compare the statistics of players' performances from season to season and generation to generation. From that perspective, the use of illicit performance-enhancing substances is perceived as spoiling those records much more so than the equally significant technological, nutritional, and equipment advancements that have helped baseball players perform better than in the past. In addition, entry into baseball's hallowed Hall of Fame is not based on athletic merit alone, but includes subjective and somewhat vague, arbitrary, and often hypocritical notions of moral character. These morality standards seem to tolerate racism, wife beating, and driving while drunk, but reject players who are widely perceived as having used performance-enhancing substances.

This type of drug or substance cheating—or the perception that a player may have cheated in this way—has come to matter much more to baseball fans and the baseball media than in other major sports, such as football and hockey, where criminal-like behavior on the field is not unexpected. Ultimately, though, baseball has been tarnished because of Major League Baseball (MLB) and its players union. For a very long time, they refused to acknowledge—and actively denied—the widespread use of performance-enhancing substances in their sport, and many fans went along with that pretense. Moreover, both the league and union took steps to cover it up—or obscure its presence—with myths and platitudes about America's national pastime and the presumed integrity of its teams and players.

## THE BROAD SCOPE OF THE PROBLEM

As the somewhat self-serving Mitchell Report—conceived of and financed by MLB—acknowledged, "For more than a decade anabolic steroids and other performance-enhancing substances were widely used by players." It was so well known that team management made possible substance abuse one of the accepted criteria for evaluating players. As for the players themselves, using performance-enhancing substances became "the key to unlocking the door to statistical and lifestyle riches."[1] What the report judiciously failed to mention, though, was how that drug use contributed to wealth generation for the owners and media covering the sport.

Additional evidence suggested that this type of substance abuse had been going on in baseball for more than fifty years, beginning with the rampant use of amphetamines in the 1960s. Reportedly, literally thousands of players took performance-enhancing substances over the years. "By 2000, about half [the players] . . . were taking steroids or something similar."[2] Yet, under the leadership of former baseball commissioner Bud Selig and his underlings, including current commissioner Rob Manfred, nothing meaningful was being done to address the situation.

Professional baseball was prospering for the leagues, the teams, the players, the agents, and the media. It also was becoming more pleasurable for fans, who enjoyed all the additional home runs and other offense that this bulking up seemed to produce. Harvey Araton of the *New York Times* concluded that the worst aspect of this scandal was not the athletes who were cheating, but rather "management's willful neglect . . . for the sake of profits, along with an obstructionist [players] union."[3]

The league looked the other way for compelling financial reasons. At the same time, the union was overprotecting the rights of its members, who were violators, at the expense of its members who never used those substances. This reinforced the suspicion and belief that the former must have been more numerous than the latter. Once it became clear, due to the public uproar, that something had to be done, even the Mitchell Report acknowledged that "the league's response was slow to develop and initially ineffective."[4]

## MISLEADING PRONOUNCEMENTS OF STRONG ENFORCEMENT

Today, baseball's "cat-and-mouse" game of detection with all its fanfare and increased lengths of suspensions appears to be only incrementally and circumstantially effective. Although considerably better than in the past, the new approach probably has more false positives than ever before. Until recently, occasional, highly publicized punishments substituted for widespread compliance. It was not until the spring of 2016 that there was a significant movement toward incrementally increasing the number and length of suspensions.

That increase occurred after a number of high-profile baseball players were named in an Al Jazeera documentary, which had implicated quarterback Peyton Manning and other athletes. The only athlete receiving an immediate punishment, though, was journeyman catcher Taylor Teagarden.[5] MLB said that the other allegations would be investigated, but offered no timetable or other relevant details. Transparency in all our major sports continues to be a problem.

In the meantime, MLB handed out lengthy suspensions to several other players based on their having failed drug tests. Most notably, the Miami Marlins' Dee Gordon, the 2015 National League batting champion, was suspended for eighty games. Apparently the major concern for the Marlins was not that they had a potential drug problem in their midst, but rather the effect of the suspension on the team's wins and losses.

Despite MLB's well-publicized efforts, many observers, including some major-league baseball players, continue to question the effectiveness of baseball's system—and for good reason. Designer drugs, particularly various forms of testosterone to improve strength, recovery time, and "tissue repair . . . can become undetectable by routine drug tests in as little as 24 hours."[6] They include drugs such as boldenone, clenbuterol, formestane, and stanozolol. In addition, players are taking the anabolic steroid known as Turinabol, which in the 1960s "became a foundation of the East German sports machine."[7] It, too, is a form of testosterone.

As former league MVP, Cy Young Award winner, and longtime Detroit Tigers pitcher Justin Verlander pointed out at great risk to his own reputation among his fellow players, "Guys are finding ways around the system. It's pretty evident, pretty well-known that the people who are making these illegal substances are ahead of the testers."[8] Testosterone knockoffs are available without prescription in "health" and "nutrition" stores throughout the country.

Despite more frequent testing, players are still able to use many of these quick-acting designer drugs after they are tested because "baseball rarely, if ever, tests the same player on back-to-back days . . . or before an off day."[9] One New York Mets pitcher was so brazen that in 2016 he received a third strike for using illicit substances while he was serving the suspension for his second violation.[10] As a result, he received a so-called lifetime suspension, which he is appealing as unfair, even though he can be reinstated after serving a minimum of two years. The potential lifetime suspension is a punishment intended to placate the media and fans, more than a deterrent that is likely to lead to a permanent ban of any players. In fact, it is questionable whether an actual lifetime ban would even be enforceable, if it were challenged in a court of law, which is why there is a mechanism for reinstatement.

Reinstatement and appeals are part of the collective bargaining agreement (CBA) between MLB and the players union. As is true in all our major team sports, the CBA governs what professional baseball may do in terms of testing and enforcement. For this reason, the Harvard Law School Study recommended that health issues not be the subject of collective bargaining. These limitations typically reflect fundamental notions of due process, but they also tend to muddle public perceptions about what is really going on behind the scenes.

Even with these new compliance efforts, a relatively small percentage of players are actually caught cheating. Moreover, as with Dee Gordon's punishment, players typically sit out their suspensions without pay and then are welcomed back by their organizations to complete their contracts, often for millions of dollars. Nevertheless, the length of the suspensions has been increasing. When MLB began its compliance campaign more than a decade ago, the penalty for a first offense was only ten days, thirty days for a second offense, and sixty games for a third offense. [11]

## PLAYERS' DUE PROCESS CONCERNS ARE REAL

Because the legal standard of proof is high and many prosecutors reflexively defer to MLB, criminal prosecutions, much less convictions, of baseball players for using illegal performance-enhancing substances are relatively rare events. Despite having all the resources of the government behind them, in high-profile cases federal prosecutors failed to convict either Roger Clemens or Barry Bonds for using illegal substances. Clemens was acquitted outright. Bonds was initially convicted of being evasive to federal investigators, but not for using illegal drugs. [12] Later, on appeal, even that tenuous conviction was thrown out. A legitimate question may be asked whether, given the available evidence, those prosecutions should ever have been pursued. Also, it seems fair to ask whether Clemens and Bonds should be denied Hall of Fame membership where the evidence is equivocal enough to lead to acquittals and reversals.

The administrative "just cause" standard of proof required for the MLB to issue a suspension, however, is much, much lower than what criminal courts require, which is proof beyond a reasonable doubt. Just cause is the civil standard used in most employment disputes. It is more like probable cause, which is the relatively low criminal standard used to decide whether or not there should even be a trial. Thus, MLB's administratively determined punishments, like most employment-related sanctions, only require that there be substantial evidence. That leaves a great deal of ambiguity and room for injustice.

After a suspension is issued, players do have the right to appeal—both the finding of lack of innocence and the duration of a suspension—to an independent arbitrator. These arbitrators are lawyers who tend to embrace

due process, or at least want it to appear that due process is being followed. At the same time, they enjoy the benefits of a generous payday
from MLB, which can disappear if they are replaced because they are too
player oriented. Yet, even if a suspension is overturned, often the damage
to the player's reputation—and corporate marketability—cannot be re-
paired.

The most prominent due process problem with regard to performance-
enhancing substances is that testing in all sports, including baseball, remains flawed, and testing positive once—or never testing positive—can
be enough to lead to a suspension. What appears to be substantial evidence may only be a mirage. Too many athletes are accused of cheating
for incidents in which they were innocent or in which proof was lacking.
On the other hand, a significant percentage of athletes who continue to
use these illicit drugs are never identified.

Testing may be packaged to the public as a predictable "science," but
in reality it is far more subjective and ambiguous than that. The tests tend
to be more comparable to medical screening tools. What is done with the
results becomes more important than the validity of the tests themselves.
Their reliability is limited, even when organizational incompetence and
self-serving manipulations are not involved. Scientifically, a positive test
result is only one sign that a more comprehensive investigation, including
retesting, is required before a reliable determination can be made. What
happens once a positive test is thought to exist is veiled in secrecy. This
lack of reliability is an important reason why many baseball suspensions
are reduced or overturned on appeal, and why a number of others appear
to be unfair.

Without corroborating evidence, a single test result should rarely, if
ever, be used to establish guilt or be grounds for sanctions against any
athlete in any sport. The medical and statistical evidence regarding the
accuracy of these tests, in the environments in which they are administered, normally would not support their scientific reliability or validity.
The public is being asked to trust the experts, who typically are hired and
fired by the very organizations that conduct the tests and interpret the
results. Moreover, how those experts arrive at their conclusions also tends
to be veiled in secrecy, so it is difficult for those conclusions to be
properly evaluated by independent experts.

## GUILT BY ASSOCIATION AND OTHER SUBJECTIVE BELIEFS

The mere belief that substance abuse has occurred, even without a positive screening result, can seriously harm the reputations of baseball players and other professional athletes. What the media collectively thinks is true becomes a substitute for clear and convincing evidence. For the most talented major-league baseball stars, this can mean that they will never be voted into the Hall of Fame, even if they have more than enough of the necessary athletic accomplishments to be enshrined.

Barry Bonds is arguably one of the two most productive offensive players in baseball history, while Roger Clemens has been recognized as being no less than one of the top ten pitchers of all time. Yet, the odds of either of them reaching the Hall of Fame appear to be remote, unless attitudes about accusations of cheating without convictions or without other official findings of guilt substantially change among the baseball writers who control the selections. All the while avowed racists remain enshrined, even though there is no doubt about their lack of moral character.

The eligibility criteria allow candidates to be blackballed based on suspicion alone. The criteria have been aptly described as both "vague" and "draconian."[13] For all players, though, this type of presumed guilt based on mere suspicion has meant that if their statistics improve significantly, there may be whispers that they are cheating, rather than simply enjoying a particularly good season. Statistically, given baseball sample sizes over a single season, there can be large fluctuations in measured performance over a year's time, especially when pitchers are involved. Furthermore, good or bad fortune may play a significant role in creating the appearance of cheating. Thus no one knows whether the substantial increase in homeruns during the 2016 season was due primarily to juiced baseballs or players.

In sports talk radio especially, and other sports media outlets as well, innuendo substitutes as evidence of wrongdoing, while repeated or multiple accusations with no basis in fact may be embraced as substantial proof. The Baltimore Orioles Chris Davis, whose home run and RBI totals went way up in 2013, became the subject of rumors and innuendo, which seemed unfair, or at least disproportionate to the reality that he had taken a banned but lawfully prescribed medication—Adderall—without baseball's proper permission. Even worse, the spring after Jake Arrieta won the 2015 National League Cy Young Award, there were media "rumblings" that he must have been juiced. Yet, there was "not a shred of evidence . . . that Arrieta ha[d] used anything artificial."[14]

Similarly, highly publicized accusations have been made against baseball players, who have been presumed to be illegal dopers because they have associated with players or other people who have been found or presumed to be guilty in the court of public opinion. Guilt by association may be known by philosophers and other academics as a prominent logical fallacy, but that does little to deter the sports media from incorrectly assuming it constitutes substantial proof. It is one thing to recognize that as a group it appears that many baseball players continue to be using performance-enhancing drugs. It is quite another thing to leap to the conclusion that a specific individual must be cheating because he is a member of that group or associates with other people who have been accused of cheating.

If guilt by association were substantial evidence, then virtually every major-league baseball player over the past fifty years should be presumed guilty. As Michael Powell of the *New York Times* wrote about those in the media who had stated or implied that Mike Piazza had fueled his stellar career with steroids, "To turn suspicion into indictment into conviction should require some proof."[15] Fortunately, cooler heads prevailed and Piazza was eventually inducted into the Hall of Fame in 2016, despite accusations and lingering belief that he must have been cheating.

Washington Nationals pitcher Gio Gonzalez was linked to Biogenesis, a Florida antiaging clinic that was known to have dispensed testosterone and human growth hormone to older men, but the company also had a long list of clients who were professional athletes, including Tiger Woods. MLB suspended a number of players who appeared on that list, including Alex Rodriguez. None of the disciplined players actually tested positive for an illicit substance. Gonzalez was exonerated legally, but not necessarily in the baseball world.

While the presumption of innocence remains in the courtroom for baseball players, no such presumption exists in the media, in MLB investigations, or on ballots for the Hall of Fame. In those venues, the freedom of writers and investigators to believe what they want about an individual player, no matter how spurious or undocumented—and to freely express their opinions and beliefs—tends to be viewed as more important than any due process considerations for those who are being accused. A gang mentality tends to predominate, often shrouded by expansive notions of freedom of the press, distorted organizational responsibilities, and distrust of the lawyer-embraced notions of due process.

Many players continue to be caught violating baseball's drug rules, including an unusually high percentage of players from Central and South America. There is every reason to suspect that discrimination in testing may be part of the reason for this discrepancy. At the same time, many Latinos return to their homelands during the off-season to vacation and train. Thus, they appear to have the opportunity to use these prohibited substances in protective environments in which the likelihood of disclosure is reported to be much less than in the United States. These players come from poor—or relatively poor—countries in which the incentives for cheating appear to be higher because the athlete's potential to earn even a modest income, much less one equivalent to professional baseball, is remote.[16]

For similar reasons, the vast majority of minor-league players who do not garner big signing bonuses are more susceptible to being caught and disciplined. For them the driving incentive is doing whatever is necessary to make the big leagues, although which individual players will succumb—or have succumbed—to such temptations tends to be very difficult to ascertain accurately.

At the same time, superstars—such as Barry Bonds, Roger Clemens, Alex Rodriguez, and Ryan Braun—also are more likely to be identified as cheaters. Not only do they have greater financial incentives to take banned substances in order to earn mega salaries, but the media and prosecutors are more likely to monitor and track their private lives, since the perceived career-enhancing rewards for catching high-profile players cheating tend to be much greater. In addition, MLB can use these high-profile investigations to support the impression that it is taking the issue of performance-enhancing substances seriously.

Current superstars, though, with the notable exception of Braun, rarely have been conclusively identified as cheaters because they failed a test. Nor have many star players been suspended for having positive results. Dee Gordon and Braun having been tested and caught still remain as exceptions, rather than persuasive evidence of a new trend. Alex Rodriguez was sanctioned based on other supposedly persuasive evidence in what appeared to be a concerted effort by baseball to punish him in particular.

## THE RELATIVELY LOW RISK OF BEING CAUGHT COMBINED WITH PLAUSIBLE DENIABILITY

The fact of the matter, though, is that most violators are never detected or, if they are, their punishments tend to be much less than what their potential rewards will be should they be caught. Outside the Hall of Fame players' reputations can be rebuilt, especially if they remain popular or even famous. Barry Bonds and Alex Rodriguez may have been widely disliked in baseball circles, but both of those former superstars were hired by teams—the former as a hitting coach, the latter as a player—despite a presumption or finding that they had used performance-enhancing substances in the past.

Reputation rehabilitation for many of these baseball players begins by pretending or suggesting that their testing positive was due to accidental circumstances. The two go-to excuses of athletes who are accused of cheating in this way are that (1) they ingested the banned substances unintentionally, or (2) the illicit substances were introduced into their food or supplements without their knowledge. Such explanations have become almost second nature for professional athletes who are caught. When sprinter Tyson Gay tested positive on a drug test and did not use such a defense, his candor was hailed as being "refreshing, somehow," at least compared to "the array of lies and fabrications and fantasies offered up by [other] athletes . . . [who have] tested positive."[17]

While this type of plausible deniability defense may be useful in establishing reasonable doubt in a court of law, it no longer has much currency, if it ever did, in avoiding suspensions or convincing the general public of one's innocence. As one columnist opined, "The idea that . . . players didn't know they were doing anything wrong is laughable."[18] Only hard-core fans of the accused are apt to take this type of excuse seriously. Nevertheless, that type of defense may be better than doing nothing, especially if the player is actually innocent.More importantly, no one knows what percentage of professional baseball players continue to use prohibited drugs, nor how many are inappropriately identified. It remains a matter of conjecture.

Most baseball fans, if the media and talk radio are any indication, appear to believe—with a great deal of justification—that enforcement against baseball players who take performance-enhancing substances is weak. The collective bargaining agreement is believed to be at fault since it prevents contracts from being voided "because of little things such as drug suspensions. Nor can awards be rescinded."[19] More importantly, though, the suspensions have been viewed as being too short. One highly publicized exception was Alex Rodriguez, who received a 162-game suspension. His situation was unusual because he was regarded—and thus treated—as a pariah by MLB, the players union, fellow players, and the fans. Nonetheless, after resuming his career in 2015, even Rodriguez was warmly embraced by Yankee fans, if not opposing spectators.

For many baseball players, the relatively low risk of being caught is worth the potential rewards. Even after being suspended, most players continue to receive substantial contracts, often for millions of dollars. This suggests that their teams either do not believe the drop-offs in their performances without banned substances are likely to be substantial, and/ or it is unlikely that the players will be caught again. In addition, for minor-league players who are convinced that performance-enhancing substances are the means for them to make it to the major leagues, be pampered, and receive a big payday, the incentive to cheat is immense.

There is much to be said for better and more frequent testing of players, rather than harsher punishments for those who are caught. Players who cheat are mostly hurting themselves and arguably their fellow competitors. Nonetheless, those competitors are the ones who generally oppose greater punishments. This suggests the use of such drugs is commonplace, rather than rare. Teams are protected from the effects of those punishments because players are not entitled to salaries during their suspensions. In addition, team complicity in cheating is almost never subject to investigations or sanctions.

## AN UNSETTLING RECONCILIATION MARRED BY HYPOCRISY OF THE HALL OF FAME

With respect to testing, baseball has beefed up its enforcement apparatus sufficiently to generally comply with World Anti-Doping Agency (WADA) standards. By 2014, George Mitchell was praising the enforcement efforts of Commissioner Selig and MLB. Mitchell also may have been using that praise as a means to lobby baseball, behind the scenes, to revive his failed bid to become the next commissioner.

As one testing expert has observed, however, baseball is no "cleaner or dirtier than Olympic sports, and they have the so-called gold standard of testing."[20] Given the number of Olympians who cheat and are never caught, as well as all the innocent Olympic competitors who are sanctioned incorrectly, meeting the Olympic standard should provide little comfort to baseball enthusiasts. Moreover, the competency and integrity of WADA itself has been called into question (see chapters 8 and 10).

Despite the flawed resolution, baseball seems to be changing. That movement is long overdue, since for many years labor, management, and the sports media were all complicit in hiding baseball's drug problems. As part of this reconciliation, testing has been enhanced to most of the affected parties' satisfaction. In addition, many of the former players who were part of baseball's drug culture are being welcomed back into the game as instructors and managers. Managers who deliberately looked the other way during this era of cheating are fully eligible for the Hall of Fame. The hypocrisy of the Hall of Fame has not gone unnoticed. Some of the greatest players of all time have been denied "their rightful place of immortality," while managers who facilitated substance abuse have been inducted, alongside racists, drunk drivers, and wife beaters of past eras.[21] "To walk the Hall and not see Barry Bonds and Roger Clemens, the two best players . . . of [their] generation is to conduct a historical mind-wipe."[22]

# 7

# FOOTBALL'S BRAZEN LACK OF COMPLIANCE

## IT APPEARS THAT ALMOST EVERY ELITE PLAYER IS USING SOMETHING

If a credible measure of deciding whether, as a group, athletes in a sport appear to be using steroids, human growth hormone, or other performance-enhancing substances is their having extraordinary, pumped-up physiques—as it was assumed to be for Barry Bonds, Mark McGwire, Sammy Sosa, and other home run hitters—then both National Football League (NFL) and major college football players should be viewed with heightened suspicion. It is important to reemphasize that publicly voicing such suspicions about individual athletes based on their having bulked-up physiques without any other corroborating evidence is overreaching and unfair. Otherwise, an athlete such as Serena Williams, who for years has dwarfed her competition, both in skills and size, should stand accused for being so much better than her opponents.

Nevertheless, while it may be improper to voice these suspicions about specific individuals, this does not mean that similar concerns about athletes in a given sport cannot be well founded. There is a vast statistical difference between drawing conclusions about individuals, as compared to relatively large groups of individuals, such as professional football players or professional cyclists. For reasons related more to perceptions of their respective fan bases, however, presumed guilt based on one's physique has been applied almost exclusively to baseball players. Those who follow football more than casually would hardly be surprised to learn that performance-enhancing substances, especially steroids or human growth hormones, appear to have been an essential part of many or arguably most elite football players' training regimens starting sometime in high school, or even earlier than that. This has been an acknowledged part of the game,[1] even though recently the NFL has been suspending a few more of its players than in the past.

Absent the use of such illicit substances, however, it would be difficult to explain the ever-increasing weight, musculature, power, strength, and recovery powers of elite football players at almost every position without a corresponding loss in speed or quickness. Even quarterbacks, wide receivers, punters, and placekickers have gotten bigger and stronger, and, with the notable exception of concussions, appear to recover from potentially devastating injuries sooner and more completely than ever before. Running backs have become so well muscled that most of the professional athletes at that position weigh between 200 and 250 pounds and have thick pistons for legs that churn out yardage while in the grasp of 300- to 350-pound titans. Bulking up and improving recovery times from injury have become second nature for football players, as have the reported—and more secret—means for doing so illicitly.

Yet, the percentage of professional, collegiate, or high school football players who are sanctioned for these types of substance abuse violations is relatively tiny by any measure—just enough to keep up appearances that the NFL, universities, colleges, and high schools are concerned enough about illicit performance-enhancing substances in football to try to do something meaningful about it. If a sport is willing to let its athletes be brain damaged from repeated concussions and brain traumas, and even goes to great lengths to cover up the true extent of that damage, why would anyone think that the negative health effects of performance-enhancing substances would be taken very seriously? Sanctioning too many athletes for such violations would be bad for business. Sanctioning a relatively small number of players continues to be a manageable cost of doing business, especially if none of them are superstars. This is how it appears to work in many different sports, not just football.

Superstars of football, like those in tennis and baseball, seem to be well insulated from being caught red-handed. Rumors may fly and accusations may surface, but no football superstar has been suspended yet. When the recently retired Peyton Manning was named in the Al Jazeera report as one of the athletes who had received performance-enhancing drugs (human growth hormone, or HGH) to aid "his recovery from neck surgery in 2011,"[2] the sports media largely dismissed those allegations even before any NFL investigation had begun. Ultimately the league's investigation of Manning and other prominent NFL players named in the documentary became an effort to show that Al Jazeera had uncovered no smoking guns, rather than to follow up on the suspicions by conducting a thorough investigation.

Manning made his public denial with the help of ESPN. Both his current team, the Denver Broncos, and the team he was with when the alleged drug use occurred, the Indianapolis Colts, gave Manning their backing. The NFL, for its part, did not even test for HGH until 2014, and then apparently halfheartedly, since not even one player tested positive.

The culture of football is such that all sorts of harmful behavior by its athletes has been tolerated, excused, and obscured by those who benefit most: the players, coaches, teams, owners, athletic departments, agents, media, relatives, friends, and fans. The major exception is when the use of performance-enhancing substances by collegiate football players and other college athletes runs afoul of the NCAA's arcane, often absurd, and usually unfair rules, which are enforced for purposes other than to protect the athletes. Otherwise, the misuse of prescription drugs to deal with pain and speed recovery from injury appears to have been rampant in both the NFL and major college football programs for years. As with cycling, wrestling, track and field, and certain other sports, performance-enhancing measures have become practically essential for football played at elite levels of competition.

## AN INEFFECTIVE TESTING PROGRAM

The general effectiveness of the NFL's testing program for illicit substances can be measured indirectly by comparing the total number of players in the league to the number of suspensions that the NFL makes public. What makes the comparison difficult is that the NFL's grudging acknowledgment of violations comes without much detail or a formal compilation of league or team totals. That would be bad for business.

There are thirty-two teams in the league and each is allowed fifty-three players on the regular roster, plus five on the developmental squad, who also are under contract. That means that during the regular season there are about 1,856 available player positions. The most comprehensive list of players who have been suspended can be found on *Wikipedia*, not the NFL's website.[3]

Each reported incident on *Wikipedia* has been referenced. Over a six-year period from January 1, 2009, through December 31, 2014, there were 107 suspensions, forty of which occurred in 2014. There were twenty-eight in 2013. Thus, even in 2014, the odds of being suspended were less than 2.2 percent (40/1,856). During the prior year the rate was 1.5 percent (28/1,856). In the previous four years, it was only about one-half of 1 percent (39/7,424). Those very low suspension rates strongly suggest that most professional football players who use illicit performance-enhancing substances are never identified, much less sanctioned as being users by NFL testing protocols that are currently in place.

Nonetheless, these football suspension rates are beginning to rival and surpass certain Olympic sports, which had the highest rates of identified offenders at around 2 percent. Furthermore, due to both legitimate and not so legitimate confidentiality concerns, the public does not know what or how many illicit substances suspended professional football players are actually taking. The NFL guarantees such secrecy by threatening with a $500,000 fine those within the league who disclose what those substances are. This privacy-obscured "lack of transparency . . . gives steroid users the cover of blaming, say, an ADHD prescription"[4] or a dietary supplement for their actual transgressions.

Not surprisingly, of those football players who have been identified as violators, many have stated that they "only" took Adderall, which is a powerful stimulant used to treat attention deficit disorder.[5] Like the now less popular amphetamines of the past, Adderall is supposed to improve one's ability to concentrate, which many college and high school students throughout the country would attest to. According to a 2012 *Washington Post* study, of the nineteen players suspended under the NFL's substance abuse policy over a period of twenty months, twelve claimed that their suspensions were due exclusively to Adderall.[6] It appears likely, however, that many—and probably most—of them were taking other substances, in addition or instead, which made them bigger, faster, and stronger.

Frequently football players, like athletes in other sports who are caught using banned substances, blame the supplements they were (or are) taking. The now familiar excuse is that the supplements contained ingredients the athletes were unaware of. As Tracee Hamilton of the *Washington Post* asked, how can anyone believe that football players who have to "learn complex playbooks every year" are incapable of reading "a simple label on a bottle of supplements?"[7]

At the same time, on rare occasions there have been well-documented instances of deception by manufacturers. A linebacker for the St. Louis Rams, for instance, won a $5.4 million judgment against a company because a natural supplement turned out to contain banned substances.[8] His unique lawsuit victory, however, should probably be viewed more as an anomaly than a pattern.

In any case, as noted earlier, until recently the NFL did not even bother to test for human growth hormone (HGH). Its use has been particularly difficult to detect in all sports. HGH, similar to testosterone, passes through the bloodstream in a couple of days and can be altered synthetically to make detection even more difficult. In 2012, one former All-Pro quarterback reportedly estimated that 60 to 70 percent of players use HGH.[9]

Frequent testing is a potentially effective way of identifying users of these quick-acting performance-enhancing substances. Yet, the NFL has been particularly slow to incorporate blood testing into its substance abuse protocols. One reason may be that HGH has proven to be useful in treating injuries to help athletes recover more quickly. Thus, there is a therapeutic and business-related justification for largely ignoring its use, which could be the underlying theme of the unproven allegations against Peyton Manning.

In July 2013, under pressure from Congress, the league finally began HGH testing, but only anonymously to determine "what a 'normal' HGH level is for an NFL player."[10] Given the strong reluctance of the players and the league to formalize such testing, suspicion arose that what was "normal" would either turn out to be suspiciously high, or the results would be manipulated behind the scenes to make the actual results appear less damaging, as is alleged to have been done by Russia's Sports Ministry to support its Olympic athletes. As it turned out, however, the first year of NFL testing detected no players using HGH,[11] strongly indicating that the applied testing protocol had been woefully—and perhaps purposefully—deficient all along.

Also, unlike baseball, which can control testing in the minor leagues, the NFL has no authority over collegiate programs where most NFL players learn their trade, including new and better ways to bulk and speed up. The NCAA "shares the responsibility of promoting a drug-free athletics environment with its member institutions."[12] Nevertheless, the NCAA, which uses the much-maligned WADA protocols, only handles drug testing in championship games and in meets involving multiple schools. Otherwise the testing is conducted by the affected institutions of higher learning themselves, using their own procedures and issuing their own self-serving sanctions.

Thus, there are substantial variations in the substance abuse policies for different college football programs. Not surprisingly, there have been numerous instances of illegal drug use in major college football programs, but most of these violations go unreported. It would seem reasonable to presume that a vast majority of these schools try to protect their programs as much as plausible deniability will allow, since that is what those institutions have tended to do whenever scandals involving elite athletes have emerged.

The pressure for transparency in football about the use of performance-enhancing substances would seem to be minimal. "Unlike baseball, football engenders far less public concern about its drug culture."[13] Nonetheless, the anecdotal evidence and informed perceptions of knowledgeable people on the inside strongly suggest that such cheating is endemic to professional and big-time collegiate football. It also appears to be widespread in many high school football programs, especially those that funnel players to major college teams. All the evidence suggests that performance-enhancing drugs have become an integral part of America's favorite spectator sport.

## HARSH PENALTIES FOR MEDICALLY NECESSARY MEDICATIONS

On the other hand, occasionally collegiate football players are unfairly scarred for using medically necessary medications considered to be performance enhancing. This happens when those athletes become caught up in the NCAA's nonsensical rules. Disproportionate enforcement as a way to make examples of less prominent athletes is not an unusual outcome for the NCAA, or any other major sports cartel. The story of University of Georgia offensive lineman Kolton Houston, as told by *ESPN the Magazine* journalist Chris Jones, underscores how inflexible and intolerant the NCAA can be. Houston was punished for inadvertently violating a performance-enhancing drug standard as a result of medical treatment in circumstances where there was no reasonable way for him to comply, other than to quit playing football.

When Houston first arrived at the university in April 2010, like all new recruits he was tested for drugs, which revealed a positive result for an anabolic steroid called norandrolone. He received a one-year suspension. Like many athletes who are so identified, he claimed that he had never deliberately taken any performance-enhancing drugs. Repeated testing, however, verified that Houston's body was somehow producing the drug inside him. It turned out that in high school after the young player had shoulder surgery, his physician on multiple occasions had injected the site with norandrolone to promote healing. Unfortunately, the steroid was improperly injected into body fat with no way to remove it, which ensured that the drug remained inside him. When Houston tested positive a second time, the NCAA banned him for life.[14]

Although Houston successfully appealed the lifetime ban, the NCAA still would not allow him to play football until tests indicated that the banned drug was completely out of his system. After "sauna treatments, an experimental antibiotic and . . . surgical removal," he still tested slightly above the allowed limit, although it was only a fraction of what the test had registered originally. It was clear that he had made every good faith effort to comply. Because the NCAA continued to refuse to grant him a special exception for his extraordinary situation, and convinced that he probably would "never play a down of college football," he gave up and quit the team.[15]

Perhaps the most galling aspect of the whole sad episode was that after Houston had spent thousands of dollars to purge most of the drug from his system, there was no significant advantage that the steroid residue could provide him in terms of enhancing his performance. Nevertheless, the NCAA punished him to make a point about the supposed strict enforcement of its drug rules, presumably because so many other college football players, like their NFL counterparts, were taking these substances without ever being caught.

# 8

# CYCLING, OLYMPIC SPORTS, AND WADA

**M**any elite American athletes go to college or earn their livings in sports governed by international organizations, which have adopted somewhat different approaches—as compared to major American professional sports leagues or the NCAA—with regard to establishing and enforcing bans against performance-enhancing substances. Summer and winter Olympic sports and cycling, which all use the World Anti-Doping Agency (WADA) protocols, have tried to appear to be the most invasive, if not the most effective, in identifying and sanctioning suspects. Much of the public relations hoopla has been an anti-doping charade to benefit those affected sports and WADA.

Unfortunately, these international sports organizations also have been demonstrably unfair with regard to protecting due process and other rights of many athletes who register false positive results. Part of the reason is that there has been a push to make WADA protocols appear to be more effective than they are. Ultimately, though, despite the violations of the rights of the innocent, most cheaters still go undetected, and apparently bribes, extortion, and other conflicts of interest to clear the names of accused athletes may not be that uncommon. Except for the U.S. Justice Department's (DOJ) well-publicized—but atypical—initiatives, there has not been much to worry about for leaders of these international sports cartels when they break the law and engage in other acts of corruption. Since its creation, WADA has been more complicit than enforcement oriented, as the Lance Armstrong and, more recently, the Russian state-supported cheating scandals have revealed.

# LANCE ARMSTRONG AND CYCLING

## The Biggest Individual Target in WADA History

Lance Armstrong's sad saga generated the most widespread and enduring global media attention involving performance-enhancing substances to date focusing on an individual athlete. He became a bigger target than Barry Bonds, Roger Clemens, and Alex Rodriguez combined. As a cancer survivor, who had won seven Tour de France titles and was generous with his time and money in support of cancer patients, Armstrong was a global icon much like Tiger Woods or Michael Jordan.

Yet, he competed in a sport in which it appeared virtually certain that most of the athletes, including Armstrong and his top competitors, were using banned substances. For years, however, he brazenly eluded detection. Before his initial retirement in 2005, Armstrong had been the exemplar in avoiding detection. Reportedly, he viciously bullied those who came forward to tell the truth and used his fight against cancer to convince members of the media to provide him with the cover of a global hero's plausible deniability. He almost never tested positive and the one time he did, Armstrong faced no discipline.

After he first retired, though, the anti-doping forces began targeting the most high-profile cyclists for testing. "Nearly every top cyclist on the Tour got caught using banned substances."[1] While there were many cheating accusations lodged against Armstrong, which raised significant questions about his Tour de France victories, nothing substantive could be proven.

His ultimate fall from grace probably could have been avoided or at least have been substantially mitigated if he had not returned to cycling in 2009. Apparently his ego would not allow him to stay retired or to recognize that if he persisted in doping, eventually he might be caught, especially if sufficient resources were directed at catching him specifically. As alleged in the documentary *The Armstrong Lie*, the world's best cyclist appeared to have too much faith in his "absolute cunning" and too little control of his "win-at-all-costs ambition."

During Armstrong's reign, WADA's credibility and testing methods were criticized, and for good reasons—the reputation of drug testing, in truth, far exceeded its actual capabilities.[2] Thus, it became imperative for WADA, working with the U.S. Anti-Doping Agency (USADA), to do everything possible to bring Armstrong down in order to restore confidence in a badly flawed detection apparatus. Since all of Armstrong's test results had been inconclusive, it was necessary to find individuals who would assert that they had seen Armstrong cheating and to convince them to become witnesses against him. Cyclists who were being threatened with prosecution and wanted leniency were much more likely to cooperate, and some might even be willing to do more than that.

Furthermore, since testing alone had proven to be inadequate in accurately detecting most of these banned substances, WADA wanted to demonstrate that there were weapons other than testing to fight against doping. Hiring experienced investigators, who were not overly encumbered by due process safeguards, was the strategic next step. Armstrong provided much of the motivation and justification for these attempts to give new life to failed testing methodologies throughout the world, but especially in the United States where baseball had suffered such highly publicized embarrassments.

## A Witch Hunt Is Launched

Armstrong's last Tour de France in 2009, and the first since he had initially retired, greatly enlarged the target on his back, particularly after he finished third and widespread rumors began surfacing that once again the top finishers had been cheating. Alberto Contador, who was on Armstrong's team and won the race, had been implicated in the use of performance-enhancing substances in the past. Not surprisingly, there appeared to be compelling reasons to anticipate that a thorough investigation would demonstrate Armstrong had used performance-enhancing substances and had been helping his teammates do so as well. Thus, what Armstrong later would describe—with considerable justification—as a "witch hunt"[3] was set in motion. Ultimately, though, while the investigation was far from being properly conducted, Armstrong's downfall seemed well deserved. The evidence against him continued to mount. His own self-serving acknowledgments on *Oprah* backfired not only by verifying that he had cheated, but demonstrating that he had lied and intimidated his critics and accusers.

For nearly three years there was a stalemate between Armstrong and the WADA-USADA alliance, as the two contentious sides utilized the media to imprint their respective points of view. The anti-doping faction did well in convincing most of the interested public that Armstrong had probably doped repeatedly. Armstrong's contingent, however, presented enough doubt the allegations might be false and had violated basic due process that the USADA chose to wait to bring formal charges. In addition, Armstrong utilized his cancer foundation and media team to convince many potential critics that he was entitled to the public's sympathy, regardless. Yes, he may have cheated like everyone else in the sport. However, he was a truly heroic and decent human being, who had devoted his life to helping people with cancer, which he could not have done without his seven Tour de France victories.[4]

The *Washington Post*'s gifted columnist Sally Jenkins, who cowrote Armstrong's autobiography, vigorously argued—even after much of the damning evidence had been made public—that Armstrong was a good man. In an article titled "USADA's Campaign Is Far from Fair," Jenkins wrote, "There's nothing short of murder that would alter my opinion."[5] However, for many people that story line was "as dishonest as the man himself."[6]

## Public Opinion and Evidence against Armstrong Shifts

In the summer of 2012, public opinion about Armstrong began to shift as more information was revealed about his blemishes. Fewer people were willing to come to his defense. The USADA notified Armstrong and the American media, simultaneously, that it would bring charges against him that could result in his losing all seven of his Tour de France victories. In addition, he could be banned for life from participating in cycling and any other sports that participated in the World Anti-Doping Code. That notification accused Armstrong of being "at the heart of systematic doping programs that began in the 1990s." Furthermore, the USADA opined that "blood tests done on Armstrong in 2009 and 2010 . . . [were] fully consistent with blood manipulation 'including EPO use and/or blood transfusions.'"[7]

However, being "fully consistent with" is far short of convincing— much less conclusive—evidence. Nevertheless, Armstrong, through his lawyer, did not deny the truthfulness of those charges. Instead he chose to attack the unfair process that the USADA was using to investigate, present, and weigh the evidence, which was the investigation's other obvious deficiency. The presiding federal judge was sympathetic to that line of defense, going so far as to question the USADA's motives. In particular the idea of using plea deals to coerce testimony against Armstrong from his close associates was disturbing, although not atypical in high-profile cases in the American legal system.

What made the USADA-WADA administrative process even more pernicious, however, was its administrative appeals process known as the Court of Arbitration for Sport (CAS). This international tribunal has little resemblance to a court of law since it is funded by the sports it is supposed to preside over. In its flawed appellate proceedings, too often due process has been sacrificed in favor of getting tough on those who are thought to be using performance-enhancing substances. Athletes almost always lose. In appeals involving Americans, for example, fifty-eight of sixty were denied.

Making matters worse, it is almost impossible to convince judicial authorities to intervene once the CAS has ruled. In 2016 a German court unexpectedly held that the nation's "most decorated Olympian," ice-skater Claudia Pechstein, could bring a civil action against the CAS. She alleged that her two-year suspension from competition had been based on flawed blood doping evidence.[8] A German appeals court, however, reversed, not because Pechstein had presented inadequate evidence, but because she, like all Olympic athletes—including cyclists—had been compelled, as a condition of being allowed to compete, to sign an arbitration agreement that waived her right to sue in her "home" country. [9]

In another high-profile CAS appeal, cyclist Alberto Contador lost his case and had to serve a two-year ban, even though it was reported that the clenbuterol found in his urine had been "miniscule . . . and its ingestion was almost certainly unintentional." Based on his past reputation as a doper, the burden of exoneration appeared to have been on him. Similarly, in many of the denied appeals involving American athletes, the evidence against them had been viewed as equivocal or even exculpatory.

In Armstrong's case, the legal evidence being compiled against him was far from airtight but was damning to his reputation nonetheless. The USADA report focused on two threads of evidence, neither of which depended on the flawed WADA testing protocols that, over many years, Armstrong had only failed once.

First, the USADA hired a reputed expert to reexamine thirty-eight blood samples from tests Armstrong had taken in 2009 and 2010. That expert boldly concluded, without providing any public documentation, that when viewed collectively—as opposed to each test individually—the likelihood of those blood levels "occurring naturally was less than one in a million."[10] In an American court of law such testimony would have been subject to cross-examination and the blood samples would have been made available to Armstrong's defense for retesting and a separate expert analysis of the results.

Second, and more damning, though, the report relied on Armstrong's own associates, including Tyler Hamilton, a former Olympic cycling champion and Armstrong teammate, as well as other figures in the cycling world, to demonstrate that Armstrong had taken performance-enhancing substances. Those associates testified, under the threat of federal prosecution, that Armstrong had been the mastermind behind a "sophisticated doping program . . . to beat the sport's drug-testing system."[11]

### The Witch Was Dead and Its Aftermath

Based largely on this evidence, Armstrong was banned from cycling and all other sports that use WADA protocols. Yet, controversy persisted. On the one hand, it was accurate to state that the champion cyclist had been part of a "sport in which needles were so deeply embedded that the choice was simple to use them, or quit riding."[12] Beginning in 1995 through 2012, only two Tour de France victors were not implicated in doping transgressions. Thus, it was reasonable to conclude that the USADA and WADA were acting unfairly by focusing exclusively on Armstrong to the exclusion of the many other cyclists who had been directly involved in this widespread doping scandal. A year after the USADA report had been released, the identities of the other cyclists accused of doping were still unknown and only Armstrong had been subjected to punishment.[13]

On the other hand, it was no longer credible to believe that Armstrong was innocent. Armstrong's statements in his own defense were viewed by many as being even more damning than the USADA report, particularly to his all-American nice guy image. His brand was in shambles. In both his interview with Oprah and in the film documentary about what had happened, Armstrong came across as a particularly nasty and corrupt human being, who had done whatever was necessary to cheat, just like most of his colleagues in cycling. Everything about him, the Tour de France, and the testing and enforcement protocols that existed in the cycling world had been besmirched almost beyond redemption.

Despite Armstrong's comeuppance, suspicions about widespread cheating in cycling have continued. Chris Froome, the 2015 and 2016 Tour de France winner, has had to answer many questions about his extraordinary athletic accomplishments. To many observers Armstrong's lifetime ban may have been deserved, but there also seemed to be a pernicious double standard. While some are barred for life, others ride on.

After the 2015 Tour de France Froome released test results, arranged for by his wife, purporting to demonstrate that he had achieved peak fitness properly. Those self-serving results, however, did little to quell suspicions that Froome either had been doping or been given an unfair mechanical advantage. Instead of convincing the media that doping had been curtailed in cycling, new concerns were now being raised that these athletes were engaging in the ultimate form of cheating by hiding tiny electric motors inside their bicycles. [14]

Those new suspicions grew more pronounced after the French network, which broadcasts the Tour de France, "suggested that motor doping is . . . at the highest levels of the sport." Ian Austen, who covers cycling for the *New York Times*, reported on April 19, 2016, that these miniature motors were being widely used based on an "ever-growing library of videos . . . [of] suspicious performances and actions by riders as well as teams." [15] Fortunately, this type of mechanical cheating does not have the negative health consequences—clots, strokes, or heart attacks—that occur when there is blood doping.

## OLYMPIC SPORTS GENERALLY

Similarly flawed WADA testing procedures, protocols, and administrative appeals are used to monitor and deter athletes from doping in all Olympic sports. Based on test results, cycling may not be the worst in terms of its athletes cheating by using performance-enhancing substances. More positive test results have been compiled for athletes who compete in weight lifting, boxing, and archery. In addition, serious doping scandals have repeatedly marred track and field, swimming, wrestling, and winter Olympic sports, especially the biathlon and cross-country skiing.

The use of performance-enhancing substances appears to be prevalent in most—and arguably all—Olympic sports now that the athletes involved can establish their careers and make substantial incomes through commercial endorsements and hefty prize money. The athletes in the major Olympic sports have the greatest opportunities to reap those rewards. This includes so-called amateur competitors, who receive deferred payouts through the use of trust arrangements but are allowed to pay for reasonable living and training expenses. The notable exceptions are athletes who want to maintain their eligibility for American collegiate sports, which the NCAA oversees with its draconian, self-rewarding, and often absurd rules on amateurism.

Whether doping rates in Olympic sports are actually higher than other professional and major intercollegiate America sports is unclear. Many testing insiders believe that these American sports would have much higher positive results if they operated under WADA's more "rigorous" protocols. On the other hand, those insiders probably have a vested interest in promoting the questionable and largely undocumented virtues of WADA.

Regardless, higher is a relative concept since a 2.4 percent fail rate for wrestlers is the highest on record, which is now being rivaled by the recent unofficial rates from the NFL. These low percentages suggest that with respect to athletes using illicit performance-enhancing substances, even in the sports with the most failed tests, only a small fraction of the offenders are accurately identified, much less sanctioned. This certainly has been true in cycling, baseball, and American football.

In addition, anecdotal evidence indicates that in Olympic sports in which time, height, or distance are all important and margins of victory can be razor thin, measured in seconds or inches, the incentives to cheat are further accelerated. Thus, swimming and track-and-field sports in particular have been linked to performance-enhancing drugs. An investigation by the *Sunday Times* of London and a German television station, for instance, which relied on twelve thousand blood tests from five thousand track-and-field athletes, found the doping in track and field to be "rampant."[16] This type of cheating is not a Russian government–inspired phenomenon. It is a widespread occurrence among elite track-and-field athletes from many nations.

Doping scandals have marred the Summer and Winter Olympics, and the many competitions leading up to those seminal events. In recent years, most of the publicized evidence seemed to indicate that this drug cheating was individualized to teams and athletes. This type of cheating has thrived due to free-market ingenuity and deliberate neglect and mal-feasance of the organizers, who richly profited by holding these competitions. Moreover, this free-market view of doping adequately explained the widespread use of PEDs. In order for athletes to perform their best, typically it is necessary to have all the known advantages possible, in addition to prodigious talent. Such advantages include having access to whatever performance enhancements are commonly available to the very best athletes in a sport.

The free-market view of individualized or team-inspired cheating had to be revised, however, to account for two major developments. First, in November 2015 WADA released a 323-page report accusing Russia of promoting "what is very likely the most extensive state-sponsored doping program since the notorious East German regime of the 1970s."[17] Much of the early evidence for that type of state-inspired cheating centered on preparations for the 2014 Winter Olympics in Sochi, Russia. Both money and national pride appeared to have been involved, but the mounting evidence later indicated that Russian government–facilitated cheating was not limited to those Winter Games (see chapter 10).

Second, another WADA report released in 2016 found "corruption and possible criminal behavior at the top levels of the International Association of Athletics Federations—the world's governing body of track and field."[18] Allegedly those officials had received bribes and engaged in extortion in exchange for allowing athletes who had tested positive for banned substances to continue competing in major events. Thus, criminal wrongdoing at the highest levels of the sport's governance had contributed to widespread doping.

These two seemingly independent revelations would become interrelated when the IAAF decided to try to camouflage its own wrongdoing and malfeasance by taking the unprecedented action of banning all Russian track-and-field athletes from the 2016 Summer Olympics. WADA and the IOC, which were also to blame for allowing this widespread cheating to thrive, supported the ban with only a few minor exceptions (see chapter 10).

# FEMALE SWIMMERS ACHIEVE EXTRAORDINARY TIMES

In swimming, two stories about alleged PED use stood out at the 2012 London Summer Games. Both were perpetuated by widespread suspicions involving the extraordinary physical accomplishments of the female athletes involved, rather than on any specific evidence that those who were accused had failed properly conducted tests. Oftentimes such suspicions are what exist in lieu of conclusive evidence because doping by athletes is difficult to prove, clearly and convincingly. Unless those who are actually guilty decide to confess their transgressions—perhaps for substantial media paydays after their athletic careers are over—it becomes unlikely that their suspected violations will ever be fully corroborated.

Typically, there is sufficient room for either credible deniability and/ or innocence because the testing protocols, in the circumstances in which they are administered, remain relatively crude. Thus, rumor, innuendo, self-interest, and subjective beliefs in the media have become substitutes for fairness and due process through properly conducted hearings.

Members of the media always have the right to express their opinions, which they are quick to point out. Unfortunately, the idea that they have a greater responsibility to be accurate and relatively certain has been watered down, along with journalistic standards more generally. Sometimes these accusations of doping seem justified; other times they are not, or are only partially justified. Most of the time, however, only the accused athletes themselves and members of their training teams are likely to actually know which characterization best fits the accusations against them.

## American Olympic Champion Dara Torres

American swimmer Dara Torres was a former national and Olympic champion who at age forty-five became the oldest Olympic swimmer in history, by many years, when she qualified for the 2012 Games. Even more impressively, she did this against strong American competition. In terms of an athletic achievement it was comparable to what Bob Beamon did in smashing the long-jump record at the 1968 Summer Olympics. Her performance was astounding.

Suspicions about Torres's training methods had been raised in 2009 when she was treated by Canadian doctor Anthony Galea, who the FBI had been investigating for illegally transporting and administering banned substances. Dr. Galea was accused of providing his patients—many of whom were elite athletes—with performance-enhancing substances and treatments including human growth hormone; Actovegin, an illegal drug that promotes oxidation in mammals thought to enhance stamina and endurance; and platelet-rich plasma therapy, which speeds recovery from injuries and initially was deemed to be an illegal form of blood doping. Implicated in the Galea investigation as well were Tiger Woods and baseball superstar Alex Rodriguez. [19]

Torres claimed that the only reason she had seen Galea was so that he could drain her knee after she had suffered a torn tendon. [20] Nevertheless, Torres's being a patient of the tainted Canadian physician was viewed as inherently suspicious, if not conclusive of wrongdoing. Her extraordinary swimming accomplishments at an advanced age required a brutal training regimen and improved oxidation, both of which would have been enhanced if she had used Galea's illicit treatment methods. The next oldest person to have participated in the Olympics as a swimmer also was Torres, who at age forty-one had represented the United States in the 2008 Beijing Summer Games. Before that the oldest Olympic female swimmer had been the great Jenny Thompson, who was thirty-one when she competed in the 2004 Games representing Australia. [21]

Torres's explanation for her unique ability to do what no other female swimmer in her early forties had come close to doing before focused on her very special training regimen and diet. According to experts on physiology, there are four elements in the natural aging process that need to be overcome for an older athlete to compete as if she were much younger: declining oxidation rates, which decrease because the "heart and lungs are less efficient"; loss of lean muscle mass, which melts away without heightened exercise; loss of flexibility; and longer "recovery [times] from a tough workout," or nagging injuries. [22]

The illegal treatments that Galea was accused of administering to his patients were designed to provide athletes with the types of performance-enhancing benefits that would allow Torres to help counteract the aging process as an Olympic swimmer. Galea's supposed methods could substantially improve her ability to regularly engage in extreme exercise and expand her oxidation capacities. Torres readily admitted—and even bragged—that she had employed various legal performance-enhancing measures to remain supremely fit at her age.

According to Torres, three times a week she received special massages to knead and stretch her muscles. She had her own personal trainer and rehabilitation specialist. In addition, she elevated her hormone production with "neurological stimulation" and improved her ability to respond to moving patterns through eye stimulation. She also used "an oxygen concentrator . . . to breathe pure oxygen while riding a stationary bike," and a "magnetic device . . . to induce a more restful healing sleep."[23] Furthermore, she took supplements designed to boost energy and increase the production of hormones such as testosterone.

Whether Torres employed anything other than legal performance-enhancing measures to help her attain Olympic glory and substantial endorsements has remained conjecture and shrouded in suspicion. What was clear is that her extraordinary physical feats were due in large part to extraordinary measures that had enhanced her times, which gave rise to two cynical questions: Would this performance-obsessed athlete, who went to such lengths to improve her swim times, use banned substances that she knew other swimmers were taking, if there was only a small chance of being caught? And, of all the doctors in the world, why had she chosen Anthony Galea to provide her with a treatment—draining her knee—for which he had no particular expertise?

As damning as the implications of those two questions might appear to be on the surface, the USADA acted appropriately in not pursuing any potential sanctions against Torres. All the evidence against her that became public seemed to be based on conjecture. There was no smoking gun.

## Chinese Swimmers at the 2012 London Olympics

Somewhat similar, but clearly different, suspicions dogged Chinese swimmers at the 2012 Olympics. As with Torres, the controversy had originated at the 2008 Beijing Games, after Chinese swimmers made remarkable advances in reducing their pool times. In 2009 those suspicions were intensified because "five Chinese swimmers were banned after testing positive for clenbuterol."[24]

Politics, particularly China's human rights record, certainly played a role in magnifying suspicions. As one bioethicist concluded, China had replaced East Germany "as the target of Western condemnation of state-sponsored doping"[25]—that is, until Russia assumed that mantle in 2015.

This scholar was not contending the accused Chinese athletes might not be cheating, but rather that the United States and its allies were overreacting because, after the Soviet Union fell, China had become the primary threat to the United States on the world stage. Chinese athletes appeared to have done nothing more than what a number of other Olympic athletes had been doing, including swimmers from the United States.

At the London Games, members of the Chinese swim and badminton teams faced scrutiny that centered on sixteen-year-old swimmer Ye Shiwen. Her chief accusers were members of the American women's swim team and their supporters, after Ye unexpectedly won gold medals in the 400- and 200-meter individual medleys. John Leonard, the executive director of both the American and World Swimming Coaches Associations, used those platforms to publicly opine, without providing any supporting evidence, that the swimmer's results were "unbelievable" and "disturbing."

Ye was being condemned because she was a member of a swim team of an unpopular nation that had been caught cheating in the past. When combined with her vastly improved times, it gave the charges a certain amount of credibility with those in the media who wanted an interesting story. At the same time, there seemed to be a double standard at play. A number of American women swimmers had failed drug tests and their team had an even younger competitor who had improved her time even more substantially in winning her first gold medal. At age fifteen Katie Ledecky won the 800 freestyle by shaving five seconds off her personal best, which represented an eleven-second improvement in about a month's time.

Both of these teen swimmers had posted jaw-dropping results, but only the Chinese girl was expected to defend her improvement. A Chinese swimmer after winning a gold medal explained his team's remarkable success: "It's because of hard work and training. Chinese are not weaker than Americans."[26] That certainly appeared to be true, but it raised the question about how many members of both swim teams—and other teams as well—had been using banned substances before or during the London Games.

# TRACK AND FIELD: A TENTH OF A SECOND OR AN INCH CAN MEAN VICTORY

## Doping Is Found to Be Widespread

Another Olympic sport that has seen more than its share of doping violations and related suspicions is track and field, particularly the marquee performers in the sprints, who have been sanctioned for this type of cheating repeatedly. Weight lifters, wrestlers, and biathlon participants probably have been punished more often, but there is much less public concern about them because their sports are less popular and, as a result, receive less media scrutiny. Sprinters, however, are at the top of the Olympic food chain in terms of popularity. Also, performance-enhancing substances can boost their times in events that are decided by hundredths of a second. Similarly, athletes who participate in field events can secure Olympic medals by improving their performances by an inch or two, but those events are not in the spotlight.

Perhaps the most notorious American track scandal in this century led to a prison sentence for Marion Jones, one of the greatest sprinters in our history, who was caught in the Balco investigation lying to federal agents about "her use of designer steroids."[27] At the 2000 Olympics she won five medals, including three gold. Seven years later she was stripped of all five. Even though she had passed "more than 160 [drug] tests during her career,"[28] she confessed to perjury in order to avoid a potentially much longer sentence if she asserted her right to a trial. Like many world-class sprinters, Jones probably was very adept at not failing drug tests.

Subsequently, the premier U.S. sprinter Justin Gatlin was suspended from 2006 through 2010 for doping. Gatlin raised new suspicions about his use of performance-enhancing substances in 2015 when, at age thirty-three, he was "running the fastest times of his life," regularly beating the world's best, including Usain Bolt. After Bolt responded by improving upon his fastest time to win the 2015 world championship, allegations about continued doping among world-class sprinters became more intense.[29]

Tyson Gay, who was the American-record holder in the 100 meters, was found guilty of using performance-enhancing substances as well. In 2013 he tested positive for taking banned stimulants. He was joined by two Jamaican sprinters: Asafa Powell, who once held the men's world record in the 100 meters, and Sherone Simpson, who had won both a gold and a silver Olympic medal. [30]

Gay admitted that the USADA's test had been correct, but claimed that he had placed "his trust in someone and . . . was let down." Powell categorically denied that he was "now—nor . . . ever [had] been—a cheat," perhaps because he thought almost every world-class sprinter was doing the same thing. Simpson ambiguously contended that she "would not intentionally take an illegal substance of any form." [31] Around the same time, Jamaican Olympic 200-meter sprint champion Veronica Campbell-Brown tested positive for a banned diuretic. Brown's agent vaguely claimed that his client was "[not] guilty of willfully taking a banned substance." These unconvincing, but difficult to disprove, excuses have become routine whenever elite athletes test positive for a banned substance.

In track and field, doping appears to be widespread. The aforementioned WADA-sponsored survey, involving more than two thousand track-and-field athletes, concluded that nearly 30 percent who participated in the world championship and a whopping 45 percent who attended the Pan Arab Games admitted doping during that past year. [32] That figure probably was low because even with promised anonymity it is doubtful whether all those athletes would be truthful in their responses.

## Flawed and Corrupted Enforcement Efforts

One might have expected that WADA would be proactive in trying to respond to this much evidence of wrongdoing in track and field, especially given the way it had gone after Lance Armstrong. Yet, two years after the WADA-sponsored study had found widespread cheating, the report had not been officially released because the IAAF was still reviewing the findings. Despite the researchers' protests, track and field's governing body—with the apparent imprimatur of WADA—was in the process of supplementing the report with its own "information" to cushion the likely bad publicity somewhat.

By that time, however, a number of anti-doping experts had already seen the original document. Professor John Hoberman stated that the results "dispelled the notion that doping was a deviant behavior among a few athletes." Similarly, Don Catlin concluded that the findings were "disturbing." [33] Thus, under public pressure, WADA decided to move forward by enhancing the penalties for doping violations in all sports under its jurisdiction, including track and field. By doubling the length of the sanctions from two to four years, offending athletes would be ineligible to compete in at least one Olympics. The harsh penalties appeared to make those "levied by the professional leagues in the United States . . . pale in comparison."[34]

Nevertheless, there still were two major stumbling blocks. First, greater penalties would not necessarily substantially decrease cheating. Actual effectiveness largely depends on testing frequency and surprise. Second, the harsher penalties would be no less difficult to implement, if providing persuasive proof that athletes have been deliberately doping was required before such a sanction could be levied. In addition to an overall lack of fairness and due process in the WADA procedures, there have been remarkable variations in how different countries, different labs, and different Olympic sports have managed their enforcement procedures. Reportedly, many nations have much worse procedures for monitoring their athletes than do the pro leagues in North America.

Juliet Macur, who covers these doping issues for the *New York Times*, warned that the new WADA penalties would be ineffective in many countries because the anti-doping agencies have "little interest in . . . administering drug tests. It is difficult to find something wrong if no one is looking."[35] Politicians, fans, and the various sports themselves want to glorify their national athletic heroes, not make them objects of disgrace, or put them in jail.

This bias intensifies if a country is hosting the Olympic Games. Before the Sochi Winter Games, for instance, major problems were found with Russian labs. Norway assumed the role of "Russia's antidoping mentor,"[36] a response that turned out to be too little too late and camouflaged the true extent of the problem (see chapter 10).

Nevertheless, this type of cheating by athletes, which is facilitated by nationalism and the profit motive in sports, is a pervasive problem that includes many more nations than just Russia or China. Despite their history of violations, "Jamaican athletes . . . weren't tested even once out of competition in the three months leading up to the 2012 London Olympics." Usain Bolt and Jamaica's other world-class athletes won twelve Olympic medals at those games, including four gold. Subsequently, after a number of Jamaican athletes tested positive for banned substances, the nation's lead drug testing official explained to the BBC that those who had been caught "were only the 'tip of the iceberg'" because athletes are rarely "stupid . . . enough to use drugs in competition," at least not any drugs that might be detected.[37]

Another problem is that the testing capabilities of many nations are inadequate due to financial and administrative shortcomings and corruption. During the 2014 World Cup, Brazil had to send its tests to a lab in Switzerland. Even though Brazil was the host country, it had no labs that had been properly accredited by WADA. That deficiency became even more embarrassing for all concerned after the lab that the Brazilians established for the 2016 Rio Summer Olympics was sanctioned for "'nonconformity' with international standards" only a few weeks before the games were to begin.[38]

In Kenya, which is famous for its superb long-distance runners, credible reports surfaced that "the blood booster EPO was readily available for Kenyan athletes."[39] Yet, even after numerous Kenyan athletes had tested positive for EPO, and WADA had made a formal request that its anti-doping agency conduct an investigation, Kenyan officials took no substantive actions. Instead, eighteen months after the WADA request was made, Kenya created a task force to look into the matter, providing few indications that there would be a serious investigation before the 2016 Summer Games. Kenya then won thirteen medals in Rio for long-distance running, including six gold. As one Kenyan writer opined, his nation's Olympic committee should have been given a "gold medal for corruption."[40]

Kenya's transgressions underscore an important anti-doping reality. Outside the Olympic Games themselves, WADA rules and protocols have only as much impact as the affected nations are willing to guarantee and effectively implement in circumstances where politics inevitably affects the outcomes. Having nations investigate their athletic heroes makes about as much sense as having professional and college teams investigate their star athletes.

Furthermore, as noted earlier, officials who run and benefit from the various Olympic sports, most recently those associated with track and field, have been accused of bribery, extortion, corruption, and other conflicts of interest. Unlike FIFA, whose officials were finally investigated and prosecuted by the DOJ, to date there has been almost no law enforcement presence to deter Olympic and related international federation officials from engaging in criminal behavior.

## THE BIATHLON AND CROSS-COUNTRY SKIING: BUILDING UP ENDURANCE

The biathlon has been described, quite beautifully, as a "thrilling sport that draws on the endurance needed to cross-country ski along steep tracks and idiosyncratic Zen needed to target shoot while gasping for air."[41] Given those required skill sets, it should come as no surprise that the sport has been a hotbed of doping accusations. The 2014 Winter Olympics proved to be no exception.

After serious discrepancies with tests in Russian labs were revealed just before the beginning of the Sochi Games, two of that nation's world-class biathlon competitors were suspended for doping violations. One of their coaches admitted that he had known for several months before the suspensions were issued that at least one team member had been cheating. A Lithuanian biathlete also was suspended. All three "tested positive for a 'nonspecific substance' . . . which . . . involved a designer version of the endurance-boosting drug EPO." These violations were nothing new, however. "The biathlon has long had issues with doping because of the unusual requirements of endurance for skiing [and] . . . a low heart rate for . . . shooting."[42]

Apparently many of the biathletes were taking PEDs at the Salt Lake Winter Games in 2002. Five tested positive. However, Jacques Rogge, the IOC president at the time—without any objection from WADA—decided not to pursue two of those cases because "it would raise a huge stink around the world."[43]

Similar doping problems seem to have infected cross-country skiing. As with the biathlon, endurance is a key ingredient of success. At the same time, the national federations and Olympic committees in the countries where those sports are most popular reportedly have neglected their anti-doping responsibilities. Thus, in biathlon and cross-country skiing this type of cheating has been widespread for many years. Those sports have been labeled "the Winter Games' version of cycling."[44]

## OLYMPIC HOCKEY PLAYER SUSPENDED FOR TAKING ALLERGY MEDICATION

While the failure to adequately identify and control drug-related cheating has been a prominent part of Olympic sports, the tendency to be too quick to condemn athletes based on tenuous evidence has been a serious problem as well. The suspension of Nicklas Backstrom—a gifted member of the Swedish hockey team on loan from the Washington Capitals—hours before he was to play in the finals of the hockey championship in Sochi illustrates the lack of basic fairness in the testing and disciplining of Olympic athletes under WADA protocols.

Due to the widespread doping scandals associated with past competitions, organizers performed 2,631 drug tests—"the most extensive testing program in Winter Olympic history."[45] Somehow those tests only detected six alleged violators (.02 percent), of whom the most notable was Nicklas Backstrom, who should not have been suspended. He had "an elevated level of pseudoephedrine, which was found in his prescription allergy medication Zyrtec-D."[46]

Although drugs with pseudoephedrine are commonly used in various cold and allergy medications, specified levels in the blood are not allowed by the IOC and WADA. Swedish team doctors, however, had approved Backstrom's medication, assuring him that its use would not violate any Olympic rules. Backstrom had been using the over-the-counter drug "for seven years to treat sinusitis"[47] and had never encountered any testing problems.

His test at the Olympics revealed a relatively minor discrepancy. The highest permissible level of pseudoephedrine is "150 micrograms per milliliter and . . . Backstrom's level was 190." A recommended dosage is 120 micrograms not more than twice a day, but that is for the average-sized person, not a relatively large professional hockey player. Normally in these situations when Olympic athletes are taking a prescribed medication, which exceeds permissible levels and there has been no evidence that they were intentionally trying to enhance their performance, the athletes have been permitted to retake the tests. If they achieve an acceptable test result, they have been allowed to compete in the Olympics.

Backstrom was never given that opportunity. He was tested after playing in Sweden's quarterfinal game, but the results were not disclosed until "hours before the gold medal game four days later." Consequently, he had to be a last-minute scratch from what was widely described as one of the most important hockey matches in Sweden's history. According to the glib IOC officials, the lab "had too many tests to process to deliver the results any sooner."[48]

At the 2010 Winter Olympics, after a provisional suspension was issued against another NHL player who had tested positive for pseudo-ephedrine while playing for the Slovakian team, a retest was conducted and the athlete was allowed to play. Two theories soon emerged as to why there had been no retest in Backstrom's situation. One theory proposed that the testing system was a "debacle";[49] the second posited that the IOC had wanted to make an example of the NHL player to deter cheating and create the impression that cheaters would be caught. Both explanations were plausible given the circumstances.

An official for the NHL Players' Association embraced the first theory. "At some point common sense should have prevailed, and it clearly did not."[50] The general manager (GM) of the Swedish hockey team embraced the conspiracy theory. He opined that the IOC had "destroyed one of the greatest hockey days in Swedish history." He believed that Backstrom's test results had been purposefully delayed "to generate the most publicity."[51]

In any case, as the chief medical officer of the International Ice Hockey Federation explained, there had been no substantial evidence of doping. Backstrom was an innocent victim of circumstances. Thus, any value that the suspension could have had as a warning to other athletes or for demonstrating that the IOC's procedures were effective was largely negated. Backstrom's suspension was an example of bureaucratic incompetence.

Throughout, the IOC refused to comment on the widespread criticisms about its actions. It continued to maintain that the suspension was "fully justified." Nonetheless, the IOC allowed Backstrom to receive a silver medal with his Swedish teammates. The IOC Disciplinary Commission acknowledged that there had been "no indication" that Backstrom had intended "to improve his performance by taking the prohibited substance."[52] Yet, like many other Olympic athletes over the years, he was a victim of overreaching by anti-doping officials.

# 9

# THE LAISSEZ-FAIRE APPROACH TO DOPING IN TENNIS

**P**rofessional tennis arguably remains the least effective sport in terms of testing, even worse perhaps than cycling or American football. Tennis's testing protocols have been criticized as being halfhearted at best, even though athletes in that sport, both male and female, have been bulking up, increasing their stamina and injury recovery times, being linked to performance-enhancing drug use, and claiming publicly that they want closer scrutiny to identify cheaters. The sport embracing the badly flawed WADA protocols and procedures appears to have been a reflexive attempt at a quick fix to try to improve the public's perception about drug cheating. If the IOC and WADA have been frequently overzealous, yet ineffective in their enforcement protocols for performance-enhancing substances, then professional tennis has been conspicuously underzealous and ineffective.

With the notable exception of Maria Sharapova, who appears to have been the high-profile scapegoat tennis was looking for, underzealous and ineffective still aptly describe doping enforcement under the auspices of the newly formed Tennis Integrity Unit. As a *New York Times* headline proclaimed early in 2016, tennis still "seems to operate in the dark," not only about performance-enhancing drugs, but also "match-fixing."[1]

## FOR YEARS IT SEEMED AS IF "THE FIX" WAS IN

Those directly associated with professional tennis have not wanted to know whether the extraordinary physical endurance, recovery capacities, increased size, or improved strength of Serena Williams, Rafael Nadal, Novak Djokovic, Samantha Stosur, Andy Murray, David Ferrer, Maria Sharapova, and many others might have been due in part to doping, as well as better nutrition, training, and other legal performance enhancements. In the words of Howard Bryant of *ESPN the Magazine* in 2013, when it comes to doping enforcement in tennis, "the fix is in."[2]

For many years, it was commonly believed that "the skills required in tennis d[id] not lend themselves to doping."[3] If that ever was true, it certainly proved to be a fallacy once the players bulked up, increased their endurance, and improved their recovery times after matches and injuries. What raised suspicions that tennis testing had been mostly a sham was that only a few marginal tennis players were ever identified as having doped. No marquee player had failed a drug test for PEDs, which is reminiscent of the way football is now and baseball used to be before selective testing was introduced.

The International Tennis Federation (ITF) reported in 2011 that only "21 out-of-competition blood tests" were conducted on the men and women players combined.[4] Notably, "whether by blood or urine, the ITF did not test the Williams sisters once out of competition." Not seriously testing the superstars of tennis appears to have been a common practice. Unfortunately, out-of-competition tests are essential since the players "are more likely to use performance-enhancing drugs during training and recovery from injury,"[5] and then let it wear off before they play their first match of a tournament.

Unlike baseball players, though, major tennis stars, at least on the men's side, including Novak Djokovic and Andy Murray, "called for increased blood testing and more frequent out-of-competition testing." Yet, professional tennis responded by actually "cut[ting] back on blood tests, especially for EPO—the one test tennis need[ed] because [EPO] helps increase endurance and recovery."[6] In December 2012, Roger Federer, who also has called for greater transparency, reported that he was "being tested [even] less . . . than six or seven years ago."[7]

Of the superstars of men's tennis, only Rafael Nadal seemed to be expressing a dissenting view. According to him, the sport needed to "clean up its image . . . [while] respecting the athlete,"[8] whatever that might mean or suggest.

In March 2013 the media pressure on the players became intense enough that the ITF decided to adopt WADA's "biological passport program." That new but controversial approach has been used to create a blood profile for each athlete, which supposedly allows for a more sensitive interpretation as to whether a test result is abnormal for each player. The problem is that this type of expert interpretation, done behind closed doors, is inherently subjective, as compared to applying exactly the same criteria to every player. The due process controversy regarding the suspension of speed skater Claudia Pechstein took place mainly because she was punished for discrepancies in her passport profile, even though she had not failed a drug test.[9]

Such organizational discretion also makes it easier to favor the stars and superstars over the marginal players or to allow certain players to be the designated scapegoats. In 2012 the ITF agreed to increase out-of-competition testing without specifying what that would mean in terms of how frequently players would be tested or whether every athlete would be subject to the same testing frequency. A few months later two relatively well-known players were accused of doping, but by that time their rankings had fallen so they were no longer considered major stars.[10]

## BIG-NAME TENNIS STARS CONTINUE TO AVOID SCRUTINY

Even with the supposed testing improvements, there continued to be concern that the big-name cheaters in the sport had escaped detection. Rafael Nadal has been at the center of such allegations. He disappeared from tennis and the public eye for nearly eight months with his second severe knee injury. When he returned in February 2013, he was playing better than ever, at least for a while. After missing the Australian Open, Nadal won both the French and U.S. Opens and overtook Djokovic to become the number-one-ranked tennis player in the world. Arguably he was the most popular as well.

How Nadal's extraordinary recovery happened was kept mostly a secret. Nadal lived in a compound surrounded by bodyguards, trainers, doctors, and advisers during his treatment and rehabilitation. Nadal's representatives acknowledged that he was using platelet-rich plasma (PRP) therapy,[11] but by that time the procedure was no long being banned as performance enhancing.

That revised judgment about PRP therapy, however, appeared to have been incorrect from a medical perspective. According to articles published in the *American Journal of Sports Medicine*, PRP "may have much wider benefits to performance."[12] Scientific analysis revealed that both anabolic and catabolic growth factors were significantly increased in the blood samples of individuals who had this procedure.

In any case, despite "repeated whispers" about his using PEDs, Nadal has yet to fail a drug test. Those whispers grew even louder in May 2013 during the trial of a Spanish doctor who had been charged with "supplying cyclists with [illegal] blood transfusions."[13] The defendant "admitted" having Spanish tennis players as clients, but inexplicably the judge ordered key evidence, which could have been used to identify those players, destroyed.

In Spain, Nadal, and to a lesser extent David Ferrer, are considered national treasures, so it was surmised by many with knowledge of the situation that the judge was protecting them in particular. Andy Murray felt compelled to tweet that the destruction of this particular evidence was "beyond a joke . . . biggest cover-up-in sports history?"[14] To be the biggest cover-up it would have had to involve a superstar of tennis. Subsequently, a former French minister opined on television "that Nadal's seven-month hiatus in 2012 was probably due to a positive dope test."[15] Nadal responded by filing a defamation suit against that former minister, which is still being litigated.

This game of making veiled accusations, which Murray played with his tweet, is similar to what occurs in other sports. Athletes who say they refrain from cheating seem convinced that they can identify many of those competitors who do cheat. Yet, there seems to be a code among most American and international professional athletes not to accuse a teammate or competitor by name. Doing so typically is viewed as acting as a "rat," a label that can be extremely detrimental to a player's standing in a sport, even more so than any cheating itself. The notable exception seems to be in Olympic sports when the athletes under suspicion represent a communist nation, like Russia or China. Then disclosure becomes a patriotic duty.

In the past couple of years, the ITF, which is part of the International Association of Athletics Federations (IAAF), has made some policy changes in its testing program, which suggested that there would be greater enforcement than in the past. The inherently subjective passport program has been enhanced to include the testing profiles of many more players. In addition, the out-of-competition testing was increased in 2014 from "just 63 . . . [to] 1,139."[16] Furthermore, higher-profile players including Marin Cilic, who later won the U.S. Open, and top-ten player Richard Gasquet have received suspensions. Yet they are not superstars. Nor do they seem much affected by being caught.

As tennis expert Christopher Clarey explained in a December 2015 article in the *New York Times*, suspicions and accusations continue to surface. Both Roger Federer and Andy Murray have continued to indicate that the ITF's testing program lacks visibility and effectiveness. "The idea of a federation administering doping tests to its own athletes and meal tickets has been flawed from the start." Recently it was discovered that "Lamine Diack, president of the I.A.A.F. for 16 years, took bribes to cover up positive doping tests."[17]

## MARIA SHARAPOVA IS MADE THE SCAPEGOAT

Until 2016 no marquee tennis player had been suspended for performance-enhancing drugs, although Martina Hingis's singles career reportedly was derailed because of cocaine use a number of years ago. The pressure, however, was building on professional tennis to seriously test its big-name stars, which finally produced its first casualty. It seems more than a coincidence that she was Russian.

In March 2016 the world's most endorsed and, at that time, the highest-paid female athlete, Maria Sharapova, shocked the tennis world by calling a press conference to announce that she had failed a drug test at the Australian Open.[18] The drug in question was meldonium, which has been used to "increase blood flow and therefore . . . the amount of oxygen taken into the body."[19] At the time, the drug had been banned for less than a month.

Many "Russian teams had used meldonium regularly and openly, viewing it as a remedy for fending off exhaustion and heart problems." Thus, Russians in particular were highly suspicious when WADA elected to prohibit this drug, which had been legal for decades. Moreover, according to published studies, the evidence of the performance-enhancing effects of meldonium appeared to be "quite thin."[20]

Unfortunately for Sharapova, a 2015 WADA report had concluded that there had been a state-sponsored conspiracy to help Russian athletes dope without being caught (see chapter 10). Thus, while WADA had approved the use of platelet-rich plasma therapy, even though the medical evidence against it had been much more damning than for meldonium, the anti-doping authorities decided to ban the Eastern European drug for what appeared to be political reasons.

Sharapova claimed that she had been taking the medication for ten years to treat various health issues and did not read the one e-mail that was sent to each player stating the drug had been placed on the prohibited list. Serena Williams praised Sharapova for forthrightly admitting her mistake. It turned out later that on a number of occasions both Serena and Venus Williams, as well as a number of other American tennis players and other athletes, had been granted special waivers to take banned substances for medical reasons.[21] The drug's manufacturer, though, cast doubt on Sharapova's professed intent in using the drug when it stated that "4–6 weeks [was the] normal course of treatment."[22] The perception that she had been stretching the truth did not help her case or her public persona.

The ITF immediately suspended her, pending a final resolution of its investigation. Three months later she received a particularly harsh two-year ban, which she immediately appealed. Even though the "ITF panel conceded that she had not cheated intentionally," it "concluded she was at the highest level of fault."[23] Unfortunately for Sharapova, the athlete-unfriendly Court for Arbitration for Sport would be hearing the appeal. To obtain a significant reduction in her suspension, she would have the difficult burden of "prov[ing] that she had 'no significant fault or negligence'" in taking the banned substance. Both parties agreed that the matter should not be resolved until after the Rio Olympics, which meant Sharapova could not represent Russia in tennis. Ultimately, however, a compromise was reached reducing Sharapova's suspension, from two years to fifteen months, making her eligible to compete in the 2017 French Open.

## TENNIS AS USUAL EXCEPT FOR SHARAPOVA

After Sharapova was suspended much seems to have remained the same with respect to how the tennis community enforces the use of performance-enhancing drugs by its best players. Sharapova received virtually all the media's attention, while testing of other stars of tennis remained shrouded in secrecy and ambiguity. At the 2016 French Open, Richard Gasquet reached the quarterfinals, but his doping violation was barely mentioned during hours of coverage of his matches on the Tennis Channel; nor was the issue of doping discussed in any serious manner.

More surprisingly, though, none of those television commentators questioned Nadal's shocking decision to drop out of the French Open only hours after overwhelming his opponent 6–3, 6–0, and 6–3. Nadal claimed he had a wrist injury, which was accepted without any scrutiny. This lack of media follow-through occurred in spite of suspicions about Nadal's faking injuries due to drug use in the past and accusations by a former French official that Nadal had been doping for years. No one in the media—even respected journalists—bothered to ask Nadal or the ITF what many of them must have been thinking: Had Nadal been informed or somehow discovered that he was about to be tested under the new WADA-inspired protocols when he made his decision to retire from a grand-slam event he had won nine times?

The answer may have been difficult to verify, since the ITF's testing process remains so nontransparent. Nonetheless, respected journalists and commentators should have at least posed the question. Despite all the hoopla surrounding the new WADA doping standards in tennis and the scapegoating of Sharapova, it still appears that no one closely associated with the sport really wanted to know the answer. This lack of vigilance seems to apply whether the player involved is named Nadal, Williams, Federer, Djokovic, or Murray. Moreover, avoidance of the tennis doping issue on American television continued that September during ESPN's coverage of the U.S. Open. Far more troubling to the commentators was the loud gong-like sound during a few key matches emanating from the newly rebuilt Arthur Ashe Stadium.

# 10

# THE IOC, WADA, IAAF, AND STATE-SPONSORED DOPING IN RUSSIA

## RUSSIAN DOPING AT THE SOCHI WINTER GAMES

In a documentary aired a few months before the 2014 Winter Olympics were to be held in Sochi, Russia, Russian athletes were accused of widespread doping.[1] A German television station, based on the "accounts of athletes, coaches and antidoping officials" in Russia, accused that government of helping "procure drugs and cover up positive results" of athletes.[2] In response, WADA established a special three-person commission led by former WADA president Dick Pound.

As it turned out, however, this was not WADA's first opportunity to address charges of state-sponsored doping in Russia. According to the *Washington Post*, WADA had learned from a "Russian whistleblower" in February 2010 that "drug cheating was endemic among Russia's Olympic athletes and how the government and Russia's anti-doping agency were complicit." WADA contended that it had not pursued the matter until January 2015 because the "agency's rules did not grant it the authority to conduct investigations."[3]

In other words, this had been a matter for the IOC to address. As the scandal unfolded, the IOC allowed preparations for the Winter Games to continue without taking any special precautions or measures to protect the integrity of the athletic events. In Sally Jenkins's biting words, the IOC members looked the other way "while they dined from the ice-sculpture buffet and sipped their aperitifs."[4]

Eleven months later, well after those games had concluded, WADA's special commission issued a lengthy report that "confirm[ed] many of the film's charges, but also accus[ed] the Russian government of abetting in the doping program."[5] Among the more serious allegations were that the Russian secret service had "intimidated workers at a drug-testing lab to cover up top athletes' positive results."[6]

In addition, it was alleged that "top sports officials routinely submitted bogus urine samples for athletes who were doping." The commission "claimed that Russia ha[d] maintained an organized national doping programme of the sort that was thought to have ended with the cold war."[7] They found that "for decades . . . the Russians maintained a secret lab at the Ministry of Sport dedicated to the development of 'undetectable' drugs."[8]

Despite the scope and grandeur of the accusations and the apparent outrage of the three commissioners, the IOC-approved WADA sanctions were remarkably restrained, at least initially. They focused instead on rescinding the accreditation of a lab in Moscow at the center of the scandal. This lab not only had destroyed hundreds of drug samples of Russian athletes, but had produced undetectable drugs for athletes to use.

In addition, WADA prevailed upon the IAAF to indefinitely suspend the entire Russian track-and-field team, with no determination whether the sanction would effectively bar those athletes from the 2016 Summer Olympics in Rio de Janeiro. Russia was given the opportunity to make changes in its doping detection program that could lead to the lifting of the ban well before those games began. There were no sanctions against any of the other Russian sports federations or the Russian officials, who had directed Russia's Olympic sports apparatus. Nor were there any negative sanctions aimed at President Putin, who appeared to have been directly involved in all important Russian Olympic sports matters.

Underlying this jarring variance between the incendiary accusations and the relatively mild sanctions appeared to be four considerations. To begin with, as has been typical with many—and arguably most—of these international doping investigations, the well-publicized charges seemed to extend well beyond the actual evidence that had been collected. The *Economist*, which has been a strong advocate for addressing doping in sports, observed that the WADA commission's report had only one "main smoking gun involv[ing] . . . the chief medical officer of the All-Russian

Athletics Federation [ARAF]." Otherwise, the report lacked "specifics . . . and seem[ed] to rely on hearsay."[9]

Furthermore, there was the familiar speculation that the specter of suspending Russia for the Summer Olympics might send financial shock waves through the Olympic community, especially to those organizers who would stand to lose money if revenues to be generated by the games were substantially diminished. Banning Russia also might have long-term negative political and economic repercussions, if it pushed Putin toward a return to the days of the Cold War in international sports.

Lastly and perhaps most importantly, the IAAF, which had imposed the provisional sanctions upon the Russian track-and-field federation, was itself mired in scandal. The IAAF's former president, Lamine Diack, had accepted more than a million dollars "in bribes, reportedly paid through ARAF, in exchange for not taking action against Russian cheaters."[10]

Making matters worse, when the IAAF's new president, Sebastian Coe, officially visited Russia prior to the WADA report being issued, he "repeatedly expressed his support for engagement with Russia instead of suspension."[11] Apparently Coe had assumed—or hoped—that the Russians would be more compliant going forward, and attempted to avoid destabilizing the IAAF and Olympic sports by antagonizing one of its most powerful members. To much of the sports world, however, this seemed to be collaborating with the enemy.

## CHARGES OF RUSSIAN DOPING BOIL OVER MONTHS BEFORE THE RIO GAMES

Coe's assumption or hope appeared to be misguided at best. With the games only half a year away, Travis Tygart, the head of the USADA, reported that it was too late to ensure that Russian athletes "in the state-supported doping program [would be] clean."[12] Tygart opined that due to politics, it would be extremely difficult to monitor those athletes.

In January 2016, WADA began to flex its muscles by placing meldonium on the banned drug list, even though for years it had been openly used by Russian soldiers and many elite athletes, especially from Russia and Eastern Europe. As described in chapter 9, Maria Sharapova was the most prominent Russian athlete to be caught in the cross fire. Sharapova contended that she did not realize the drug, which she supposedly took for a heart condition, had been banned. She too was suspended, provisionally, and faced a lengthy suspension, as much as two years, which if carried out probably would end her professional career as a top-notch singles player.

As Patrick Reevell reported in the *New York Times*, the Russians began to mount a two-pronged defense of meldonium users. They argued that the drug had specific health-related benefits in protecting the hearts of athletes who were pushing themselves to the limits of human endurance, and, regardless, the testing protocols were deficient because it was impossible to know with any reasonable degree of certainty the length of time meldonium takes to leave the body.[13] Thus, it was premature to conclude that those who tested positive in the weeks following the ban had been using it afterward and not before.

In addition, the Russians implied that enforcing this ban against their athletes would have negative financial consequences for various international sports and the Olympics. To emphasize that point, the Russian minister of sports pointed out that entire teams were not competing in various events "over fears that they would test positive for meldonium."[14]

Less than a week later WADA apparently recalculated the political and financial implications of its policy. It issued new guidelines to respond to this "'unprecedented situation' caused by the banning . . . of meldonium." Those doping tests occurring before March 2016 that showed meldonium concentrations under one microgram would be given a free pass. If the concentrations were between one and fifteen micrograms, then there would be a further lab review to calculate "excretion times more precisely." The onus would be on the athletes to explain their particular case. The Russians held that these changes in policy were an opportunity for athletes who "had been unfairly trapped by the meldonium ban . . . to seek amnesty."[15]

In May 2016, American—and presumably most Western—attitudes toward the Russian doping scandal shifted dramatically after the *New York Times* published an interview with Grigory Rodchenkov, the director of the major Russian lab that had been in charge of processing the tests "for thousands of Olympians." He claimed to have been part of "one of the most . . . successful . . . doping ploys in sports history." According to him, members of the government's secret service worked with Russian anti-doping experts to dispose of urine samples that tested positive for PEDs by replacing them "with clean urine collected months earlier."[16]

While this revelation was hailed as persuasive proof of a state-sponsored conspiracy, there was no actual smoking gun and no convincing corroborating evidence. In addition, Rodchenkov's credibility was called into question because he already had left Russia and signed a deal with an American documentary producer who was doing a film on doping by Russian athletes. Rodchenkov alleged that he had been compelled to leave Russia after two other unidentified Russian doping officials had "died unexpectedly."

A key part of Rodchenkov's narrative was that Russian officials, with the assistance of state security operatives, had somehow managed to tamper with the tamper-proof bottles that were used to store athletes' urine for testing purposes, although he did not know how it had been done. According to experts, the bottles had been meticulously designed by Swiss manufacturers to protect the samples once the lids were closed. A former head of an American Olympic laboratory said, "I tried to break into these bottles [myself] . . . and couldn't do it. . . . It's shocking [to believe that someone else did]."[17]

Furthermore, no one had been able to corroborate Rodchenkov's hearsay evidence that the bottles were tampered with. Nor could anyone replicate a procedure that demonstrated how it could have been done. The best working theory was the fragile argument that the Russian security operatives must have figured it out, since Rodchenkov had alleged that he had seen them tampering with those bottles.

Nonetheless, given the mounting accusations against the Russian Olympic apparatus and the Russian government's low status in the United States, the American media were ready to pounce. Juliet Macur of the *New York Times* called for Russia to be barred from the Rio Olympics. Yet even she was not optimistic that her recommendation would be followed. The "WADA and the I.O.C. have a record of going soft when dealing with Russia," she noted.[18]

A *New York Times* editorial took a somewhat more nuanced position. It recommended that the Russian athletes be banned from competing in Rio unless there was "tangible and convincing proof that Russia has cleaned up its act."[19] The burden would be placed on the Russians to disprove allegations, which had never been conclusively proven in the first place but were presumed to be true by most Americans who strongly believed Putin and his government were corrupt.

In response to all the bad publicity and calls for banning Russian athletes from the Summer Games, representatives of the Russian Ministry of Sport admitted that there were doping problems, but blamed "coaches and athletes [who] made 'serious mistakes.'"[20] The ministry added that it would be unfair for all the "clean [Russian] athletes . . . [to] suffer for the behavior of others."[21]

Tim Layden of *Sports Illustrated* reminded Americans in his article "Bear Down" that "while it's tempting to demonize Russia, it is not the only nation with track and field athletes under suspicion." The United States, Kenya, Ethiopia, and Jamaica all have had multiple athletes test positive in recent years. "One victory has been won in the fight against doping. But many more lie ahead."[22]

## THE IOC AND WADA HYPOCRISY

The crux of this ongoing controversy soon became whether all Russian athletes, those representing the very worst Russian sports federations, or individual Russian athletes should be barred from participating in Rio. As Will Hobson reported in the *Washington Post*, there would be several hurdles for the IOC to overcome "to ban all of the country's athletes from the upcoming Summer Games."[23] To begin with, there were other countries, besides Russia, suspected of widespread doping violations facilitated by their government officials, including Kenya and Ethiopia. Jamaica and China probably should be on such a list as well. Moreover, as Michael Powell of the *New York Times* observed the "list of American runners and bikers and skiers who have doped is long and desultory. . . . The Salt Lake Winter Olympics in 2002 was a festival of bribes and doping."[24]

In addition, there were a number of geopolitical reasons why Russia was an important country to the Olympics, not the least of which is that in the past, athletic competitions with the United States have generated large television audiences and revenues. Furthermore, the evidence to date had fallen short of being convincing. In part that was because, as the *New York Times* reported later, WADA was playing its own politics by not acting on "detailed tips from Russian whistle-blowers" and "pass[ing] along word of one such whistle-blower to the same government officials accused of running the doping program."[25]

Before the threshold question about the IOC's and WADA's true intentions toward Russia and its athletes could be revealed, however, two new developments, reported on the same day, further complicated the enforcement calculus. Both developments made the Russians look worse in the court of public opinion, but each provided the IOC with an excuse to delay its ultimate decision. First, the IOC announced it had tested "454 urine samples from the 2008 Summer Olympics . . . [that] revealed suspicious samples from 31 athletes from 12 countries." In addition, the IOC said that it would "soon test 250 samples from the 2012 Summer Games." Although athletes from several countries were facing potential bans from the Rio Olympics, the emphasis was on "retesting" the Russians due to the mounting allegations against them.[26]

Second, the Department of Justice (DOJ) had "opened a criminal investigation into possible state-sponsored doping by top Russian athletes." Although this development made for a great news event, obtaining criminal convictions would be very difficult. Even convincing a judge to hear the case would require the DOJ to establish a tangible connection to U.S. law, such as the use of a bank in the United States by the Russian officials to commit "conspiracy" or "fraud."[27] Whatever happened, though, it would be virtually impossible for the DOJ to complete its investigation and prosecute any charges before the games were held.

In the meantime, the focus would continue to be on punishing individual Russian athletes who may or may not have cheated in order to help quell the public furor. Sally Jenkins railed at the IOC's anti-doping hypocrisy. Blaming Russian athletes "whose choice was to either participate in doping . . . or face angry state authorities, maybe even a gulag . . . conveniently diverts attention from the IOC's own misdeeds, the offenses they either commit themselves or enabled and ignored."[28]

From a health and security perspective, the IOC's mishandling of doping at the Rio Games seemed almost inconsequential when compared to the hazards posed to athletes, their families, and significant others by the Zika virus, the disease-causing pollution at the sites where water sports were to be held, and the possibility of injuries or disruptions in medical services due to Rio's professed bankruptcy and the growing potential for civil unrest. As a Brazilian columnist opined, these "Olympic

Games . . . are an unnatural disaster . . . [which was] man-made, foresee-able, [and] preventable."[29]

## RUSSIAN TRACK-AND-FIELD ATHLETES
## BANNED FROM RIO

While the IOC contemplated what should be done, the pressures on the IAAF to do something became immense. Athletes from around the West-ern world—who would likely benefit from the absence of Russian ath-letes at the Olympic Games—and the American, British, and European media insisted that strong actions should be taken, even before a compre-hensive and thorough investigation could be completed. More important-ly, the IAAF was already under fire. As discussed earlier, its former president had participated in the alleged Russian cover-up and corruption, while its new leader, Sebastian Coe, had appeared to be cozying up to the Russian track-and-field federation. Thus, appearing to be strong advo-cates for strict sanctions became "an institutional necessity."[30]

After its initial weak response, the IAAF unanimously voted to take the unprecedented step of barring Russia's entire track-and-field team from competing in Rio. Russian track-and-field athletes, however, would be given the opportunity to petition to participate as individuals, but they would have to prove "clearly and convincingly . . . they [were] not tainted by the Russian system." According to Rune Anderson, an anti-doping expert from Norway, this very limited opportunity existed "because we 'are living in a world of lawyers.'"[31]

The onus would be placed on individual Russian athletes, however, to prove that they were not guilty of cheating under a standard that was far more onerous than the one that WADA, the IOC, and the IAAF used to supposedly prove that athletes were tainted. The double standard was remarkable. Even the USA Track & Field president conceded that an unknown number of Russian athletes were being made to "pay a [stiff] penalty for the serious transgressions of their federation"[32]—not to men-tion the incompetence and corruption of the IOC, WADA, and the IAAF. With some justification one Russian athlete, pole-vaulter Yelena Isinbay-eva, said that "the decision was a violation of human rights,"[33] or, per-haps more accurately, reasonable expectations of due process.

Ultimately, though, as much as the decision was hailed as something the Russians under Putin deserved and a welcome indication that finally WADA and the IOC were getting tough on dopers, the outcome appeared more like a face-saving gesture spurred on by a public relations crisis. IOC president Thomas Bach "acknowledge[d] that the current [WADA] structure was rife with conflicts . . . [and] has some deficiencies." He recommended that the international anti-doping system be made "independent from sports organizations" it serves. This separation would avoid the "politics and possible conflicts of interest" of the past, he argued.[34]

Bach and the IOC also publicly disagreed with WADA and the IAAF as to whether the Russian athletes, who would be allowed to compete in Rio—including those track-and-field competitors who had proven their innocence—should be competing as representatives of Russia. Bach stated that they should be. Not surprisingly, the Russian sports minister was in favor of the IOC's decision, which suggested that an IOC-Russia accommodation regarding the Rio Games might be in the offing. As Roger Pielke, a University of Colorado professor who studies the governance of sports organizations, explained, "The last chapters of this saga haven't even begun to be written yet. . . . It's still unfolding."[35]

In the meantime, just weeks before the Rio Games were to begin, WADA had to suspend the Brazilian laboratory that was set to handle drug testing at the games "in a new escalation of the doping crisis in international sports."[36] Fortunately for the IOC, WADA, the IAAF, and NBC Sports, contrary to the doomsday scenario that had been expressed previously, it seemed likely now that American television ratings and revenues would not be negatively affected by the absence of the Russian track-and-field team. Dick Ebersol, the former chairman of NBC Sports, explained that "the removal of a major rival might help the United States win more medals. . . . 'Anything that helps you win more medals is a help [for the ratings].'"[37] Regardless, with the exception of the men's 100-meter sprint, track-and-field events are not among the most highly watched Olympic competitions anyway.

Ratings, it turned out, was a non-issue as compared to the political fall-out. After the summer games, Russian hackers decided to embarrass U.S. anti-doping officials by revealing that a number of famous American Olympians, including the Williams sisters in tennis and multiple Gold Medal winner Simone Biles in gymnastics had received secret medical exemptions that allowed them to compete in the Rio Games, even though they were taking banned substances.[38] The IOC and WADA responded to that attack by announcing that after retesting urine samples from the Summer Olympics in 2008 and 2012, they found that 75 of the competitors were guilty of taking banned substances. Not surprisingly, most of those athletes were Russian and Eastern European.[39] In addition, certain U.S. athletes competing in winter sports threatened to boycott the February 2017 world championships in Sochi, Russia.

Thereafter, the WADA released a report overseen by Richard McLaren a Canadian lawyer, alleging that state-sponsored doping by Russian officials encompassed more than 1,000 Olympic athletes. That report, however, created the misleading impression that doping in the Olympics is primarily a Russian phenomenon and also raised more questions than it answered. To begin with, if, as many in the U.S., Great Britain, and other western nations contend, government-controlled activities are inevitably less efficient than those carried out by individuals in the so-called free market, it begs the question about what is going on behind closed doors where governments take a laissez-faire approach to doping? Baseball, football, cycling, track and field, and tennis are all well-documented examples of sports in which individualized doping has flourished because government involvement has been minimal.

Second, if Russian cheating was so widespread and the suspicions of cheating so well-known, why were the IOC and WADA so willing to ignore what had been going on right in front of them for years? The levels of incompetence and corruption in both those organizations in order to allow this to occur must have been palpable and should be thoroughly investigated. And finally, if the state delivered mechanisms for doping in Russia compelled many of those athletes to participate whether they wanted to or not, is this not a far more serious issue? Assuming almost every elite Russian Olympic athlete was given these performance-enhancing substances, it would appear that there may be a potential public health crisis brewing, much like what happened to the East German female Olympic athletes during the Cold War. What is the IOC going to do to protect the health of those athletes now and in the future?

# II

# REGULATING PEDS TO PROMOTE ATHLETES' HEALTH

## THE SUBJECTIVE NATURE OF AN UNFAIR COMPETITIVE ADVANTAGE

According to the American Academy of Pediatrics in 2008, a substance should only be viewed as performance enhancing if it is "taken in non-pharmacologic doses specifically for the purposes of improving sports performances."[1] That health-promoting definition allowed for drugs and other substances to be prescribed in accepted dosages for medical treatments, even if its usage would enhance an athlete's ability to perform. This is a healthy way to proceed.

Nevertheless, most of the sports cartels and affiliated organizations—including WADA, MLB, IOC, IAAF, NCAA, NFL, and ITF—focus on whether substances provide athletes with unfair competitive advantages instead of emphasizing their health risks and benefits. Focusing on and then determining what is competitively unfair has become a slippery slope with many arbitrary, self-serving, vague, unfair, and ambiguous detours on the path toward perceived morality. The primary reason for this chaos is the strong inclination to protect the specific financial and competitive advantages of the business enterprises governing each sport, as well as the long-established myth that sports provide every athlete with an equal opportunity to develop their skills and talents.

In addition, even though many of these sports seem to rely on WADA, its organizational structure—as explained by IOC president Bach—lacks the independence to counter these economic and other biases. In this environment, anti-doping measures and their implementation have been very different depending on the sports authority that is ultimately in charge. The only broad area of agreement seems to revolve around the tacit acknowledgment that protecting the health interests of athletes should only be a secondary consideration.

While there are many ethical and practical concerns aired about performance-enhancing substances and the rules that should prohibit their use, the dichotomy between how health care providers view performance enhancements compared to these sports organizations is both instructive and disturbing. Regardless, that dichotomy is expanding as increasingly science, medicine, nutrition, and pharmacology are able to provide enhanced living opportunities for everyone, not just athletes. These advancements, which do have risks, continually improve equipment, treatments, and rehabilitation for injuries and diseases, allowing human beings to be healthier, bigger, stronger, and faster. Collectively they have increased human endurance to such an extent that a sixty-four-year-old female athlete (and shrewd self-promoter), Diana Nyad—with some sanctioned, performance-enhancing assistance—was able to swim from Cuba to the United States, after several unsuccessful attempts. [2]

Yet, like nuclear power, this enhanced living is accompanied by the potential for abuses with devastating results that need to be regulated in rational ways. Unfortunately, there is an inherent unfairness and irrationality when sports organizations impose arbitrary limits on athletes, with respect to the medical, nutritional, and other scientific and technological assistance that they may receive, merely because those athletes might benefit competitively. Even assuming these sports cartels and WADA would be willing to redefine what constitutes illicit performance enhancement, the challenge is separating legitimate medical and nutritional interventions from improper and fraudulent performance enhancements in an environment in which health care is inherently subjective.

As has been noted frequently elsewhere, medicine—and by extension health care and nutrition—tends to be more of an art than a science, meaning by nature it is partly or largely subjective. That underlying subjectivity places an extreme burden on athletes when it is up to them to prove that the medical and therapeutic assistance they are receiving does not—or should not—violate a particular sport's guidelines. In Olympic sports, even the basic human question of who is eligible to compete as a female has been the subject of a discriminatory controversy fueled by irrational notions of anti-doping and competitive advantages.[3]

## A PUBLIC HEALTH PERSPECTIVE WITH ATHLETES' INPUT

In the United States and many other industrialized nations there is an accepted general standard governing whether a drug or health care intervention should be used or not. That broad standard asks whether the intervention is potentially harmful to the patient or client and if so, does the potential for improved health justify the risk, both to that individual and society? From this perspective, the suitability of a performance-enhancing substance should focus very little on whether it provides an athlete with an unfair advantage, and much more on whether it creates an unjustified health risk to the athletes who use—or are encouraged to use—that substance to compete.

At the same time, the approved use of new substances should be delayed, until the health risks can be properly evaluated, scientifically. This may be almost immediately or after extensive experimentation and study. In America, however, these common threshold health care decisions have been—and should continue to be—made by the Food and Drug Administration or similarly constituted scientific, medical, and regulatory governmental bodies in the public interest. There is little benefit to the American public in allowing these decisions to be made by biased, self-interested, and too often ill-informed national and international sports enterprises that are making huge amounts of money for themselves and their members and constituents off the athletes they neglect.

While this public health approach will not eliminate cheating, it will improve the rules that are being enforced, making them more fair and rational for everyone involved. It also will reduce the number of circumstances and situations that will constitute cheating. Catching this type of cheater is difficult anyway, unless those who view the cheating up close are willing to report their observations to the proper authorities. Generally athletes, coaches, and trainers are not willing to do this, except perhaps in golf. Yet, even in that sport, players and their caddies reporting suspicions about the use of performance-enhancing substances is frowned upon.

Ultimately, there has been too little scientific evidence to support most investigations and sanctions about illicit doping, which has meant that false accusations are too frequent, while the percentage of actual cheaters caught has been way too low. Thus, once a list of illicit performance-enhancing substances has been compiled, scientifically, by a federal regulatory body, it would seem reasonable to allow adult athletes in a given sport to have direct input into the regulatory implementation of the rules and punishments against this type of cheating through sound collective bargaining (see the conclusion in this book). After all, it is the athletes who are the ones that suffer most from the consequences of cheating and unhealthy lifestyles.

With respect to intercollegiate, scholastic, and youth sports, parents and responsible educators and community leaders should help make and enforce these rules on behalf of underage athletes. There also should be input from the young athletes themselves, and the applicable governmental authorities, to ensure that the rules are being prescribed and enforced in healthy ways. For older juvenile athletes in high school and college, the input should be greater than for younger athletes, which is consistent with how we treat minors in other risk-creating situations.

The primary emphasis in all such regulatory efforts should be safety and good health care, rather than unfair competitive advantages to those who use medical prescriptions and treatments appropriately. The presumption should be that a legitimate treatment or properly prescribed medication is permissible, until it is demonstrated that the treatment or prescription, or how it is being used, creates an unjustified health risk for the athletes involved.

The distinction in sports between doing everything possible to be physically and mentally able to perform well, and addressing a physical or mental impairment, disease, or athletic limitation with legitimate medical interventions, is thin at best. All of these proposed medical interventions should be part of the same life-enhancing continuum that benefits all Americans, and should be evaluated as such. Once a sophisticated and targeted method of identifying what should be allowed and what should be banned in terms of performance-enhancing substances has been agreed upon scientifically and medically, then it makes sense to expand the testing protocols to more accurately identify and increase the testing frequencies for these properly banned substances to ensure compliance, particularly out of competition.

Currently, almost all the organizations that oversee anti-doping in sports, and the testing protocols and enforcement procedures that they use, remain largely a mess. Collectively they provide little reassurance to the public, insufficient fairness and due process to the athletes, and unacceptable scientific and statistical reliability. The protections in place today are dictated much more by self-serving organizational and financial objectives than sound public policies that protect the health of the athletes involved. Regulation of PEDs is an essential component of the governmental structure that should be created to oversee health-related matters in sports (see conclusion).

# Part III

# Physical and Mental Impairments

# 12

# A LITANY OF SPORTS-RELATED IMPAIRMENTS

**W**hile misusing drugs and playing with pain and injuries have caused or contributed to life-changing mental and physical impairments in our most popular contact sports, unintended injuries, hyperaggression, violence, neglect, and overexertion can be equally or more devastating for athletes, both initially and long term. Traumatic events by themselves, or in combination with other events or problems, can diminish or end athletic careers, diminish the quality of life, and even cause death. Making matters worse, health-care- and disability-related benefits in our major sports, which one might think would be top notch, tend to be worse—and oftentimes far worse—than in other American corporate businesses, especially after the once-prized athletes are no longer able to perform at elite levels.

Furthermore, children who practice and play these sports with the small hope that they, too, will become elite suffer the same types of injuries and impairments. Typically, however, these young athletes, due to their developmental immaturity, are more vulnerable to harm, but receive relatively little medical supervision and care beyond what their families provide for them, which often is too little too late.

Today, a great deal of the injury focus has been on concussions and other head injuries, which is understandable. That focus is due in large part to the frequency of concussions; the fact that their impacts often are not obvious or appreciated; the fact that concussions have potentially catastrophic implications; and the brazen attempts of sports organizations, most notably the NFL, NCAA, and football youth leagues, to ignore or cover them up. Nonetheless, there are many other types of severe injuries, impairments, and conditions that can and do happen to athletes at all levels of competition, but especially to those who "play" these sports as a career path or a way to pay for college.

The combination of physical and mental injuries and substance abuse can be particularly dangerous for athletes in contact sports. Football, boxing, and hockey appear to have physical and mental impairment rates that probably are only exceeded by soldiers in combat. As All-Pro NFL cornerback and part-time social critic Richard Sherman said in explaining why he didn't need to watch the film *Concussion*, "I see a concussion movie every Sunday."[1] In collision sports, the intent to harm—or at least aggressively overwhelm—one's opponent(s) can be palpable, as well as a source of great pride.

As has been true in the military, effective prevention and treatment strategies normally come only after there is organizational acknowledgment of the true prevalence rates of these injuries and their likely long-term effects on those who are impaired. Unfortunately, when generating revenue or winning wars or games are the prime directives, the incentives weighing against candidly acknowledging impairments become substantial, both in sports and the military. Moreover, the bad practices and lack of candor at the professional level tend to filter down to collegiate, scholastic, and youth sports programs in very unhealthy ways.

Our athletic role models inculcate values, both good and bad, but in today's world the overall impact has been mostly negative. With regard to physical and mental health, as opposed to just athletic fitness, the record is disturbing, and sometimes unconscionably so. With regard to mental impairments, stigma and various stereotypes within the sports world tend to make the health care neglect much more profound.

Football, hockey, boxing, lacrosse, soccer, wrestling, many skiing events, and even baseball and softball are among the most popular American sports that—to a greater or lesser extent—expose their athletes, and sometimes even the fans and coaches, to heightened risk of serious and even catastrophic physical and mental injuries and impairments. Males participate in all the most dangerous sports and thus are most likely to become the victims of their athletics.

Females do not tend to participate in football, boxing, wrestling, and baseball, except in relatively small numbers. In sports that females do actively participate in, however, such as soccer, ice and field hockey,

softball, and skiing, the injuries and impairments may be generated somewhat differently, but often are no less frequent or severe as compared to
males who participate in those same sports. In fact, evidence is mounting
that females are more susceptible to certain types of injuries, including
concussions, migraines, and knee problems, than are males.

At the same time, the greatest health risks are in sports in which males
tend to dominate, such as football, boxing, wrestling, and ice hockey. In
ice hockey, which is played by both sexes, women and girls were thought
to be at much less risk because fighting and stick attacks have been
legislated out of their game. The commonsense perspective, which can be
misleading, is that because of physiology and natural selection, men and
boys tend to be bigger, stronger, faster, more aggressive, and more violent, all of which contribute to greater physical impact when they play
contact sports. Nonetheless, women and girls appear to have special vulnerabilities that may be exposed when they play those sports, which, due
to Title IX and changing attitudes, they do with increasing frequency and
rewards.

## BOXING: THE CANARY IN THE MINE SHAFT

Historically, boxing, even more so than football, has been the canary
dying in the mine shaft with respect to mental and physical impairments
associated with contact sports. What happened to boxing is what terrifies
those who benefit most from professional football, hockey, rugby, and
other violent contact sports. Boxing went from being near the mainstream
of American life and immensely popular to largely a fringe sport due in
part to mismanagement, criminal involvement, and racial stereotyping,
but more fundamentally due to its brutality. What was once admired and
enhanced by journalists and intellectuals as the "sweet science" became,
as Richard Hoffer has intoned, a "bittersweet science . . . [which argu-
ably] prepar[es] its players for nothing more than dysfunction or death."
Hoffer has described boxing as a "sport in which concussion is not merely an available outcome but the preferred, cleaner one,"[2] as compared to a
prolonged barrage of blows to the head and other vulnerable body parts,
such as the kidneys and testicles.

In its purest form, "boxing is more democratic than any other sport,
encouraging ambition without the organizational constraints and hypocri-

sies others impose."[3] That is why traditionally, even more so than base-ball, boxing has been viewed as the sport that best allows men—and now a few women—to climb the social ladder out of poverty or to be "res-cued" from fates apparently worse than the aftereffects of boxing. Mu-hammad Ali may have been riddled with the pains and diminished mental and physical capacities from the early onset of Parkinson's disease—which was probably due to his being hit in the head so many times—but almost everything he was able to accomplish outside the ring can be traced to his boxing career. On the other hand, while Mike Tyson was immersed in the boxing culture, he was mostly a lost and violent soul. Now that he has moved on from the sport, Tyson is performing one-man shows on Broadway.

Ali and Tyson, however, are the exceptions that help support the argu-ment that the sport of boxing should have a greatly diminished role in a civilized society. For the few boxers who have achieved social success, there are many, many more who have experienced carnage and devasta-tion. Perhaps no one illustrated the brutality of the sport more vividly and publicly than the great Emile Griffith. During his early years as a profes-sional beginning in 1958—which, due to television, coincided with the height of the sport's popularity for nonheavyweights—he won six world championships across three weight classes.

Griffith was the embodiment of the sweet science of boxing, as well as a ferocious puncher, who unfortunately will be most remembered in his illustrious twenty-year career for one round of unrelenting violence. In 1962, at the height of his boxing prowess, he hit Benny "Kid" Paret with "a series of 29 unanswered punches before Paret slumped to the canvas [never to regain consciousness]." Afterward, Griffith revealingly ex-plained that he "'didn't go in there to hurt no one.' [H]e was only going for the knockout," as if rendering someone unconscious was no big deal. Apparently his dying opponent was unable to escape because he was pinned in the corner. For years most knockouts, like ringing someone's bell in football, were frequently marginalized as being discrete and tem-porary incapacities that usually had no lasting physical or mental impact beyond losing the bout.

Despite what he said about his fight with Paret, Griffith's career took an extended nosedive, suggesting that the winner had profound misgiv-ings. Griffith would box for another fifteen years, but he was never the same fighter, nor was his damaged sport ever the same. Griffith lived until he was seventy-five, but died "of kidney failure and complications from dementia." Both those conditions were part of his laurels in becoming a Hall of Fame fighter. Beyond those personal tragedies, however, his athletic career was viewed as a rousing success compared to most professional boxers. After having grown up as an abused child living in poverty, it is doubtful that he would have wanted to forgo his distinguished life as a world champion boxer.[4]

By the 1970s, boxing had begun a steady decline. In 1982, the horror of the Griffith-Paret tragedy was reprised when "Duk-koo Kim . . . died after taking a pounding from Ray Mancini in a lightweight title match." The turning point for boxing was January 1983 when the *Journal of the American Medical Association* "denounced boxing as 'an obscenity' and said it should be outlawed."[5] Today, those same types of violence concerns center on football.

## CONCUSSIONS AND OTHER TRAUMATIC BRAIN INJURIES

Historically, the only American sport other than boxing to be widely condemned for its brutality and the physical and mental impairments that it causes has been football, although in more recent years North American ice hockey has had many detractors because of its needless fighting and violence. Campaigns to ban football first occurred at the turn of the twentieth century, spurred on by President "Teddy" Roosevelt. Nearly one hundred years passed, however, until concerns about concussions gained enough momentum that abolishing the sport became a serious issue again.

While professional football has been the lightning rod for most of the criticisms and concerns about head trauma and its care and treatment, the public health threat and liability posed by similar injuries in other sports have become widespread, both in the United States and Great Britain. It is the one serious injury to athletes that has been steadily increasing, while the prevalence rates for other injuries have been falling.[6] Whether that is because identification has become more conscientious and routine, collisions in certain sports have grown more forceful and frequent, or a combination of factors, remains uncertain. Whatever the full explanation, this increase in the perceived prevalence of these traumatic incidents has been identified by medical experts as a serious public health problem. It has been referred to as a "'silent epidemic' [in sports generally and] the NFL's quiet career killer" more specifically,[7] and those sentiments may be understatements.

Internationally, especially in countries that were once part of the British Commonwealth, rugby—which is a violent contact sport played without protective gear—is believed to have a higher concussion rate than football.[8] Unfortunately, a mythology has evolved in the United States and elsewhere that because there is little protective equipment, the players are more conscientious about not deliberately injuring their opponents. Thus, the risk of impairment from brain traumas is presumed to be reduced as compared to American football. Whether that is true or not, making this comparison seems to be the international version of marginalizing mental and physical dangers in order to promote the virtues of an inherently dangerous sport.

## Causes, Prevention, and Treatments

Like many other medical conditions that have multiple causes and impacts, the term "concussion" encompasses a wide range of symptoms and degrees of severity. Two common definitions focus on trauma that affects the individual's brain or mental status, but does not necessarily involve the loss of consciousness, although it may. One of those definitions refers to "traumatically induced alteration in mental status," the other "a complex pathophysiological process . . . induced by traumatic biomechanical forces."[9]

These head traumas are substantial enough to be compared to impacts from a motor vehicle accident. They arise when "collisions, falls, or . . . a whiplash force is applied to the body."[10] One of, if not the, most common whiplash concussion in sports is from crack-back blocks in football, which for years has been taught and retaught to players beginning in the youth leagues, but can no longer be executed below the knees in the form of a chop block.

Another way to examine the effects of a concussion, explains the *Economist*, is by distinguishing it "from blunt-force trauma . . . [in which] the injury is caused by directly transmitted shock from the impact. Concussion, by contrast, is caused by the internal movement and distortion of the brain as it bounces inside the cranium after an impact." This bouncing "stretches and deforms bundles of axons that connect different regions of the brain," which "shears some axons directly, releasing their protein contents, including tau, which with time can form abnormal tangles similar to those found in Alzheimer's disease." Thereafter, these "damaged axons . . . trigger a process which releases protein-breaking enzymes that destroy the axon, further disrupting the brain's internal communications." Furthermore, repeated head traumas of this sort "could set the stage for a continuous autoimmune-type attack on the brain" as the body responds by fighting the various proteins and enzymes that are being released. [11]

The immediate symptoms that concussions produce are somewhat different for each individual. According to the National Association of Sports Psychologists, symptoms include "various types of headaches," "light and noise sensitivity, slowed information processing," "impaired concentration, difficulty remembering," "ringing in the ears," "blurry vision, depression, anxiety, personality change, lack of motivation, fatigue, sleep disturbance," "loss of balance," "nausea," and "inappropriate social responses." As described earlier, the most devastating damage for many athletes involves a "long term process where primary and secondary brain injury occurs . . . [causing] . . . a potentially diverse range of lifelong negative consequences." They include "altered cell functioning and cell death along with . . . physical, cognitive, and emotional impairments." [12]

Permanent impacts and symptoms are more likely with repeated concussions and/or more traumatic concussive injuries. Devastating diseases such as depression, Parkinson's, Alzheimer's, and chronic traumatic encephalopathy (CTE) have been linked, through medical diagnoses and statistical associations, to more severe and repeated concussions. A groundbreaking study published in 2012 found that routine blows to the head that occur in sports like football and hockey might cause long-term cognitive impairment. Autopsies on brains of eighty-five athletes found that 80 percent of those who had experienced "repeated mild traumatic brain injury . . . showed evidence of chronic traumatic encephalopathy . . . a degenerative and incurable [brain] disease." [13]

Yet, even one concussion can cause lasting damage. A University of Illinois study found that two years later "children who had sustained a single sports-related concussion still had impaired brain function." [14] Since then, the scientific and medical evidence about the severity and seriousness of these sport-related brain injuries has been accumulating. A small 2016 study involving high school and college football players aged fifteen to twenty-one who had a concussion found that 80 percent of them "continued to have visible damage in their brain six months after their injuries." The implication is that "the effects of a [single] concussion can be permanent."[15]

Unfortunately, as with tobacco and lung disease, it continues to be difficult to prove with a high degree of certainty that concussions have caused mental impairments in specific individuals, even though many of the effects on large groups, such as football or hockey players, may be well known. Regardless, the close association between repeated concussive impacts and mental impairments should be alarming. There is overwhelming medical evidence that indicates that concussions can cause short- and long-term symptoms of brain damage and alter the neurocomposition of the brain itself.

Repeating the bias of medical science more generally, however, these studies have focused almost exclusively on men. That means discovering any possible differences in results for women and children have been obscured and delayed unnecessarily. This is an important reason why former soccer star Brandi Chastain "pledged to donate her brain posthumously to researchers studying the impact wrought by repetitive head injuries."[16] She has been joined by many of her former teammates, including former U.S. goalie and concussion victim Briana Scurry.

Reportedly some of the worst head injuries occur when repeated concussions take place before a previous concussion has been fully healed. In addition, the use of recreational and performance-enhancing drugs and alcohol while recovery is taking place "may not only impede the healing process but may . . . further damage the brain."[17] Thus, improper drug use of any kind by athletes or juveniles—which apparently is not infrequent—combined with being concussed, can be especially harmful. There is some evidence that medical marijuana might be useful in preventing and treating concussions by protecting a person's neurons, but this is based on animal research and does not negate the possibility that marijuana could negatively affect concussion prevention and healing as well.

Whatever the consequences may be for the individual athlete who suffers a concussion, it is almost always going to be much more serious than what the sports-related expressions of it's "just a ding" or having one's "bell rung" would imply. Making matters worse, "even what seems to be a mild bump or blow to the head can be serious."[18] That is because damage to the brain through the relatively fragile skull cannot be determined by measuring physical forces alone. Special vulnerabilities and good or bad fortune contribute as well. In that sense, it is like playing Russian roulette where even well-trained neurologists cannot reliably predict whether future brain impairments will occur and what they will be.

Furthermore, there is little agreement which treatment approach is best or how effective each is in helping to decide when athletes can safely resume practicing or playing their sport. Both prevention and treatment of concussions and related brain traumas appear to be very subjective, which plays into the hands of those who want to control and manage the decision outcomes to maximize their short-term objectives and profits. "The old adage 'when in doubt, sit them out'" typically is outweighed in our major spectator sports by "pressure to allow the athlete to prematurely return to competition, especially in the 'big game,'"[19] or when the outcome of the game is on the line.

## Sports-Related Concussions Are Widespread

What have been described collectively as "sport-related concussions (SRC) are not limited to specific age ranges, professional athletes, or gender," although the incidence rates differ. Including recreational activities, the total number of SRCs is at least one million each year and has been estimated to be as much as 3.6 million.[20] If only organized sports injuries in which an actual hospital admission intake form has been filed are counted, the number of SRCs would be more than three hundred thousand annually.[21]

Most concussions, though, either are never reported or result in a private physician office visit. Thus, the American Academy of Neurology estimates that more than a million athletes a year are concussed. Whatever the actual number may be, the prevalence of SRCs is a serious public health problem that even today tends to be understated, particularly in football, which reportedly accounts for the highest rate of such injuries in sports, except perhaps boxing.

While football, boxing, ice hockey, wrestling, and rugby—both anecdotally and based on the physical forces involved—appear to be the sports in which the prevalence rates are the highest, SRCs happen relatively frequently in all collision sports and many other types of athletic competition as well. Athletes who play or participate in baseball, horse racing, soccer, gymnastics, and field hockey, for example, also are at a significant risk of being concussed. At the same time, there are few if any sports that are safe from concussions, if the wrong circumstances or bad fortune are present. Physical contact between opposing athletes increases the likelihood substantially, but the absence of contact does not remove the risk. For example, the most frequent source of concussions in soccer appears to be from heading the ball, rather than athlete-to-athlete collisions.

An essential distinction, however, is whether these SRCs are accidental and rare, or relatively common because they reflect the hazardous or intentionally aggressive or violent nature of the activity involved. Merely because the equipment and playing techniques improve does not mean that sports such as boxing, football, wrestling, or hockey can reduce the incidence of concussions to a point where the risks are justified or no longer problematic. While safety measures may improve, athletes continue to get bigger, stronger, and faster, making athlete-to-athlete collisions more violent.

In addition, closely related to brain injuries are migraines, which are severe headaches that can render athletes unable to function, much less participate in a contact sport. While migraines do not seem to be due to concussive impacts alone, the two conditions appear to be related, and for some reason are "far more common in women."[22] Not only do concussive impacts seem to cause migraines, but studies show that those who suffer from them "are more susceptible to concussions, and when they do sustain one, it takes longer for them to recover."

## Informing Young Athletes and Parents of the Risks

Obviously doing something to limit these injuries and conditions is better than doing almost nothing, as was done in the past. Nevertheless, those involved in playing aggressive sports should be fully informed about the risks, especially minors and their parents. Yet, they have not been.

Certain sports may have to be altered substantially to minimize those risks to acceptable levels, whatever those levels may be. Even then certain sports and leisure activities, such as football or skateboarding, may no longer be appropriate for children, including adolescents, and even for many adults. The point is that much more relevant health- and safety-related information about these injuries should be disseminated to the public by health providers and educators, who do not have a vested interest in promoting or condemning specific sports.

In a society in which the regular consumption of large sodas or other calorie-laden foods is viewed by many as unhealthy and inappropriate for minors, how can playing certain sports that regularly lead to permanent brain injuries be acceptable? Unfortunately, concussions tend to be far more serious for children than adults. Children's brains have not fully developed and they have a more pronounced "physiological response to mechanical stress" because their skulls and brains "have a different geometry."[23] Counterintuitively, children can absorb a much greater physical impact than adults without showing clinical symptoms. This means children are at considerably higher risk of not being properly diagnosed, especially when they sustain repeated blows to the head.

Furthermore, essential preventive measures, medical supervision, and treatment interventions tend to be lacking in contact sports played by youths and at most high schools. That is primarily due to the additional costs involved, but also to the reckless notion that such risks are manageable or overblown. Parents should be more concerned when their children are "playing sports. Taking one for the team is all very well. But the price of doing so may be paid over a lifetime."[24]

## OTHER CATASTROPHIC INJURIES, SOME OF WHICH ARE NOT SO RARE

While many of the more serious negative health consequences of impairments to athletes involve long-term physical or mental conditions that present themselves later in life, potentially devastating or even lethal outcomes can occur immediately, especially for children. Many of these catastrophic events are due to neglect or lack of proper supervision, including (1) preexisting conditions in athletes that were never properly diagnosed; (2) diagnosed conditions that the athletes—and their parents—chose to assume or ignore the risk for, so the athlete could play that sport; (3) injuries that were not properly treated; and (4) excessive exercise and/or the lack of proper hydration during practice and training sessions. Spinal injuries, heart defects, and heatstroke lead the parade of relatively rare but potentially catastrophic harms, which could be reduced or made less devastating through prevention, superior equipment, and/or better treatment and supervision.

## Spinal and Head Injuries

Spinal and head injuries can occur in many different sports, but they are relatively rare. The most publicized examples are in football. Unlike the long-term effects of repeated concussive impacts, these devastating injuries are more preventable with better headgear, improved tackling techniques, and rules to minimize the delivery of the type of physical force that is likely to cause the most immediate damage.

Despite taking modest precautions, these unexpected tragedies still happen, both in the NFL and college, because of the violent nature of the sport. Darryl Stingley of the New England Patriots, Mike Utley of the Detroit Lions, Eric LeGrand of Rutgers, and Devon Walker of Tulane are all former football players whose athletic careers ended, and the rest of their lives were disrupted, after they became paralyzed.

More recently, a Naval Academy football player died from "swelling and bleeding on his brain"[25] sustained during spring practice in 2014. It was unclear whether a specific hit had caused his injury as his father initially tweeted, or it was a result of "carrying the football normally, doing what he truly loves," as his mother explained. What was clear is that as a senior in high school he ruptured a blood vessel after being hit in the head during a football game.

According to his mother, for nine months after being injured he had avoided football "just to be safe." Both the navy and his parents wanted to avoid any dangerous situations, she explained. Apparently, he had plenty of high-tech medical care, including "four to six CAT scans and MRI exams," and numerous visits to neurosurgeons. Ultimately, though, "more [was] going on in his brain than . . . could [be] . . . detected,"[26] which is a substantial risk confronting every athlete who has sustained significant trauma to the head. There are no guarantees of safety once an athlete's brain is severely traumatized.

## Cardiac Arrest and Heatstroke

In youth sports "the No. 1 killer . . . is sudden cardiac arrest, typically brought on by pre-existing, detectable conditions that could have been treated"[27] but were never identified. Heatstroke is another "completely preventable" condition. While sports-related concussion deaths rarely happen, indirect-trauma deaths from either cardiac arrest or heatstroke are more common. During the decade in which the last such study was conducted—2000 through 2009—"indirect-trauma deaths" outnumbered head and spinal-cord fatalities 108 to forty-one.[28]

Yet, lethal and catastrophic indirect traumas are almost nonexistent in professional or major collegiate sports, primarily because the money required for effective prevention and immediate response is not a significant expense for these very profitable business enterprises. Many young athletes, however, who experience these types of death could have been saved if more money had been available to implement sensible precautions, diagnosis, and treatment.

For instance, it has been argued that adding an electrocardiogram to physical examinations "would detect about two-thirds of the deadly, concealed heart trouble aggravated by exercise in competition."[29] Unfortunately, requiring electrocardiograms presents certain complications and liabilities. Routine physical exams are required for high school sports, but not necessarily independently operated youth leagues. In addition, the advisability of mandating electrocardiograms remains somewhat controversial, not only because of the added expense but also because normally that procedure is not covered by insurance.

Furthermore, electrocardiograms produce a significant percentage of false positives, which leads to needless testing. As with many medical screening protocols, such as PSA tests for prostate cancer or mammograms for breast cancer, identifying additional people at risk may not be a good thing, unless the accuracy and reliability of the screening tool is high enough to justify testing everyone. The necessary benefits could be attained more readily by employing a more targeted approach, which identifies the sports that make particularly high cardiovascular demands on athletes, such as basketball and soccer,[30] as well as the individual athletes who have a higher risk of encountering cardiac-related problems due to hidden physical vulnerabilities.

The less controversial, and arguably more effective, approaches for addressing cardiac risks and heatstroke in all sports, at all levels of competition, have focused on proper training and exercise and the ability to respond immediately when one of these potentially tragic events occurs.

Most of the time that young athletes spend participating in a sport involves training and practices, not games or competitions.

One of the most dangerous times is the preseason workouts that get athletes conditioned for games that count. This has been a problem in football, especially if the initial practices are less structured or unsupervised, take place in high temperatures, or do not encourage proper hydration. According to one expert who directs athletic training at the University of Connecticut, too often in these practice sessions there is no proper oversight. "Many coaches 'just run willy-nilly' trying to make men out of boys."[31]

Between 2000 and 2011 in college football alone, twenty-one players experienced fatal events during summer workouts. Many more high school players died in this way. Yet, there were no deaths among top-level college football players in regular practices or games. The primary reason for this difference in death rates has to do with taking the necessary precautions to stress safety. To begin with, conditioning drills should be phased in for "every sport . . . rather than start[ing] at maximum intensity on day one." In addition, punishments should never involve additional exercise. Most importantly, the coaches who organize these workouts need to be well trained "in health and safety issues [and] . . . be present during all conditioning sessions" or ensure that an athletic trainer is present to handle health and safety matters.

Much of the advice regarding conditioning workouts applies to practices and training. Heatstroke involves high temperatures but is common enough in sports activities that it has its own name: "exertional heat illness." Especially in hot climates, at the beginning of a sports season there should be "gradual levels of exercise."[32] Throughout the season, athletes should drink plenty of water, have "proper warm ups," and "avoid sudden, intense exertion."[33]

Overexertion should be strongly discouraged. "Working athletes longer and harder is not exercising smart,"[34] nor is the practice of withholding water to build their endurance and fortitude. The bottom line is that no healthy young athlete should die from a routine practice.

The other major factor in preventing deaths and long-term impairments to athletes is being prepared to deal with critical situations should they arise. Minimally, there should be someone present who is properly trained in first aid. Otherwise it's comparable to dropping a kid off at a swimming pool even though there is no lifeguard. That person should also be certified in resuscitation and heart defibrillation, and the necessary equipment including a defibrillator should be on-site. In a medical emergency involving heart attacks or heatstroke, minutes become critical.[35]

When sudden cardiac arrest occurs, every minute that goes by before an automated external defibrillator (AED) or CPR is used reduces the athlete's survival rate by 10 percent. Athletic trainers or comparable personnel should be present who know how to administer CPR and use an AED, and can teach others in a sports program to do the same. For this reason, "many sports medicine experts argue . . . that every high school [should] employ at least one full-time trainer."[36] Hiring a properly certified trainer would be cheaper and more effective than administering regular electrocardiograms.

Currently, considerably less than half of our high schools have done so. Such a trainer also would be able to recognize signs and symptoms of heatstroke and provide treatment immediately. Ultimately, though, the most effective approach for heatstroke is preventing it from occurring in the first place by enforcing strict workout precautions. "Exertional heat illness . . . [is] 100 percent preventable . . . and . . . solutions can be very low-tech and inexpensive."[37]

Another major factor that would improve safety for kids' in sports is encouraging their parents and guardians to be more involved in monitoring the coaches and other athletic program staff. In the words of *New York Times* columnist Frank Bruni, "Some [parents] question the amount of homework more readily than the number of laps [their young] athletes run on a 95-degree day. . . . It's . . . [this] unquestioning worship of sports that puts young lives in jeopardy."[38] Too many parents further increase the health risks to their athletically inclined children by "shopping" for doctors who will allow their child to compete in a sport before he or she is fully recovered or medically ready.

## KNEE AND OTHER LEG INJURIES, PARTICULARLY FOR FEMALE ATHLETES

Leg injuries can derail athletic careers, permanently limit an athlete's effectiveness, and have long-term health consequences. In the NBA, for example, knee, ankle, and foot surgeries have impaired the careers of many gifted players who depend on being able to leap and spin, much like ballet dancers. Former All-Stars, including Danny Manning, Tim Hardaway, and more recently, Derrick Rose, are all marquee players who experienced career-diminishing injuries to their knees. Similarly, Greg Oden, the number one draft pick in 2007, has suffered a series of knee injuries, which undermined what initially appeared to be an All-Star-caliber NBA career. Now he is a role player at best.

Knee injuries in football are particularly common. In large part this is due to the aggressive nature of the sport and to low blocks and hits that are deliberately designed to attack the opponent's knees. One of the more original arguments used against outlawing hits to the head has been that football players would be inclined to injure opponents in other ways, especially by targeting their knees. Serious leg injuries are so common in football that being "'carted off' [the field] is . . . jargon, familiar enough . . . to fans to need no further explanation."[39]

While head and spine injuries also require the use of these "injury carts," the more common use is for players with leg injuries that leave them unable to walk even with the assistance of others. Yet, not so long ago, there was resistance to using those carts because doing so was viewed as being unmanly. In 1985 Hall of Fame coach Bill Parcells reportedly told one of his frequently injured players that "the next time [someone] had to go and get him on the cart, he better be dead."[40]

Similarly, young female athletes experience knee damage frequently enough that, like concussions, it has been referred to as a "national epidemic." Remarkably, though, a majority of those knee injuries have not been due to collisions. According to the American Orthopedic Society for Sports Medicine, women and girls are "two to eight times more likely than young males to tear their anterior cruciate ligaments." This is a very serious knee injury that requires surgery followed by a long rehabilitation period that may or may not fully repair the damage. A majority of these ACL tears to females—about 70 percent—occur without athlete-to-athlete contact.[41]

ACL tears are most common in women's lacrosse, soccer, and basketball, which involve a great deal of running and changing of direction. There appear to be sound physiological explanations as to why young female athletes are more likely than young male athletes to sustain ACL tears. As a result, doctors and trainers recommend that through drills and exercises the muscles of young female athletes be retrained when they engage in these sports in order to make tears less likely. Unfortunately, less likely does not mean unlikely. Those anatomical differences may be due, at least in part, to the fact that young boys are more apt to be encouraged to play sports at an earlier age and thus to train their muscles to respond more protectively. This type of muscle training is like learning a foreign language. The earlier it begins the better.

Regardless, even elite women athletes are vulnerable to these leg injuries. In 2013, Maryland's vaunted women's basketball team lost three of its players to ACL tears, including two starters. Typically, these tears take more than a year to heal. One of the more publicized knee injuries in recent years involved Lindsey Vonn, the world's best female skier until she sustained "torn anterior cruciate and medial collateral ligaments and a lateral fracture of the tibia" in a violent fall a year before the Sochi Winter Olympics. Her "ski buried and stopped dead, [while she was] moving downhill at 50 or 60 mph."[42]

Hers was not a typical injury, nor was Vonn a typical athlete. She continually pushed herself to the edge of disaster, which was a key to her prodigious success. Apparently, she did not fear injury as much as losing. Not surprisingly, she attempted to accelerate her rehabilitation so she could compete in the 2014 Olympics. Instead, Vonn came back too soon, reinjuring her knee in the process. By the fall of 2015, she was consistently winning races against the world's best competition until she severely reinjured her leg.

## MRSA INFECTIONS, ESPECIALLY IN FOOTBALL

A less recognized danger of playing team sports, especially football, has been a potentially fatal bacterial infection that is resistant to "penicillin-based antibiotics." This potentially deadly superbug is known as MRSA (methicillin-resistant *Staphylococcus aureus*), and athletes have been a prime target because it "thrives in steamy locker rooms and enters the body through nicks, abrasions, and cuts." This is an infectious disease that appears "in clusters," especially football teams.[43]

An increased incidence of MRSA has been associated with artificial turf from the abrasions that playing on it causes. This danger was an important reason why women international soccer players, led by the American team, complained to FIFA so vociferously about being compelled to play on artificial turf rather than on sod like the men. Football, however, is where most of the publicized cases of MRSA have occurred.

In 2003, five members of the St. Louis Rams came down with MRSA infections, along with ten players at a Connecticut college. The following year, Texas high school football teams reported eighty-one cases. After the Texas outbreak there was a great deal more public education about the infectious disease, but cases have continued to surface.

According to a Vanderbilt University Medical Center epidemiologist who studied these types of infections in that university's athletes, "Staph is a common bacterium that colonizes most people, which means it lives in them unnoticed." MRSA, which is a more serious type of staff infection, "colonizes at least 5 percent of the people in the United States."[44] In team sports those rates rise to between 8 and 31 percent, with football players being the highest rates.

While the disease can exist in the human body without complications, infections can "occur if there is a pathway for the bacteria to enter the body through an open wound, cut or abrasion." The Centers for Disease Control and Prevention says "MRSA can also spread by skin-to-skin contact, exposure to contaminated surfaces used by a carrier or exposure to someone who already has a full-blown infection." Thus, MRSA infections are more prevalent in locker rooms because open wounds are being dressed and the athletes share shower, toilet, rehabilitation, and other facilities. Football teams, because of the large number of athletes crowded into one locker room, appear to be particularly vulnerable.[45]

In the NFL, MRSA infections have been infrequent, but not rare. According to a survey by NFL doctors, at least thirty-three were identified from 2006 to 2008. In 2013, three members of the Tampa Bay Buccaneers came down with the disease. This motivated the Atlanta Falcons to use "a cleanup crew wearing hazmat suits . . . to disinfect the visitors' locker room after Tampa Bay played at the Georgia Dome."[46] Two of the infected players became sick enough that their careers were threatened. Both of them sued the Bucs for compensation, but the NFL convinced the courts involved that the collective bargaining agreement with the players preempted those lawsuits, resulting in dismissals of their claims.

The NFL and its teams tend not to talk about these infections publicly and do not compensate affected players for lost income as a result of their playing careers being curtailed because they become infected. Even more disturbing, there is no formal league policy on preventing the spread of MRSA, much less helping those athletes who are stricken. As the New York Giants explained in October 2015 when their former tight end Daniel Fells almost died from MRSA, "Each team is responsible for their own infection control guidelines."[47]

Fells's bout with MRSA resulted in multiple surgeries that took parts of his foot, which in all likelihood ended his football career. Fortunately, it did not take his life or lead to amputation of his foot or leg. Although in public the Giants supported Fells throughout much of his recovery, the team cut him, which meant he no longer had a job, a salary as a football player, or health benefits. What happened to Fells is typical of how NFL teams respond when one of their low-profile football players loses his elite athletic ability to injuries. Fells became a distant memory.

# 13

# CONCUSSIONS IN THE NFL

## Myths, Deceptions, Denials, and Lies

**P**rofessional boxing was the precursor to what can happen to an immensely popular North American contact sport, should its organizers ignore, downplay, and/or cover up severe brain damage to its athletes. Nevertheless, professional football—because of its enormous popularity, influence, media attention, aggression, and violence—has evolved into the new exemplar of a sport in serious trouble by failing to make effective changes to protect, treat, and rehabilitate its elite athletes from life-altering mental and physical impairments. Moreover, this seismic cultural shift undoubtedly will envelop collegiate, high school, and youth football as well.

What has made the NFL's injury situation such a monumental saga for the media, fans, and critics—beyond the fact that anything compelling about professional football is going to be of interest to a large American audience—is its tragic, soap opera nature:

- life-changing mental impairments to former star players that were largely ignored or covered up, despite numerous warnings
- human failings, particularly the superman complex and bad behavior of the athletes and coaches, along with the avarice and duplicity of the league, team owners, and management

- acts of treachery by players and teams alike in order to physically or psychologically injure their opponents and even their own team-mates
- disgrace and condemnation for America's most popular spectator sport

Much of what has made football so popular in the United States—violence; aggression; military-like tactics, strategies, and precision; obedience to rules; and its secrecy and tunnel vision when it comes to cheating, winning, bad behaviors, and making money—has enveloped players in a highly pathological environment. Year after year, game after game, practice after practice, hit after hit, and block after block, elite (and not so elite) football players are being physically and mentally impaired by a sport that most of them say they love to play.

As a result of a uniquely American form of cognitive dissonance, the football establishment and its fans have ignored what should have been obvious for many decades: that repeated hits to the brain and other vulnerable parts of the body will inevitably lead to serious, debilitating—and possibly catastrophic—health problems. Such consequences include death, shortened life expectancy, dementia, lack of mobility, substance abuse, and excruciating pain. To a certain extent these devastating outcomes—like fighting in hockey or causing opponents to crash at high speeds in NASCAR—are what make the game special.

The potential physical and mental damage to athletes who play football was widely known at the beginning of the twentieth century, if not fully appreciated. Nevertheless, even as those harms should have become more transparent, they were being shielded behind a veil of ignorance, feel-good myths, duplicity, and preparations for war, which increasingly became more impenetrable. A century later, however, the images of our football heroes being transformed into middle-aged men whose memories and bodies had been destroyed, who could no longer think or walk like normal human beings, and were wracked with constant pain was too much to accept for the general public and most fans. This grim reality has been broadcast into American living rooms and onto our electronic devices through twenty-four-hours-a-day sports coverage, which has created an almost insatiable demand for stories about damaged athletes, especially those human tragedies with an emotional edge.

It was one thing for teams and fans to ignore and attack the views of reputable doctors, researchers, and other experts about what was happening to football players. Anti-intellectualism has a rich history in America as our politics and sports teach us almost every day. On the other hand, it has become increasingly painful to watch our football idols die premature deaths, or fail when they try to speak, think, and walk like normal middle-aged and older men.

## THE EARLY WARNING SIGNS

Once football became the nation's most popular spectator sport in the 1970s, it should have been far more difficult to obscure the pathologies that had become an integral part of the professional, collegiate, and even high school competitions. Increasingly, the dark sides of football were poking through the rose-colored cameras and were even being mentioned in the early days of sports talk radio. Since the 1890s, there had been "an endless history of football at once inflicting and ignoring brain trauma."[1]

For many decades the most damning evidence against football was player deaths. Those tragedies were emblematic of the crushing hits that players regularly delivered and absorbed to the delight of themselves and their coaches, teammates, and fans. Statistically, though, the totals were relatively small, even though those death rates were disturbing when compared to most other sports, except perhaps for the carnage in boxing.

The smoking gun turned out to be the accumulating impact of brain injuries, but for years such revelations were obscured and covered up. The sports media—especially talk radio and its television equivalents— and coaches, along with the NFL and NCAA, continued to embrace the myths, deceptions, and even the lies that insulated the business of football from serious scrutiny. Until recently there was little popular understanding, much less acknowledgment, that over their football careers a high percentage of players sustained brain injuries that would transform them into replicas of punch-drunk boxers. Somehow the anecdotal evidence about former professional football players with severe mental incapacity was not widely shared or appreciated.

In part this was due to the extreme social stigma and negative stereotypes involved in having a mental disability (see chapter 24), especially in a macho sport like football. In addition, an overwhelming majority of the people who had access to this key information about individual football players were failing to make, ignoring, or even hiding the connection between the mental impairments they observed and the fact that these patients and loved ones had played professional football. Famous—and not so famous—football players and coaches consistently downplayed the seriousness of concussions, which were typically referred to as "dings," rather than brain injuries or traumas.

Nonetheless, there were highly publicized incidents that should have been scrutinized more deeply but were quickly marginalized as exceptional, rather than as symptomatic. Perhaps the most famous violent hit in football history occurred on November 20, 1960. New York Giants Hall of Fame running back and receiver Frank Gifford "was flattened by Chuck Bednarik, an Eagles linebacker and future Hall of Famer, himself. . . . Gifford dropped the ball and lay motionless as Bednarik wave[d] his arms and shook his fists,"[2] like a conquering barbarian.

That one blow was devastating enough that Gifford not only was knocked unconscious and had to leave the field stretched out on a cart, but he was unable to play the rest of that season and chose not to play the next season as well. For years the thoughtlessly embraced image of Bednarik violently gyrating over Gifford's motionless body was a symbol of the manliness of the NFL, rather than of a serious public health problem.

Gifford would go on to gain even more fame as an announcer, alongside Howard Cosell and Don Meredith, on *Monday Night Football*. In his final years, however, he remained out of the media spotlight. When he died at age eighty-four in 2015, his media-savvy wife, Kathie Lee Gifford, and the rest of his family announced that their suspicions that he had been experiencing "the debilitating effects of head trauma [had been] confirmed." A medical diagnosis after his death revealed that he too had the now infamous brain disease called chronic traumatic encephalopathy (CTE). Gifford was not the only football player turned announcer to become cognitively impaired due to symptoms that characterize CTE. Gifford's teammate and fellow Hall of Fame member Sam Huff, who for years broadcast football games in Washington, can no longer care for himself.

In 1980, on the eve of his retirement, former Dallas Cowboys quarterback, Heisman Trophy winner, and Naval Academy hero Roger Staubach became one of the first players to publicly voice his concerns about possible brain damage playing football, citing a "string of concussions" that he had endured.[3] Yet, it was not until the early 1990s that the danger of concussions began to gain traction as several other players, including Al Toon and Merrill Hoge, retired due to repeated head trauma.

## THE NFL-ORCHESTRATED DECEPTIONS BEGAN WITH TAGLIABUE AND PELLMAN

One of the most auspicious concussion-related events involving professional football occurred at a 1994 panel program moderated by Pulitzer Prize–winning journalist David Halberstam. It included then NFL commissioner Paul Tagliabue as a featured speaker. When questioned about the NFL's growing concussion problem, he referred to it as a "pack journalism issue."[4] The usually astute commissioner claimed that concussions were relatively rare in the NFL, only occurring once "every three or four games." This was only true, however, if being dragged off the field unconscious was Tagliabue's definition of a concussion.

Tagliabue continued to manufacture support for his misleading assertion. Being a highly skilled corporate lawyer, he should have appreciated the long-term consequences of his duplicity in a business that was constantly in the media spotlight. This appears to have been the genesis of the NFL's decision to publicly deny that concussions were a serious problem and the beginning of the league's irresponsible and well-funded subterfuges.

As Mark Fainaru-Wada and Steve Fainaru chronicle in *League of Denial*, it was not long before Tagliabue convinced NFL owners to hire a handpicked panel of experts to supposedly study concussions. Their obvious intent to protect the NFL and the game of football was captured in the panel's name: the "Mild Traumatic Brain Injury Committee (MTBI)." Committee members were "made up almost entirely of NFL insiders . . . [n]early half [of whom] . . . were team doctors." This included its "chairman (Elliot Pellman) . . . who had not produced a single piece of scientific evidence on the subject [of brain trauma.]"

Despite his obvious lack of expertise, Pellman was not shy about issuing authoritative public statements "perfectly aligned with NFL doctrine," especially that concussions should be viewed as "an occupational risk."[5] In other words, brain injuries were part of the game and a calculated hazard that every player willingly accepted. More importantly, if the legal establishment accepted that assertion as being true, it would create an overwhelming hurdle for players to clear in trying to establish the league's liability for any long-term impairments that football-related concussions had caused.

With the league's able assistance, the ill-informed Dr. Pellman would magically transform himself into one of the nation's foremost medical advisers on the subject of concussions and brain traumas, becoming a consultant for the NHL and MLB, as well the NFL. Unfortunately, puffery was not Pellman's worst sin. He apparently exaggerated and falsified his medical credentials, which the *New York Times* revealed just after Pellman had testified before Congress in 2005.[6] Beginning in the 1980s his resume reflected that he had graduated from the State University of New York at Stony Brook and was an associate clinical professor at Albert Einstein College of Medicine.

Neither assertion was true. Due to his less than stellar college grades, Pellman had attended a medical school in Mexico and never taught at Albert Einstein. The primary reason he had been appointed chair of the committee seemed to be that he was the New York Jets' team physician. Later, he became Tagliabue's personal physician as well.

On its face both the NFL's MTBI Committee's composition and name, which used the word "mild" as a point of emphasis, suggested that the league either was hoping to marginalize and contain the concussion issue, and/or did not really appreciate its potential gravity. At the same time, the use of such transparent tactics was not surprising. Many American corporations would have dealt—and did deal—with this type of negative publicity similarly.

Assembling a task force of experts to study the matter in a way that would be favorable to its interests was what General Motors did in 2014 when faced with a safety-recall scandal. Sometimes a long delay can be enough to diminish such a problem or even make it go away. The NFL's MTBI Committee did not publish its first research until October 2003, nine years after it had first been convened and six years after Tagliabue had become "Pellman's patient."[7]

## THE NFL-CONTROLLED RESEARCH AND TESTING PROGRAMS

While the NFL was trying to proceed slowly and continued to deny that concussions posed a special risk, attitudes among players began to shift noticeably. In 1995, Leigh Steinberg, the well-respected sports agent, tackled the concussion issue from the point of view of the famous players he represented.[8] Steinberg invited six quarterbacks, including Troy Aikman, Warren Moon, and Steve Young—who would all be inducted into the Pro Football Hall of Fame—as well as a panel of neurologists, to make recommendations to the NFL's Competition Committee about how to better protect quarterbacks from concussions and other serious on-the-field injuries. Even though the NFL largely ignored those recommendations, the proceedings publicized the palpable dangers involved in playing professional football, especially for quarterbacks, who in those days did not play in a protective cocoon.

Dings to the head and getting one's bell rung, which had been casually dismissed as nothing to worry about or even had generated laughter in the past, were being seen as far more serious by players and coaches alike. As onetime New York Giants safety Maurice Douglass explained in 1996 after teammate Tyrone Wheatley had been knocked out, "Concussions are funny . . . unless they happen to you." In an article about that incident, *New York Times* columnist Dave Anderson warned, "Concussions are football's silent career killer." Anderson then chided the NFL, observing that while "teams often let knocked-out players return the next Sunday," many states won't allow boxers who have been knocked out to "compete for 60 days."[9]

In response to this growing bad publicity, the league authorized one of the members of its MTBI Committee to establish a "neuropsychological testing program" for the league. He was "the chairman and co-founder of ImPACT, a baseline [concussion] testing company that does big business with the NFL." By 2001 most teams were using this program in some form.[10]

Furthermore, the MTBI Committee, which had conducted its own "research" on the concussion problem, was ready to publish some of its closely manicured results. Apparently the NFL committee selected the medical journal *Neurosurgery* as potentially the most cooperative publication because its editor was Michael Apuzzo, who was a "consultant" with the New York Giants. Apuzzo created a special section in the journal "on sports and the brain." He then made neurosurgeon Bob Cantu, "King of Concussions," the editor. In 2003 the special series of NFL papers were released to the public.[11]

The first two articles were illuminating, but both seemed to deliberately shift potential legal liability from the NFL to football helmet makers. The emphasis was on the lack of "effectiveness of football helmets in preventing head injuries." Neurosurgeon Julian Bales, who had sounded the alarm about signs of dementia in NFL football players he had examined, congratulated the NFL for "usher[ing] in a new era in the study and analysis . . . of these high-speed bodily collisions." As was described in *League of Denial*, however, the NFL also was using that journal to disseminate articles that "portrayed NFL players as superhuman and impervious to brain damage."[12]

The medical community, including Apuzzo himself, generally panned those articles. Several were of such poor quality and so biased that the papers "were rejected by peer reviewers and editors and later disavowed even by some of their authors."[13] Years later a *New York Times* investigation revealed the NFL researchers had deliberately excluded "more than 100 diagnosed concussions" from those studies. That breach of ethics substantially reduced the concussion rates, making them "appear less frequent than they actually were."[14] It allowed the NFL to claim that "professional football players do not sustain frequent repetitive blows to the brain on a regular basis."[15] This assertion was widely condemned by the medical community. It also ignored compelling anecdotal evidence, which indicated that most NFL players, coaches, teams, and owners did not disclose, had ignored, and/or tended to minimize the impact of concussions. Furthermore, it was contrary to what any football fan could see on the television screen every Saturday and Sunday, from August through January.

Shortly thereafter the NFL claimed that based on league data about how "quickly players went back on the field . . . , they were at no greater risk than if they had never been concussed." This second conclusion contradicted compelling medical evidence that each additional brain injury increased the health risks substantially. When neuroscientists reviewed the NFL's study, they found that the methodology was empirically deficient. The NFL had preselected a small percentage of the available baseline measures of concussed players to study, "throw[ing] out thousands of . . . tests," which presumably would have produced damning results.[16]

Making matters worse, Riddell, the maker of the NFL's helmets, used this corrupt research to claim that its helmet, which it marketed to youth football, "significantly reduced concussions in children." The implication appeared to be that its equipment would make this dangerous sport safe for these young players. After a thorough investigation, though, the Federal Trade Commission determined that the available evidence did not support such a claim.[17]

Undeterred by the negative reactions to its research in the scientific and medical communities, the league's MTBI Committee released another paper in *Neurosurgery*. This time the NFL drew the dubious conclusion that the type of brain damage associated with boxers "has not been observed in professional football."[18] That assertion turned out to be false and deliberately misleading, if not an outright lie. By carefully parsing its words to focus on what their researchers had chosen to observe, rather than what all the available evidence indicated, the NFL was trying to create the impression that football head injuries were much fewer and less serious than they were.

## THE NFL'S RESEARCH IS DISCREDITED

As powerful as the NFL was in trying to control information about concussions and brain damage to its players by influencing the sports media who covered football and by conducting its own research, two other factors proved to be more dominant in the long run: (1) the scientific method as applied to brain injuries through well-funded research; and (2) the ingenuity of plaintiffs' lawyers, who would soon find ways to use the legal system, the media, and medical and scientific research to obtain compensation for former players, who had suffered—or appeared to have suffered—serious brain injuries while playing professional and collegiate football.

The turnarounds, both in the public sentiments and legal assessments of liability, regarding football head injuries were similar—in a more limited way—to what had happened to Big Tobacco in the United States. Eventually those who had contracted lung and other cancers related to smoking began winning lawsuits as the science—and what is known in the law as proximate causation—caught up to the denials and deceptions. These same types of legal victories would reprise themselves in concussion lawsuits against the NFL, and then spread to professional hockey and the NCAA.

But first the science had to advance far enough to substantially impact public perceptions and the legal establishment. Of all the spurious assertions that the NFL made through its MTBI Committee, what ultimately would hurt the league the most was the claim, backed by flawed NFL research, that there was no evidence that professional athletes sustained long-term brain damage playing football. This patently false conclusion helped to galvanize neuroscientists to prove that the assertion was wrong. The new research focused on the potential effects of single and repeated brain traumas on NFL players at a time when research was being conducted on soldiers and veterans who had experienced somewhat similar types of traumas in combat. Substantial federal and private funds were available for brain researchers, far more than the NFL could provide for its own tightly controlled "research" initiatives.

In addition, by the time the league had made its unsupportable assertion about the absence of long-term mental impairment from playing football, the NFL's retirement board already had grudgingly awarded ongoing compensation to several players based on impairment from those types of brain injuries. Nevertheless, the league's retirement board continued to try to either deny or hide the fact that these mental disabilities probably originated while the claimants had been playing professional football. More importantly, from a public relations standpoint, damaged athletes and their loved ones and friends began coming forward with tragic stories of how former NFL players were succumbing to the symptoms of brain injuries and other severe mental and physical impairments.

## THE MIKE WEBSTER TRAGEDY CHANGES PUBLIC PERCEPTIONS AND THE LAW

One of the worst, most publicized, and legally significant football-related, health, and human tragedies involved Pittsburgh Steelers Hall of Fame center Mike Webster. He died prematurely in 2002 at age fifty from drug-induced "heart failure . . . [after a long] odyssey of bizarre behavior and . . . homelessness."[19] His failing condition had been intensified by isolation, severe mental impairment, seizures, and chronic pain. Webster would soon become the poster man-child for the types of disabilities, torment, addictions, and lack of services that could and did destroy many NFL players' lives once their football careers were over. Webster was a near-perfect plaintiff for a lawsuit challenging the league's stingy and duplicitous retirement compensation apparatus.

As ESPN writer Greg Garber vividly described several years after Webster's death, this once-superlative athlete became "a tormented soul . . . , a worst-case scenario for physical and emotional well-being [of a former football player]." He compulsively and repeatedly took "a numbing cocktail of medications." This included "Ritalin or Dexedrine to keep him calm. Paxil to ease anxiety. Prozac to ward off depression. [And] Klonopin to prevent seizures."[20]

Furthermore, Webster regularly ingested powerful opioid painkillers—Vicodin, Ultram, Darvocet, and/or Lorcet—as well as a medication for patients who suffer from Parkinson's disease, the disease that eventually killed Muhammad Ali. In addition, he suffered from "dementia . . . [constant] head throbb[ing] . . . hearing loss . . . frayed and herniated discs [in his vertebrae] . . . damaged right heel . . . right shoulder . . . [and] right elbow . . . knees [with barely any] . . . cartilage . . . [and] fingers [that] bent gruesomely wayward."[21] Because of football, Webster had become a broken man in many different ways.

Webster's downfall, after retiring from football in 1990, was both immediate and lengthy. According to his lawyers, only months after his last game, Webster had become "completely disabled." Yet, his mental and physical impairments continued to grow much worse. By the time Webster died eleven years later, "he was bed-bound in a haze of pain and narcotics, a bucket of vomit by his side."[22]

Through this agonizing health deterioration process, however, Webster had established a legal precedent, which the league would not be able to erase, although it would try to limit its reach. In 1999 the NFL, through its retirement board, agreed that "Webster had suffered irreparable brain damage from repeated concussions."[23] Nonetheless, he was only awarded compensation for conditions that arose after he had retired.

The grim circumstances surrounding Webster's death provided the circumstances for Pittsburgh coroner and pathologist Bennet Omalu to discover "tau-deposits" in the football player's brain.[24] In 2005, this led to the discovery that football players, like boxers, could die of CTE. Dr. Omalu's discovery was the subject of the 2015 movie *Concussion*.

Around the same time, two other professional football players received "permanent benefits" due to "brain damage."[25] Their names were withheld on grounds of confidentiality, which meant the media, the public, and various plaintiffs' lawyers could not easily identify who those former players were or what their compensation was for. The league's convenient embrace of confidentiality in this situation, however, did not extend to the care and treatment of active players where team physicians frequently breached player confidentiality (see chapter 4).

Despite this veil of secrecy, enough leaked out that a viable legal precedent was being established. This meant it would be easier to obtain compensation for other players who had sustained these types of brain impairments in football and other sports such as hockey as well. After Webster's death, lawyers successfully filed for additional compensation for his family. Eventually his estate received more than $600,000 in disability payments, but only retroactive to 1996.[26]

Webster's family sued for additional retroactive compensation on behalf of the player and his children. They contended that the NFL's retirement board had improperly concluded Webster did not have a disability within six months of his retirement, even though consulting experts, including one hired by the league, had found that he had been substantially impaired as a player. A federal court awarded the plaintiffs about $2 million in damages, which the Fourth Circuit Court of Appeals upheld in 2006.[27]

## THE GOODELL ERA BEGINS

Around the time of the finalized verdict, Commissioner Tagliabue, who was now sixty-five, decided to return to his corporate legal practice. Whether he was nudged out or wished to leave remains unclear. Despite notable success in building league revenues and bargaining with the players, the concussion controversy would mar his legacy. Being saddled with a major share of the responsibility for the accumulating bad concussion publicity appears to be a major reason why he has not been inducted into the Pro Football Hall of Fame after being nominated five times.

The NFL chose one of his chief lieutenants to take his place, but the appointment signaled a change in tactics if not direction. The new commissioner, Roger Goodell, was not trained as a corporate lawyer. As the son of a distinguished congressman and U.S. senator from New York, Goodell seemed to know politics well. For many years he had focused on public relations for the league, had developed a cozy relationship with the media, and was nearly twenty years younger than Tagliabue.

Minimizing damage to the NFL and the sport of football from concussions and related controversies would become a key component of the new commissioner's mission, which was to "keep the labor peace and the good times rolling for a . . . nearly $6 billion-a-year business."[28] Success would be nearly impossible to achieve, however, if players, the fan base, and corporate sponsors perceived the sport to be unsafe and uncivilized.

The Webster family's lawsuit and its unanticipated outcome turned out to be the genesis for much expanded litigation against the league, which many former players would join. At the same time, the conclusive evidence needed to prove brain trauma liability in the courts was still evolving. In 2007, a few months into his tenure, the league decided to bring Roger Goodell "up-to-speed on the developing crisis," hoping that Goodell's appointment would represent a clean slate. The league organized a summit featuring an assembly of experts, including members of the NFL's MTBI Committee. Some in the media suggested the new commissioner had "inherited a cover-up," even though Goodell had been knee deep in defending the league as Tagliabue's chief lieutenant and its lead publicist.[29]

Among the experts invited to the summit were two distinct groups: those who could be counted on to continue to spew the NFL party line, and those "dissenters" who regarded the MTBI Committee "as a sham." Among the dissenters was neurosurgeon Julian Bailes, who had seen a number of football players with brain damage in his practice. Their symptoms included "depression, dementia, even suicide." By then Bailes had become "almost certain" that the cause was "repetitive head trauma related to football." He too had examined the brain scans of dead players and found the telltale "brown splotches" from damaged brain cells that demonstrated the presence of CTE. [30]

In response, the new chair of the NFL's MTBI Committee, Ira Casson, reportedly "rolled his eyes" and scoffed at Bailes's presentation, suggesting that it was not based on good science. Goodell himself expressed doubts. The new commissioner opined that examining deceased players' brains "without looking at their entire medical history . . . is irresponsible," implying that Bailes's work had been shoddy (or worse). [31] These personal attacks on Bailes demonstrated the seriousness with which the NFL now viewed the concussion threat, as well as the league's desperation.

## CTE TAKES CENTER STAGE

Two years later, in 2009, researchers at the Boston University School of Medicine's Sports Legacy Institute began to move the CTE discussion forward, beyond the control of the NFL. For the first time, respected neuroscientists had obtained a professional football player's brain to study. [32] It belonged to John Grimsley, a linebacker who had played nearly ten years in the NFL from 1984 to 1993. Like Webster, Grimsley had died prematurely with signs of emotional upheavals in his shortened life.

Similarly to many professional football players who play defense, Grimsley was known "as a hard hitter with a mean streak." He had died suspiciously at age forty-eight of a self-inflicted gunshot wound to the head, which was ruled an accident. Such a finding is not that unusual when suicide is the likely cause. Sympathetic local coroners understand that ruling a self-inflicted death as deliberate would be emotionally devastating to the grieving family and preclude the spouse from recovering life insurance.

In a newspaper story about Grimsley's death, his wife dutifully reported that he was a "happy guy." At the same time, she submitted his brain for CTE testing and described a whole set of symptoms in her husband, which refuted the earlier "happy" characterization. She readily acknowledged that Grimsley had numerous impairments, which included problems with his memory, and "mood swings" that brought on loss of his "temper without warning or provocation." [33]

Dementia and other types of cognitive impairments have a number of potential physical, social, and environmental causes, which has made it difficult to conclusively prove that brain traumas are the primary cause of these catastrophic impairments in former football players. The game changer for researchers, lawyers, and the media turned out to be advances in imaging technology to map out and closely examine areas of the brain.

That imaging process revealed the presence of abnormally high amounts of "tau" in the brains of boxers, veterans of combat, and football players who had CTE. Typically, that brain disease is triggered by concussions and other brain traumas. Tau's presence, like lung cancer in those who use tobacco, would become a smoking gun. The tau protein is known to kill and actually replace healthy brain cells.

In 2008 researchers found that Grimsley's brain had tau everywhere. That same year the Boston University researchers found tau in the brain of another professional football player. He had died of a drug overdose. As many more such heart-wrenching cases involving professional football players with CTE came to light, a consensus began to develop among neuroscientists and other brain experts. It was becoming apparent that the CTE being found in so many football players was due to the fact that they all had suffered repeated concussions and/or other concussive brain impacts during their football careers.

Eventually courts began taking notice of this consensus and created—implicitly if not explicitly—what in the law is called a rebuttable presumption that playing football was the primary likely cause of CTE in former and current players. Yet, even that presumption fell well short of establishing liability in individual cases. Once CTE was proven to exist in the brains of deceased players, that legal presumption meant the NFL would have the burden of disproving the causal link between the impairments from that condition and playing football.

The NFL would either have to present an alternative theory of causation, or demonstrate that the CTE diagnosis was incorrect or deficient. That, however, would not be so difficult to do since there could be many other intervening variables and factors at play. Even today neuroscientists caution that the science surrounding CTE remains "in its infancy" with respect to "pinpointing symptoms, risks and prevalence of the disease."[34]

## PLAUSIBLE DENIABILITY AND DELAY

For a number of years, the NFL's experts had tried to show, using their flawed science, that the researchers who had gathered and examined the brains of football players had been largely mistaken in their findings and conclusions. In 2009 the NFL was still contending that the CTE found in the brains of so many deceased former football players had been caused by other factors, including "steroids, nutritional supplements, high blood pressure, [and] diabetes."[35] The NFL continued to deny that there was a problem due to the "cognitive decline among its players."[36]

Plausible deniability had become the NFL's fallback position because persuasive proof to support their assertions was more than just elusive. It did not exist. A leading CTE researcher, in a formal presentation to the NFL's MTBI Committee, called the committee members "delusional." Beginning in September 2009, the evidence supporting concussion-related brain damage in football players began accumulating rapidly, as did the media coverage.

In a series of groundbreaking articles, *New York Times* reporter Alan Schwarz showed football fans and the general public how the latest independent CTE research "regarding N.F.L. players and the effects of their occupational head injuries" was puncturing the NFL's public relations mythology. In addition, an NFL-funded study by the University of Michigan Institute for Social Research had found that among former NFL players "Alzheimer's disease or similar memory-related diseases appear[ed] to have been diagnosed . . . vastly more often than in the national population." The league's longtime public relations spokesperson, Greg Aiello, dismissed the research as "telephone surveys," which did not involve formal diagnoses, and noted that "thousands of retired players . . . do not have memory problems."[37]

Nevertheless, as West Virginia University School of Medicine neurosurgeon Julian Bailes observed, the Michigan study would be a "gamechanger" in terms of public attitudes. Not surprisingly, the NFL tried to stall for more time. Aiello said that the NFL would be taking steps "to understand [the issue] as it relates to our retired players." Ira Casson, the cochair of the NFL's MTBI Committee, added that "there's a need for further studies to see whether this finding is going to pan out." Casson contended that while the "respondents [may] believe they have been diagnosed [with brain diseases] . . . the next step is to determine whether that is so."[38]

As it turned out, what the NFL really wanted was to have the issue put on hold until the NFL's MTBI Committee could complete its own "longterm" study about the potential cognitive decline of players. The league tried to pretend that this would be the definitive study that would make all the other research obsolete. The *New York Times*, however, contacted a number of distinguished epidemiologists and social scientists who, after analyzing the NFL study's design and methodology, all agreed that it was "fraught with statistical, systemic and conflict-of-interest problems that make it inappropriate to examine [this] issue."[39]

## THE NFL'S WOEFULLY INADEQUATE DISABILITY PLAN

Around the same time that the NFL's so-called definitive research was being panned as an emperor without clothes, the *New York Times'* Schwarz wrote an exposé revealing that the NFL's disability plan "run jointly with the players union" did not "consider dementia to be an occupational risk."[40] It was not that awards based on football-related brain disorders were nonexistent, but that they had been few and far between. This pattern had continued, despite—or perhaps because of—revelations about how common cognitive impairments in football players appeared to be.

Under the NFL's plan, compensation for any type of brain disease or mental injury was extremely limited, especially as compared to awards for physical conditions and injuries. Also, benefits were only granted for impairments that "developed within 15 years of . . . retirement." This was shortsighted from a health perspective—probably intentionally so to save money. Football-related mental impairments and some physical conditions, like severe forms of arthritis, can present themselves much later in life, or in the case of CTE not even be definitively diagnosed until after a player dies.

The NFL's sanguine response was that "playing in the NFL was a very positive experience. . . . Overall they are in very good physical . . . condition."[41] The league conspicuously avoided mentioning cognitive impairments and other mental conditions of former players, pointing out instead that the aforementioned Michigan study had found that with respect to diabetes, heart attacks, and strokes, former players reported better than average results.

It was not unreasonable to presume that a majority of former players, particularly those who had retired from the game more recently, had the financial means to purchase good health care for themselves. At the same time, it also was likely that a substantial minority could not afford good health care; incurred conditions—such as obesity, CTE, or substance abuse problems—that placed them at much higher risk;[42] or incurred mental impairments and addictions, which distorted their judgment about the need for or benefits of health care. Thus, many former players were being placed in jeopardy because the NFL's disability compensation coverage was—and continues to be—deliberately deficient.

One major reason that this health care gap has existed for so long without being addressed is that the NFL contends that any issue regarding compensation or benefits for its former players is a matter "for collective bargaining" between the league and the players union.[43] The fundamental flaw with that arrangement was—and continues to be—that retired players are not directly represented in those negotiations. Their interests have been contrary to the interests of current players, who, like the owners, want to receive a greater share of the league's revenues, rather than providing what would be a relatively small percentage of those proceeds to former players.

As a result, there were—and continue to be—strong economic disincentives to providing former players with substantially improved—much less comprehensive—disability and health care benefits. Yet, given the accumulating evidence of the health risks of playing the game and the huge revenue streams that the NFL has been generating for so long, one might have hoped for much better disability and health plans. Both the league and its players should have realized that providing former players with greatly improved health care and disability benefits had become—and continues to be—one of the essential ingredients for the game to remain viable as a civilized sport.

## THINGS GO FROM BAD TO WORSE FOR THE NFL

A similar message about the need to protect players, however, was being delivered in a different way. The threat posed by litigation, continued bad publicity, and potential congressional action convinced the NFL to reformulate its public persona on concussions. Just before Christmas in 2009, the NFL signaled a change. Remarkably, the league decided that it not only "would support research by its most vocal critics but . . . conceded . . . concussions can have lasting consequences," although it was still unwilling to admit what those consequences were. Furthermore, the NFL announced it had accepted the resignation of Dr. Casson, the cochair of its concussion committee.[44]

Greg Aiello—again speaking for the league in the noticeable absence of Commissioner Goodell—explained that it had become "quite obvious from the medical research . . . that concussions can lead to long-term problems." Aiello's statement raised the question: Had it become obvious before the NFL had trashed all the independent studies, or in the prior two and a half months? Apparently the NFL had gained the necessary clarity sometime after the House Judiciary Committee had held a hearing in October at which "the league's approach to science was compared to that of the tobacco industry."[45]

Not surprisingly, in 2010, shortly after that congressional spanking, all hell began to break loose with respect to the NFL's credibility on concussions and other related matters. First, a University of Wisconsin professor of science journalism recounted in the *New York Times* that the respected *Journal of the American Medical Association* (*JAMA*) had warned physicians and the public that "single or repeated blows on the head . . . cause multiple concussion hemorrhages."[46] That same issue of *JAMA* had published another study titled "'Punch Drunk'" that was based on a "meticulous examination" of the brains of prizefighters. The medical researcher detailed the symptoms he had found in those fighters—"loss of coordination, cognitive deficits, uncontrollable rages."[47]

What made both the *JAMA* editorial and article especially compelling was that their publication date had been 1928. The Wisconsin professor wondered why, more than eighty years later, the NFL was still contending that the long-established link between concussions and dementia was something "new, and still somewhat debatable." She was convinced, based on her own research, that America had been slow to recognize the dangers of concussions "mostly because the NFL, the National Collegiate Athletic Association and their allies have done an outstanding job . . . of ignoring and dismissing the medical record" about brain damage in athletes, particularly football players.[48]

One of the sport's most outspoken political allies, a member of the House of Representatives from Texas, proclaimed that "football as we know it could be destroyed if we move toward greater protectiveness."[49] His response succinctly captured the issue for millions of Americans. Should the health risks posed to football players be allowed to disrupt how the game has been played and enjoyed for so many years?

In May 2010, the NFL's strategically renamed Head, Neck and Spine Committee had its two new cochairmen testify before a panel of the

House Judiciary Committee. This was the same panel that had compared the former MTBI Committee to Big Tobacco and had accused it of "bias and poor science." The renamed NFL committee stumbled badly. The new chairmen sounded "like the same old N.F.L." Even worse, they could not "answer even basic questions about [football] helmets."[50]

One of the first things that the NFL did do was hire what the league would misleadingly describe as "independent neurologists for return-to-play decisions" and to promote "concussion guidelines for youth sports."[51] The NFL's two-pronged strategy was intended to help limit its liability for future injuries and redirect the discussion away from concussions in football toward sports more generally. Nonetheless, what was happening to former NFL players continued to capture most of the media's attention. Not only were these athletes compelling public figures, but by most commonsense measures—weight, strength, power, speed, aggressiveness, violence, and the number of years they had played football competitively—NFL players appeared to be in the greatest jeopardy. Between 2002 and June 2010, in the early stages of this brain trauma research, twenty-three football players already had "been identified with chronic traumatic encephalopathy,"[52] and the list was growing.

More disturbingly, around that same time there was a finding of CTE in a recently deceased current player. Chris Henry, a talented but erratic and troubled NFL wide receiver, had died after falling out of the back of a pickup truck in December 2009 during a tempestuous domestic dispute with his fiancée, who had been driving the vehicle. Henry was only twenty-six years old and at the height of his professional football career. This led many in the media to ponder "how many current players . . . may be playing with [CTE] . . . and experiencing its effects, which include depression, impaired decision-making and ultimately dementia."[53] People around the country also must have begun to wonder how much the behavioral symptoms of CTE were contributing to violence against women and other antisocial actions alleged to have been committed by NFL players who increasingly were making headlines based on such accusations.

Not long after Henry's posthumous diagnosis, the "early stages of CTE" were found in the brain of a twenty-one-year-old offensive lineman for the University of Pennsylvania "with no previous history of depression" who had committed suicide. He had hanged himself just after being named one of the team's captains. Since a disproportionate percentage of young adults commit suicide, playing football could not be reliably identified as the likely single cause. On the other hand, as a group, football players appeared to be at a considerably higher risk of suicide. This type of sudden "depression and [loss of] impulse control . . . had been found among N.F.L. players, two of whom . . . committed suicide in the last 10 years."[54]

As one Boston University doctor and expert on CTE explained, the college lineman's death "proves the disease can begin, and perhaps influence behavior, among football players below the N.F.L. level."[55] This was not even the first football suicide at that particular Ivy League school. In 2005, a University of Pennsylvania running back had killed himself just "two days after one of the best games of his career."[56] And this was Ivy League football. Whether the cause was primarily CTE, the culture of football competition, and/or depression from another source, those two suicides raised unsettling questions about the game's impact on older adolescents and young adults.

Toward the end of 2010, the NFL implemented new concussion reporting protocols. Reportedly, there had been 154 concussions through the first eight weeks of the season including in games and practices.[57] This was a 21 percent increase as compared to a similar time span in 2009 and a 34 percent jump from 2008. The Head, Neck and Spine Committee responded by issuing a self-serving warning aimed at protecting the NFL from liability.

The committee members contended that while "playing through pain is good . . . what sports are about . . . a brain injury . . . can threaten [a player's] future." They were concerned that players were hiding or marginalizing "the effects of a concussion."[58] The implication was clear that while the NFL was acknowledging what should have been evident since 1928, players—and not teams or the league—were primarily responsible.

For the 2011 football season, the NFL added a rule change that affected one isolated aspect of the game. By having a team kick off from the 35-yard line, rather than the 30, the number of "returns fell by about 32%,"[59] reducing the opportunities for concussions, especially among those who returned kicks. During that season, based on NFL-managed data, there was a 12.5 percent reduction in concussions across the league and those who were concussed tended to be held out longer than in the past. The NFL noted that these types of brain injuries had decreased during the 2010 season as well.[60] This seemed like bragging that instead of playing Russian roulette with three bullets in the chamber, from now on the NFL would use only two.

Yet, even that reported small incremental advancement in safety was called into question. After conducting an independent analysis of the NFL's figures for those two years, researchers, as part of an ongoing collaborative effort between ESPN's *Outside the Lines* and PBS's *Frontline*, concluded that the league had released "two different sets of data . . . making it impossible to evaluate the league's claims." In addition, the researchers alleged that the NFL teams had been describing concussions with "imprecise" language that distorted the actual "prevalence and severity of head injuries." Moreover, on many occasions teams continued to send concussed "players back into games despite apparent symptoms."[61]

## POTENTIAL LEGAL LIABILITY OF THE NFL GROWS

In May 2012 the professional football world was rattled again—arguably even more so than by the Mike Webster tragedy—when the forty-three-year-old, recently retired All-Pro, and certain Hall of Fame linebacker Junior Seau died after shooting himself in the chest.[62] He was a contemporary of many members of the players union and well respected among his peers. Seau had come to realize that he was declining noticeably due to brain damage, which made him subject to outbursts of rage that isolated him from friends and family. In one of his "darker moments" just after he had been arrested on charges of domestic violence, Seau drove "his sport utility vehicle off a cliff."[63] Despite all of this obvious emotional pain and upheaval, when he finally took his life he aimed his gun at his chest rather than his head. This supported the subsequent observation that Seau had wanted his brain to be studied.[64]

Seau's suicide was remarkably similar to that of longtime Pro Bowl safety Dave Duerson. In 2011 at age fifty, Duerson—the former standout Chicago Bear—realizing that he had severe symptoms of dementia and was declining physically, placed a gun to his chest and shot "himself to death." According to his family, Duerson's final words were: "Please, see that my brain is given to the NFL's brain bank." His son Tregg, who had played football at Notre Dame for one year before quitting, grieved, "I just wish he had played baseball."[65] Both Seau's and Duerson's brains revealed the presence of CTE.

In addition, Ray Easterling, a former Atlanta Falcons safety, had "died of a self-inflicted gunshot wound two weeks before Seau."[66] By late 2012 Boston University researchers had "examined the brains of 34 former NFL players. Thirty-three had CTE,"[67] which only could be diagnosed posthumously. While the sampling was far from random—most of the families who had donated brains had observed symptoms of mental impairment and abnormal behavior associated with CTE in the tested players—a staggering 97 percent of the tests (thirty-three of thirty-four) had found the presence of this neurodegenerative disease. By June 2016, the number had nearly tripled to ninety-four, and ninety of those players' brains (96 percent) had tested positive.[68]

Legally, such a high probability, especially if it could be replicated in subsequent examinations of former NFL players, would be enough to establish proof of what is called proximate causation. This is distinguished from causation-in-fact, which represents virtual certainty. Unfortunately for the players and their families, the direct connection between CTE and football-related mental impairments of individual players remained less certain. Also, while the incidence of depression was significantly higher in former players, particularly before they reached middle age,[69] a National Institute for Occupational Safety and Health study had "found fewer than half as many suicides among . . . retired players . . . as in the general population."[70]

In addition, the research on CTE had not progressed far enough to determine how much tau in the brain was necessary to significantly affect a person's behavior, or how that condition would manifest itself. Similarly, it was not possible to reliably determine which behaviors and cognitive symptoms that specific individuals had incurred while playing in the NFL were due to concussions. Still, the evidence seemed compelling that concussions and other forms of brain trauma could cause CTE, particularly if these concussive impacts were repeated frequently.

There was no denying that an unusually high percentage of NFL players had this abnormality when their brains were tested after they died, and many of them had developed various mental impairments while they were alive. Despite some medical and scientific ambiguity, former players and their families began filing multiple concussion lawsuits against the league. Yet, these were not the first concussion-related lawsuits to have a legal impact.

# CONCUSSION-RELATED LAWSUITS FILED AGAINST THE NFL

## THE INITIAL LAWSUITS

The early, slow trickle of concussion-related lawsuits involved both professional and collegiate football players but focused on mistreatment issues filed against team medical personnel. Most notably, former Pittsburgh Steelers and Chicago Bears running back and ESPN commentator Merril Hoge obtained a jury verdict of $1.55 million in 2000 against one of his former team physicians.[1] Nearly eight years later, lawyers for a La Salle University football player negotiated a $7.5 million settlement in a suit filed against that university's medical staff.[2] Each of these lawsuits was based on traditional negligence or malpractice theories, which did not involve the NFL or NCAA as defendants.

These two legal actions probably whetted the appetites of personal injury lawyers, motivating them to think creatively about the legal possibilities related to the concussion issue, especially following the verdict for Hoge. By June 2008 there were at least "85 suits involving more than 2000 former players" against the NFL. Furthermore, an assemblage of lawyers representing former players and their families had filed a massive class action suit in the U.S. District Court for the Eastern District of Pennsylvania alleging "negligence and fraud . . . , wrongful death and civil conspiracy."[3]

By August 2012 *Sporting News* was reporting that the number of concussion lawsuits had increased to 135, involving more than 3,400 former players and billions of dollars of potential liability for the league.[4] And the numbers kept growing. By November the Associated Press was reporting that "more than 3800 players ha[d] sued . . . in at least 175 cases."[5] This type of litigation was becoming so prevalent that the *Washington Times* sports department created an online database to track those legal actions.

None of those cases, however, had been resolved on their merits, although a few had been dismissed for procedural reasons. A significant portion of the complaints had been consolidated into the aforementioned class action. The unifying theme was that the NFL had been "concealing the long-term consequences of head injuries from players."[6]

In May 2012, another group of retired football players sued the NFL Players Association for "hundreds of millions of dollars in additional postcareer benefits."[7] They alleged that those benefits had been improperly lost when the union reached a collective bargaining agreement with the NFL that limited health and disability compensation for those former players. That suit was summarily dismissed because the plaintiffs had not stated a claim that was considered justiciable (capable of being decided). The players union successfully argued that it had no legal duty to protect the interests of those former players because they were not—and could not be—members of the union. Thus, all the judge could do legally was note on the record that "she was 'empathetic to [the former] concerns.'"[8]

Given what had happened to Junior Seau, it was not a surprise when his family filed suit against the NFL in a California state court alleging his death was wrongful. Like many of these suits, this January 2013 action named the NFL's helmet maker (Riddell) a defendant, alleging that those "helmets were unreasonably dangerous and unsafe."[9] The NFL had helped to create this perception of shared liability with its early research into the deficiencies of those helmets.

That same month the NFL's brain trauma problem grew worse when President Obama made national headlines by telling the media that if he had a son, he would not want him to play football. In the president's opinion, "The most popular sport in America cause[d] irreparable harm to many of its participants."[10] Clearly public attitudes about football and concussions were changing.

## THE CLASS ACTION PROCEEDS SLOWLY, WHILE THE NFL TRIES TO LIMIT ITS DAMAGES

That spring the concussion class action against the NFL and Riddell, which had been consolidated in judge Anita Brody's federal courtroom in Philadelphia, began. With all that was at stake, the two opposing "legal teams . . . were stacked with top talent, including litigators who ha[d] argued in front of the Supreme Court." The issues that were likely to be decisive boiled down to whether: "the league knew about the long-term dangers of head trauma but hid them"; responsibility for "player safety . . . [and player] injuries [was] covered by collective bargaining," and thus not subject to litigation; and the players had assumed the risks of participating in this dangerous sport.[11]

Beyond those narrow legal questions, this groundbreaking class action had much broader social implications. For many Americans the most important consideration continued to be the value-laden question: "Are concussions ruining sports?" The answer really depended on what people chose to hear.

Many fans heard the question as being whether the legal hoopla surrounding brain damage was harming many of America's favorite spectator sports, especially football. The implication was that unnecessarily worrying people about these impairments should be the biggest public concern. Most Americans, though, particularly nonfans, heard the question differently. They wondered whether what was being revealed about concussions required substantial changes to be made to high-risk sports like football, especially when played by children.

Given the divergence in these two competing perspectives, one might have assumed that there was no feasible way to arrive at an acceptable legal conclusion in this case. Yet, American law tends to embrace compromise, particularly when two substantial social perspectives or interests are in conflict. *Roe v. Wade* and plea bargaining are two important examples in which such legal compromises have been reached. Thus, it was not surprising that in asking the related question—"Will brain injury lawsuits doom the NFL?"—from the outset the answer appeared to be no. If football was doomed it probably would not be due to litigation.

Concussions and other brain injuries would not bankrupt football and other sports, but rather would likely become "a cost of doing business,"[12] which has been the pattern with other public health risks associated with tobacco, asbestos, and radon, for example. The tried-and-true corporate strategy would be for football to make changes, which appeared to significantly advance safety, without upsetting the fundamental nature of how the game is supposed to be played as perceived by the fans, television networks, and corporate sponsors that provide the revenues. Because those business costs were likely to be substantial, however, the NFL would continue do what it believed was necessary to limit its liability and expenses.

By the end of August 2013 the class action litigation, which had been consolidated in Judge Brody's courtroom, included "more than 4,500 retired players," but the NFL was hoping to convince the judge to "dismiss hundreds of [those] cases." Instead, she ordered both "sides to continue working with a mediator . . . to reach a settlement." Her approach was the very embodiment of a legal compromise, which could—and probably should—have involved billions of dollars as the NFL's reasonable cost of doing business. [13]

Despite ongoing mediation, the league still was trying to control the public discourse involving concussion safety in other ways. In a move that was more characteristic of a commissioner trained in manipulating public perceptions than engaging in litigation, the NFL apparently put pressure on ESPN to disassociate itself from its joint documentary with PBS's *Frontline* on the NFL's efforts to cover up its concussion problem. While the NFL denied any untoward involvement, ESPN's sudden decision to drop its support for the program, after being a partner in the project for more than a year, seemed to be highly suspicious. At the very least, the sudden change in priorities indicated that ESPN felt that its best interests would be served by not delving too deeply into what the NFL and the sports networks had been doing all these years.

Accusations of improper influence were fueled by the indisputable fact that ESPN had a contract with the NFL to broadcast *Monday Night Football*, a "ratings juggernaut and cherished source of revenue." [14] Thus, those tampering allegations hurt the NFL's reputation, which already was reeling from multiple revelations that it had tried to hide key information about brain injuries from the players and the public. The image of the league using its considerable power and influence behind the scenes to try to derail concussion-education projects on public television reaffirmed the basic thesis of the documentary—as well as the book upon which the program was based. When it came to concussions, the NFL was a *League of Denial*, and probably myths and deceptions—if not outright lies—as well.

## A TENTATIVE SETTLEMENT FAVORABLE TO THE NFL

Nonetheless, two days after the historic federal court case against the NFL had resumed and just before the first regular season game was to be played in September 2013, a tentative settlement was reached. In the opinion of most legal experts, the outcome represented a relatively small cost of doing business for the NFL, even though it was a potential bonanza for the plaintiffs' lawyers. Without admitting liability, the league agreed to pay "765 million . . . [as compensation to] more than 4,500 former players . . . . [and] to fund medical exams and research as well."[15] The league already was providing millions of dollars for NFL-guided research, which would help to blunt the financial impact of the settlement on the owners. In addition, over half of the total award was to be spread out over seventeen years.

Remarkably, the proposed settlement was intended to cover "all NFL retirees, approximately 16,000." This equaled about $25,000 in expenses per player. For a sports enterprise "generat[ing] more than $9 billion in annual revenues,"[16] which had been increasing almost every year, this would be less than 1.5 percent of its total revenues in the first three years of the settlement and no more than one-quarter of 1 percent for the remaining fourteen years. In other words, it would be a drop in the bucket.

As Mike Wise of the *Washington Post* exclaimed, sarcastically, "What a great day for further memory loss and long-term suffering." Wise pointed out that both parties had squandered a "real chance to make an impact [on safety]. . . . Goodell's lawyers took advantage of the immediate gratification needs of the NFL's former players." This was like taking "advantage of woozy-headed men who knew their careers might be over if they didn't go back in the game."[17]

A few weeks later, in response to *League of Denial*, Goodell earnestly postured that the "NFL is safer than ever," which was faint praise indeed. Nonetheless, the commissioner seemed to understand that in terms of public perceptions "the issue of player health and player safety [was] something the NFL . . . want[ed] to get out in front of." He pointed out that the league had "eliminate[d] the 'head slap' in the 1970s . . . the 'horse collar' in the 2000s . . . [and] hits using the crown of the helmet [more recently]." [18] For his many critics, this all seemed to be too little too late with no healthy resolution in sight, especially for children and adolescents playing the dangerous game of football.

That November the NFL took another hit when eight former players revealed, based on a relatively new testing methodology (positron-emission tomography) being used at UCLA, that they had all shown signs of having CTE. The victims included Dallas Hall of Fame running back Tony Dorsett, Buffalo Hall of Fame offensive lineman Joe DeLamielleure, and former New York Giants All-Pro Super Bowl defensive lineman Leonard Marshall. Dorsett announced that he was experiencing memory problems and "temperamental outbursts," was unable "to control his emotions," and was "clinically depressed." [19]

The UCLA story was significant in two ways. First, it meant that going forward, living players could be tested for CTE and might be able to take meaningful steps to deal with the progressive condition, such as not playing anymore, should test results and further diagnosis suggest that the disease was present and advancing. Not coincidentally, since then a growing number of NFL players have decided to retire, even though they could still play productively and earn large salaries and current players including Washington's Jordan Reed have considered the possibility.

Perhaps the most startling early retirement involved Chris Borland, the superlative San Francisco 49ers former linebacker, who in March 2015 walked away from millions of dollars after a "rookie season . . . in which he was credited with 107 tackles, one sack and two interceptions in 14 games." Borland explained that after consulting one of the UCLA researchers, he became convinced that he fit the profile of an athlete who was likely to develop CTE. [20]

Whether any of the players who in recent years have walked away from professional football received a diagnosis of CTE has not been made public, although logic suggests that at least some of those players have. Borland in particular avoided answering the question whether he had been tested while he was at UCLA. One could appreciate, however, why he would want to keep the results confidential, if he had been. In any case, it is significant that he appears to have chosen to embark on a mental health career as an intern for the Carter Center in Atlanta.

A second reason the UCLA tests appeared to be significant had to do with their potential legal implications. The fact that living players were now able to receive a more accurate diagnosis of CTE indicated that the potential pool of plaintiffs suing the NFL might increase. There also were legal grounds for arguing that the final settlement in Judge Brody's courtroom should be expanded to include current players and living former players who could reasonably demonstrate that they have tested positive for CTE.

## SETTLEMENT MISGIVINGS

Since the judge had not yet given her "preliminary approval," there was room for both sides to maneuver, which led to "growing discontent on multiple fronts,"[21] especially with former players. As often happens with large settlements, some members of the class—and others who were not part of that class—began to publicly express misgivings. Much of their angst was spurred on by the repeatedly expressed belief within the legal community that lawyers for the former players had negotiated for too little. Since a deal already had been struck between the parties, the only good faith way for the plaintiffs' attorneys to rectify any perceived shortcomings was to contest aspects of the settlement that remained in flux—or could be placed in flux—or to drop out of the settlement altogether.

The first major reported disagreement, which emerged in December 2013, involved payments to the attorneys. Normally in these types of cases plaintiffs' lawyers work on a contingent fee basis. They receive a substantial share of any award or settlement, which can be as much as 33 percent of the proceeds—and sometimes even more than that. On the other hand, those lawyers receive almost nothing, except certain designated expenses, if their client loses.

The former players and their families claimed that they had been under the impression that the $765 million award would not include attorneys' fees, which Judge Brody would add to the settlement total later. Not only was that perception incorrect, but reportedly "some lawyers st[ood] to receive multiple paydays" for the same work that they did on the case for different clients. While "double-dipping . . . [is] not prohibit[ed] . . . , courts generally frown upon the practice,"[22] and often exercise their discretion to limit such payments.

Second, a number of the "families of players who were diagnosed with football-related brain damage after they had died" and had been "cut out of the settlement" as a result decided to sue the NFL in California Superior Court.[23] This included the families of Mike Webster and Junior Seau. In addition, living former players, including former Dallas Cowboys quarterback Craig Morton, had filed separate actions, as did Hall of Fame quarterback Dan Marino soon after CBS fired him as an NFL analyst.

It was no coincidence that none of the former NFL players who were being paid by the various networks that broadcast, give opinions about, or analyze NFL football were publicly identified in this litigation as plaintiffs. One might have concluded that this reluctance was due to their loyalty to the NFL, which ultimately provided the networks with the money that was being used to hire and retain these former players. The stronger incentive, however, appeared to be that these former players feared retaliation, since the league could apply economic pressure on the networks to fire these employees or diminish their roles. That is what CBS had done to the popular golf analyst Gary McCord after the men who ran Augusta National and the Masters objected to his humorous and deprecating commentary about the event.

A third discordant note was struck just before Christmas. Only a few days after stories about the settlement had been released, it was announced that the agreed upon compensation might have to be shared with a broader pool of former players than the original settlement had specified. An "extra category, which . . . had not been fleshed out [earlier] . . . would allow retired players . . . [with] mild dementia to receive [benefits] . . . , [which could double] if they developed full-blown dementia." The maximum each member of this category would receive could be as much as $3 million.[24] As with the settlement itself, this new category was subject to the judge's approval and that approval could be appealed by any player or segment of players.

Fourth, in January 2014 concerns were raised about whether there was enough money to cover future health-related expenses for all the plaintiffs who might be part of the settlement. There were at least two good reasons to be concerned that "the $765 million could run out faster than either side . . . believe[d]." To begin with, it would be next to impossible to accurately predict how many potential class members would "develop these conditions."[25] Already there had been strong indications that the numbers would increase significantly from those initial modest projections.

Finally, according to the terms of the settlement, once a class member was diagnosed with a qualifying condition, he would be entitled to "a lump-sum payment that [would vary] with his age and career length." That money was supposed to kick in as soon as one of the class members could demonstrate he had been properly diagnosed with an eligible impairment, regardless of whether it could be proven to be football related. Unfortunately, the total available money in the settlement pool had been based on incidence rates for impairments in the general population. This assumption was both unrealistic and shortsighted because the best medical evidence strongly indicated that these players were incurring these conditions at much higher than normal rates.

For these and other reasons, final approval was unlikely to come quickly in this settlement, which is exactly what happened. It took about four months for the proposed settlement details to be worked out and for the attorneys on both sides to file their recommendations and arguments with the court. After receiving those submissions, Judge Brody slowed the process down again by asking for "more proof that the money was enough to last . . . the life of the settlement."[26]

The most palpable tension, though, was between the existing parties and former and current players who had not yet been formally identified as having eligible conditions. For the most part, the current plaintiffs and their lawyers wanted the agreement to be finalized, so that they could receive their various forms of compensation as soon as possible. Once that happened, new members of the class might not be able to recover their necessary medical and related expenses if the fund ran out of money or they did not meet the self-serving eligibility criteria stated in the settlement.

It was the responsibility of the judge to try to ensure that all the potential eligible parties were treated equitably, while avoiding expensive, time-consuming litigation. As time passed, pressures increased on the judge to finalize the settlement. Once she did, the final settlement did not end the larger concussion problem for either the league or the NFLPA.

Dissatisfaction with and criticisms of the settlement had added to the public perception that the NFL's concussion problem was more complicated than paying off the most aggressive former NFL players who had been first in line to receive compensation. Football was still being reamed by its critics as an unconscionable sport. Parents whose children might have played in youth leagues or high school teams in the past were questioning the advisability of the sport for their children.

Making matters worse for the NFL, in May 2014, shortly after the settlement had been reached, former players and their lawyers sued the league for its dangerous and irresponsible drug practices. The litigation took "aim at the way professional football teams [had] distributed drugs to players for the past four decades." Over "600 players . . . [had] filed a class action . . . alleging the league illegally supplied them with painkill-ers to 'conceal injuries and mask pain.'"[27] Those plaintiffs further alleged that the players had been administered "addictive drugs . . . without proper medical supervision . . . with little or no explanation of the risks and dangers," including "their potential side effects." This all had been done in order "to speed the return of injured players to the field and maximize profits."[28]

In addition, neither the tentative concussion settlement nor the new drug-related litigation addressed what the NFL and the NFLPA should and would do in future collective bargaining agreements to protect players' health and to pay for football-related impairments. With respect to the settlement itself, Joe Nocera wrote in the *New York Times* that it was "hard not to view the settlement as the cynical effort by the N.F.L. to contain its potential liability; indeed, once the settlement is final, it will be nearly impossible for players—past, present and future—to be com-pensated [through the courts] if they are found to have [CTE]."[29] Similar-ly, the settlement did not compensate players for the symptoms of mental illnesses or diseases that they could develop later from CTE, such as mood swings and depression. The emphasis was on long-term "cognitive impairment." Nocera concluded that the agreement was "a travesty."[30]

Feeling similarly, a few former players decided to bring their settle-ment concerns before the U.S. Court of Appeals. Based on the questions the appellate judges asked, it seemed clear that higher court was skeptical about overturning the lower court's decision. As lawyer and commentator Michael McCann wrote in *Sports Illustrated*, federal appellate courts "normally defer to settlements, in part because they weigh the conse-quences of rejecting a deal, which here would [have led] to months of litigation."[31]

## NFL DAMAGE CONTROL

While awaiting final resolution of the settlement, the NFL continued to engage in damage control on several other fronts. The first opportunity arose in July 2015 when Junior Seau was to be posthumously inducted into the Pro Football Hall of Fame and Seau's daughter had been prohibited from making a speech on her father's behalf. In 2010, as the controversy about former players with brain damage was cresting, the NFL-dominated "Hall of Fame passed a rule . . . that forbids relatives of deceased inductees to speak at the . . . ceremony."[32] By comparison, living inductees are not only encouraged to speak, but typically a relative, friend, or former player or coach introduces them as well.

In lieu of presenting the reality that had been Junior Seau after football, the Hall of Fame produced a sanitized video tribute, which scrupulously avoided any mention of his suicide or troubles due to brain disease. After media stories about Seau's daughter's quest to speak at the ceremony created a national firestorm of bad publicity for the league, Commissioner Goodell engineered a one-sided compromise. He allowed Seau's daughter to be interviewed onstage using approved questions, while still steadfastly upholding the rule that forbids relatives of deceased inductees from speaking at the ceremony itself.[33]

Another example of how the NFL does damage control came to light after the *New York Times* ran a story, based on "studio emails unearthed by hackers," documenting that Sony Pictures Entertainment had changed the underlying theme of the movie *Concussion* to "avoid antagonizing the NFL." The December 2015 film starring Will Smith was transformed into a heroic "whistle-blower story, rather than a condemnation of football or the league."[34] As a *New York Times* film critic explained in her review of the movie, the "NFL . . . remains a vague, largely anonymous presence" while its "new Commissioner, Roger Goodell . . . [is played by] Luke Wilson, in a flattering bit of casting."[35]

Around that same time, ESPN's award-winning show *Outside the Lines* aired a story on the league's efforts to influence federal concussion research by allegedly reneging on a commitment to fund Boston University's CTE study on the brains of deceased football players.[36] The NFL had made an unrestricted $30 million grant to the National Institutes of Health (NIH) in 2012, which was intended to be used to fund BU's brain research program. In 2015, when that money was supposed to be transferred to BU, NIH decided to fund the grant instead with other money. The NFL's donation was used to fund other concussion-related research.

For those familiar with federal funding involving large donations from private sources, what ESPN had revealed about the carefully managed outcome involving the NFL's donation was neither illegal nor technically improper, although it still appeared to be pretty sleazy. NIH did not violate the law or any of its internal rules in reallocating those funds. BU received what it had been promised, while the NFL was able to accomplish two objectives: avoid having to be directly associated with the results of the BU research; and ensure that additional research would be funded, which might be more in line with the NFL's perspective on concussions.

For many years now, the NFL's largely successful strategy had been to deny that there was a causal relationship between concussions and CTE, no matter what the leading research revealed. Until March 2016 the league steadfastly refused to acknowledge that there was "a link between football-related head trauma and the brain disease CTE."[37] Furthermore, the NFL had released its own questionable research, which had marginalized any such CTE association, in order to "tamp down fear among parents over football's physical toll"[38] on players of all ages.

In this damage control effort the NFL still had allies in the medical community. During the same week questions were being raised by ESPN about the league's efforts to manipulate federal CTE research, pediatric neurologist Steven M. Rothman published a shocking op-ed piece in the *New York Times* indirectly supporting the NFL's position. He warned that America's "excessive fear of concussions may discourage parents and medical professionals from letting kids play healthy team sports."[39]

The good doctor correctly pointed out that no one yet knows what the long-term health effects are likely to be for kids who play contact sports, especially football, because most of the relevant studies have not included children. He opined that it would be wiser to err on the side of taking uncertain risks with these youngsters' health. Inexcusably, Rothman ignored overwhelming medical and scientific evidence that due to their immature brains and skulls, kids are considerably more susceptible to serious injuries from concussions and other brain traumas than are adults.

## THE U.S. COURT OF APPEALS UPHOLDS
## THE SETTLEMENT

In April 2016, despite widespread criticism that the settlement did not go nearly far enough to compensate brain-injured former players or current players who might develop severe symptoms, a three-judge panel of the U.S. Court of Appeals for the Third Circuit upheld the agreement.[40] Even though the NFL had finally publicly acknowledged that playing football could cause CTE, there would be no compensation for living players who had not yet died of that condition. There would be, however, "generous payments for former players suffering from [other] debilitating conditions, such as Alzheimer's disease or amyotrophic lateral sclerosis [ALS]." Also, a relatively small amount of money—$4 million—was set aside for the families of players who had died of CTE before April 2015.[41]

This agreement, which was finalized after the U.S. Supreme Court refused to review the settlement, "resolved thousands of lawsuits and covered more than 20,000 NFL retirees for the next 65 years." Yet, the amount the NFL had agreed to pay—just under $1 billion—over many years, when compared to what the teams in the league earn, made it a great deal for (1) the NFL, (2) players who were eligible for large payments now, and (3) plaintiffs' lawyers who participated in the settlement. The criteria for determining whether the settlement should be approved on appeal was not whether it "was good or bad, but whether it was 'fair' and 'reasonable' under the conditions of the deal."[42] Under those standards, the appeals court found that Judge Brody had acted appropriately.

In addition, those former players who chose to opt out or were never part of the settlement could still sue, but they would have substantial legal hurdles to overcome. At the very least new plaintiffs would have to be able to prove that playing in the NFL caused their impairments and that the collective bargaining agreement between the league and the players did not preempt those lawsuits.[43]

Nonetheless, even assuming the NFL managed to ensure that all future personal injury lawsuits against the league and its teams were going to be part of a relatively small cost of doing business, which seemed to be likely, the league still has an extremely serious image problem among parents, parents-to-be, educators, and much of the public who now view football as a dangerous sport. Increasingly, sports fans and the rest of the public are being bombarded with stories about the NFL's bad faith and duplicity when it comes to protecting football players of every age from the severe health consequences of brain injuries.

## MANIPULATING MEDICAL RESEARCH

In May 2016, only a month after the NFL's apparent legal victory, a "scathing Congressional report . . . issued by Democratic members of the House Energy and Commerce Committee . . . charged league officials with trying to influence a major U.S. government research study on football and brain disease." This turned out to be the same NIH research to which the NFL had donated unrestricted funds. "Elliott Pellman, the league's former medical director . . . [had] sent an e-mail to . . . NIH . . . saying 'there are many of us who have significant concerns re BU and their ability to be unbiased and collaborative.'" In addition, NFL representatives alleged, without any basis in fact, that Robert Stern, the BU program's lead medical researcher, had "a conflict of interest and that the grant application process had been tainted by bias."[44]

The congressional report characterized the NFL's accusations as being "ridiculous." More importantly, the report concluded that the "NFL's actions 'fit a long-standing pattern of attempts to influence the scientific understanding of the consequences of repeated head trauma.'" "DeMaurice Smith, executive director of the NFL Players Association, called the [congressional] findings 'another example' of a league that is out of control."[45]

Sally Jenkins—quoting the remarks of noted conservative constitutional lawyer Theodore Olson—concluded that under Commissioner Goodell's leadership, with respect to both science and the law, the NFL was "biased, agenda-driven, and self-approving."[46] Goodell, rather than disputing the congressional report, complained that it had been "issued . . . without even talking to any of our advisers."[47] He added that while he had not yet read the report, the NFL's "commitment to medical research is well documented."[48]

Unfortunately for Goodell, the relevant documentation has uncovered the NFL's interference, manipulation, and bad faith in carrying out its own research and in trying to influence the research of others. Making matters worse, around that same time, BU, the Department of Veterans

Affairs, and the Concussion Legacy Foundation revealed that "Bubba Smith, an All-Pro defensive end in the N.F.L. who went on to a second career as a movie actor, had chronic traumatic encephalopathy . . . when he died in 2011."[49] He was the ninety-fourth former professional football player to be tested and the ninetieth found to have CTE. Even worse for the NFL, a New York state judge ruled that insurance companies, which underwrote policies that the league took out to protect team owners against concussion-related legal damages, are entitled to review NFL documents to ascertain whether the league intentionally withheld information about the risks of concussion-related impairments from the players. Although it was virtually certain that the NFL would appeal, that precedent was damning to the league's interests.[50]

# 15

# FOOTBALL'S UNHOLY TRINITY

Brain Traumas, Bounties, and Deliberate Injuries

## THE DELIBERATE INTENT TO INJURE

**F**ootball at its best is a spectacular, precise, and intricate team sport in which planning and preparation make focused, but explosive, aggression on every play exquisite entertainment for many millions of Americans. Controlled—and sometimes uncontrolled—violence has been a major part of the sport, especially as individual players have become bigger, stronger, faster, and more skilled at certain competitive nuances of the game. Unfortunately, football, as it has been played in the NFL, college programs, and many high schools, accepts and often teaches criminal or quasi-criminal actions in the form of deliberate attempts to injure opponents and, occasionally, teammates. Various myths and platitudes have helped to marginalize and obscure this intentional mayhem.

The boys-will-be-boys mentality off the field also tends to manifest itself in on-the-field assaults, which make most of the NBA's gang-related associations and shenanigans pale in comparison. In the self-congratulatory words of Washington cornerback Josh Norman, "I'm like a rogue savage out there. . . . I want to play the game ruthless and violent."[1]

Very few professional or collegiate football players or coaches have complained publicly about such rogue behavior, much less tried to stand up against it. Snitching or being perceived as a rat or an outsider is viewed as a far more serious offense than physical or mental assaults, and, as NFL bully victims Jonathan Martin and Michael Sam can attest, a sign of personal weakness that almost no player—or player-to-be—can completely recover from.

No one who has played or closely followed football would be surprised to learn that players are taught, deliberately learn, and/or pass on techniques that allow them to better incapacitate their opponents. For many years the debilitating results of such training drills were glorified, and the rules did little, if anything, to constrain such violence. In the 1960s and 1970s, knocking other players out by hitting them in the head, or creating a situation in which they hit their head on the cold or frozen turf, was a favorite way of making a violent impression. Those who did it the very best became football legends and, like Chuck Bednarik, members of the Hall of Fame.

Ostensibly these techniques were supposed to more easily separate the ball carrier or receiver from the football or prevent a player from making a pass, a tackle, or a block. Yet, the glory came in causing an opponent to lose consciousness, or to be so woozy, unable to run, or in such pain he could no longer play effectively or stay in the game. If that meant the player sustained a serious injury, so be it or so much the better, depending on the players and teams involved. Either way it has been an acceptable and widely emulated part of the sport that remains deeply embedded in the football culture and mentality even today.

In the 1970s and even today, for example, Hall of Fame Chicago Bears middle linebacker Dick Butkus has been beloved by the fans and feared and respected by his colleagues because of his violent nature. He was celebrated as the "meanest, angriest, toughest, dirtiest son of a bitch in football." Despite his legendary reputation, he famously tried to distinguish himself from lesser players he called "assholes" who had to resort to deliberately injuring their opponents. Butkus could hurt them simply by playing football his way, like "an animal."[2]

When the distinction between appropriate and inappropriate is as precarious as it was in Butkus's mind, and the minds of so many other football players, their superaggressive attitudes tend to foment serious behavioral problems, both on and off the field. It is difficult—albeit not uncommon—to be an animal on the field and a role model off it, which is why, when the veils of secrecy are removed from so many of our football stars, bad behavior is exposed. Duplicitous behavior may be part of our culture, but in football it is skewed toward physically overwhelming one's opponents through aggression, violence, and strategic cheating.

## TARGETING OPPONENTS' KNEES

For many years it has been advantageous—and arguably essential for football success—to learn how to cut a player's legs out from under him by hitting his knees, probably the second most vulnerable part of the player's body after the brain. Traditionally this kneecapping tactic was even more effective than causing a concussion because the opponent was more likely to be immediately incapacitated. In 2012, *ESPN the Magazine* writer David Fleming focused on the extreme damage these blocking techniques can cause. He observed that "the cut block . . . might be the dirtiest play in football," and then asked, Why "is it still legal?"[3]

In March 2016, the league finally decided to penalize players for "chop blocks," which meant that it was likely that the number of knee injuries would be reduced, although not eliminated, as a strategic weapon. Previously the NFL had outlawed those "blocks on special team plays" and then made it illegal to make such a block if "a defender is not able to see the blocker." Nevertheless, a problem remains because often the perceptual "line between legal and illegal is thin," enforcement tends to be relatively "slack," and it frequently seems more beneficial, in terms of winning and losing, to violate—or at least shade—the rules than not. Players normally avoid using such injury-causing techniques in practice against their own teammates, except occasionally when they get angry or otherwise lose control. On the other hand, coaches understand that cut blocking is effective and often encourage their offensive players to employ it wisely in games.[4]

This tactic has proven to be particularly important to teams that are trying to implement some version of the popular "West Coast offense" in order to "slow down pass rushers." It also "opens up passing lanes" by making defensive linemen "drop their hands in order to protect their knees," which is a particularly "vulnerable part of a player's body." Football "players are far more concerned about the immediacy of a blown-out knee than the long-term implications of concussions."[5] Thus, attacking the knees has become a key psychological, as well as physical, tool for offensive players, which gives them a decided edge over their opponents' defenders.

Until 2016 very little was being done to control hits to the knees of defensive players, although the NFL took a number of steps to better protect high-profile offensive players, particularly quarterbacks and wide receivers, from punishing blows to the head. Former Washington Redskins and New York Giants safety Brandon Meriweather, who was repeatedly fined and suspended for his violent hits, complained that these concussion rules made it more difficult for defensive players to do their jobs,[6] which is true, if not particularly persuasive. In addition, Meriweather argued that in order to tackle effectively under the new rules, defensive players have to "tear people's ACLs and mess up knees,"[7] implicitly acknowledging his view that the only way to play defense effectively is to deliberately injure one's opponent.

## FLAGRANT HITS

Defensive players like Meriweather have bemoaned the double standard they see, which tries to protect players on offense but leaves defensive players at the mercy of dirty football. At the same time, no one has sued the league for hits to the knees like they have for hits to the brain. Not coincidentally, improved offenses generate greater audiences and more league revenues for everyone involved. It will be interesting to see how vigorously the new chop block restrictions are enforced. Will it be half-hearted like concussion protocols?

What makes the complaints of these defensive players difficult to embrace and less worthy of sympathy is the perception, backed up by a full-blown league-wide scandal, that teams have informally placed bounties on offensive players and offered praise, and even monetary rewards, to defensive players who deliberately injure their opponents. Almost anywhere in the United States, except in organized contact sports, such a deliberate intent to injure another human being could be prosecuted as a violent felony.

Still, it is not only defensive players who initiate these violent on-the-field assaults, as the New York Giants mercurial superstar receiver Odell Beckham demonstrated on national television in December 2015. During a critical contest with playoff implications, Beckham repeatedly tangled with Carolina Panthers cornerback Josh Norman—a player who himself takes pride in employing on-the-field violence. The game's referees, Beckham's coaches, and his teammates sat idly by watching Beckham's blatant but ineffective attempts to injure Norman.

The Giants receiver remained in the game and was never counseled by his coaches, even after he was penalized for multiple unnecessary roughness fouls including "running full speed, slam[ming] his helmet into the side of Norman's [helmet]." Only after the game, once the media criticism became too loud to ignore, did the league step in to suspend Beckham for one game as punishment for his "flagrant hit against a defenseless player."[8]

While occasionally today's NFL players are fined or suspended for these types of flagrant hits and out-of-control behavior, the truth of the matter is that most of this violence goes unpunished because it normally has to be obvious to a television audience to generate any league action, beyond a penalty on the field, and sometimes not even that. The referees rarely throw players out of games, and in fact frequently draw praise from the football media and fans for exercising restraint. Then, during the week, coaches and teammates teach their own players how to break the rules without being caught. NFL sanctions are mostly about changing perceptions, rather than changing violent attitudes and tendencies that are part of the professional football culture.

There can be little doubt that this widespread intent to harm opponents has substantially increased serious injuries to football players, not only in the NFL and in major college programs, but in high schools as well. It is both a symptom and a reflection of the culture of violence that infects football and football players at the highest levels of competition. Like the use of steroids and human growth hormone, it is another way to get an edge over one's opponents. Yet players often get out of control, and in doing so, their actions become counterproductive as well as antisocial. Regardless, the violence and danger of the game, like fighting in hockey, is highly entertaining to millions of football fans.

## BOUNTY-GATE

Ironically, the full scope of what has been happening in the NFL, major college programs, and even high schools, with regard to football players deliberately injuring opponents, was actually obscured by the brazen and outrageous behavior that was nationally publicized in recent years as part of what became known as "bounty-gate." Unfortunately, the full blame for that scandal was placed on the extreme behavior of the New Orleans Saints football team, rather than attributing a major share of the responsibility to the NFL's culture of violence, bad behavior, and cover-ups.

The first documented evidence of extreme wrongdoing in the Saints' organization can only be traced back as far as 2009, shortly after Gregg Williams became the team's defensive coordinator. He instituted a high-profile system of bounties, which apparently did not raise red flags among the Saints' players or coaches, or anyone else in the league. The Saints treated those bounties like business as usual. While significant cash rewards may or may not have been typical, certainly the practice of encouraging and praising players for devastating hits was nothing new and bounties of some sort were far from unusual.

While bounty-gate was not revealed in the national media until early 2012, the timeline in which it unfolded gave context to the acknowledged misdeeds. Much of the best reporting was local, based on the work of Katherine Terrell in the *New Orleans Times-Picayune*. Not surprisingly, the identified offenses occurred during the playoffs where the rewards for winning are the greatest and the media cover for bad behavior can be the most pronounced.

In mid-January 2010 the Saints were playing the Arizona Cardinals in a playoff game. According to the NFL's subsequent investigation, Saints linebacker Jonathan Vilma had offered a $10,000 reward to any teammate "who could knock . . . Cardinals quarterback Kurt Warner out of the game." Subsequently "Bobby McCray's block . . . sent [Warner] out of the game for several plays."[9]

Two weeks later, prior to the NFC Championship Game, Vilma placed a similar $10,000 bounty on Minnesota Vikings quarterback Brett Favre. The Saints won as their defensive unit hit Favre repeatedly, injuring his ankle severely enough that it required surgery. The NFL fined the Saints a relatively paltry "$25,000 for illegal hits on Favre."[10]

Outraged Vikings head coach Brad Childress broke the unwritten rules of NFL coaching etiquette by complaining that the Saints bounty program had targeted Favre. It was only then that the NFL was compelled to begin an investigation. Once Gregg Williams found out that the NFL would be closely scrutinizing his team, he told an assistant coach "to destroy documents and lie to the NFL" about the team's bounty program.[11]

For two years nothing much happened, however, which is not uncommon in these types of internal investigations into actions and events that are potentially embarrassing to a major corporate entity. Often these long delays can help to deflect and dilute bad publicity. In mid-January 2012, Gregg Williams left New Orleans for a similar position with the then Saint Louis Rams. Initially that transfer did not raise questions because in 2010 and 2011, the Saints' defense under Williams had slipped since his inaugural year in 2009. Thus, his departure was characterized as nothing more than the NFL's coaching carousel in motion.[12]

## THE NFL-MANAGED VIEW OF BOUNTY-GATE

Six weeks later, the NFL announced the preliminary results of its lengthy investigation. The timing created a revised impression that Williams's departure appeared to have been orchestrated to put distance between him and the brewing media firestorm in New Orleans. The NFL judiciously laid out the basic elements of the story it wanted to tell, without divulging the thousands of pages of documentation that it had gathered. This NFL-managed scenario of what had happened turned out to be plenty bad enough. Making matters worse, though, the NFL's version not only appeared to be less than the whole truth, but it conspicuously avoided the broader question: Which other coaches and teams had been awarding bounties or otherwise encouraging their players to deliberately injure opponents?

According to the NFL, Williams had established a bounty program when he became a Saint that "paid $1,500 for a 'knockout' and $1,000 if an opposing player was carted off the field."[13] His defensive players had not only targeted Warner and Favre, but Aaron Rodgers and Cam Newton as well. Saints superstar quarterback Drew Brees, after a week to reflect with his closest advisers, issued a statement implausibly denying "any knowledge about the bounty program."[14]

Brees made his categorical denial despite the fact the investigation already had implicated many Saints players, the head coach, and the general manager.[15] By then it also was becoming clear that bounties were nothing new to the NFL. For someone as smart, critical to, and involved

with the Saints' fortunes as Drew Brees, his denial appeared to be prepos-
terous on its face.

At the same time, there were strong suspicions that like the banks in
managing their involvement in the mortgage crisis, the league was managing—and inevitably slanting the information it had found in its investigation—to reduce its potential liability. By then the NFL already was the
defendant in numerous personal injury lawsuits by former players alleging that the league had failed to take appropriate steps to protect them
from brain injuries.

If the evidence against the Saints had been compiled for a criminal
prosecution, it could well have been deemed, as Steve Coll of the *New
Yorker* put it, a "conspiracy to commit felony assault and battery in order
to advance a shared business interest."[16] That interest would have been
players and coaches reaping the financial rewards of winning in the
playoffs. Containing the breadth and depth of the scandal and minimizing
bad publicity appeared to be the NFL's primary concerns in writing and
documenting its self-serving report.

According to a number of NFL players and coaches, there was nothing
remarkable about the "bonus pools used by the Saints."[17] It was routine to
have these types of "side bets" and symbolic rewards. In Washington, for
instance, the special teams coach would hand out a "'hit stick" to the
player who "made the biggest hit each week."[18] As former *Washington
Post* sports columnist Mike Wise observed, "Bounties have been around
forever . . . in this musclehead subculture."[19]

Only a couple of months earlier in the conference championship game
leading up to the 2012 Super Bowl, players on the winning Giants team
admitted trying to deliberately injure one of their opponents. After being
provided with information about the "concussion history" of the kick
returner of the 49ers, Giants players acknowledged that they had "wanted
to hit him to see how he would respond." If they did their jobs correctly,
he would not have been able to respond at all. Media coverage of this
incident shed additional light on the NFL practice in which coaches brief
their players about opponents' injuries and other weaknesses based on
weekly injury reports. "Testing an opponent's weakness is a routine part
of game strategy."[20]

Between 2004 and 2007, when Gregg Williams coached Washington's defense he apparently began his practice of placing bounties on the
heads of offensive players, especially the stars. These violent hits were

called "kill shots."[21] Both in Washington and New Orleans—and probably on other teams as well—rewards or praise were being "handed out . . . for 'inflicting injuries on opposing players that would result in them being removed from a game.'"[22] As one player admitted, this was "an ugly tradition. . . . But . . . Gregg Williams isn't the only one who did this. He's . . . taking the fall.'"[23] All of this indicated the presence of "a systemic issue rather than an isolated one,"[24] which the NFL was being careful to avoid and obscure.

As it turned out, the entire Saints organization took the fall. None of them had much of an excuse, beyond making the explosive argument that what they had done was not that unusual or not unusual at all. In its report, however, the NFL protected itself and other teams as much as possible, implying that this was an extraordinary situation that was unique to the New Orleans Saints. It supposedly bore no resemblance to what normally goes on in the honorable world of professional football.

Commissioner Goodell suspended Saints head coach Sean Payton for a full year, Williams indefinitely, and two other coaches eight and six games, respectively. In addition, the Saints lost two second-round draft picks and were fined $500,000. Some league observers thought this was much too harsh, but as one team owner explained, "With all the concussion stuff . . . [h]e had to do it,"[25] presumably to protect the rest of the teams and their revenues from continuing bad publicity, the displeasure of their corporate sponsors, and legal liability to former players.

Nearly six weeks later the NFL suspended a number of Saints players as well. Linebacker Jonathan Vilma, who reportedly had placed the bounties on the heads of Warner and Favre, was initially suspended for the entire 2012 season; other Saints players received from three to eight game suspensions.[26] Player punishments took much longer to resolve because the NFL Players Association (NFLPA) had to review the proposed penalties to determine whether they ran afoul of the collective bargaining agreement. The union had a fiduciary duty to advocate for its active players.

## A BIASED APPEALS PROCESS

Not surprisingly, with the support of the NFLPA, the suspended players appealed. The NFL stunned the legal community, many journalists, and many in the football media by appointing former commissioner Paul Tagliabue to hear those appeals. To say the former commissioner had a conflict of interest, given the fact that he had been overseeing the league when Williams started his bounty program with Washington, was to state the obvious. What transpired, though, was not a simple rubber-stamping of the punishments Goodell had issued. It was more sophisticated and nuanced than that. Tagliabue, a shrewd and highly experienced corporate lawyer, used his skills and temporary position to protect both the commissioner's office and the NFL, while still giving the impression that he was independent and being fair. He also was teaching his successor a lesson about how to manage a crisis.

Tagliabue overturned all the player suspensions, finding that their cases had "been contaminated by the coaches and others in the Saints organization."[27] He concluded that team management had deliberately obstructed the NFL's investigation.[28] At the same time, Tagliabue upheld Goodell's findings regarding the four players involved who had "engaged in conduct detrimental to the integrity of, and public confidence in, the game of professional football."[29] This was another way of creating the impression that the Saints' coaches, players, and management had acted abnormally, rather than as part of a pattern involving other teams throughout the league.

The NFL did not challenge Tagliabue's findings as it has done almost reflexively whenever other hearing examiners have ruled against the league in high-profile cases involving player suspensions. Instead the league said that it respected the former commissioner's decision, but also praised Goodell's "strong action . . . to protect player safety."[30]

Undoubtedly the NFL had eliminated the system of paid bounties on the Saints, but otherwise its response appeared to be weak. The investigation and the hearings never addressed the underlying problem of a malevolent and out-of-control football culture, which had spawned the mentality that deliberately injuring opponents is part of the game, as long as it is not too blatant. Furthermore, Goodell's mishandling of this fiasco would be a precursor of things to come when other even more embarrassing football-related transgressions, involving player violence against women, would explode on his watch. Despite his charm, public relations skills, and revenue-generating successes, Goodell was demonstrating that he lacked the legal acumen and organizational foresight of his predecessor.

## CONDEMNING THE VIOLENCE

As a result of bounty-gate, concussion-gate, sexual assaults, bullying, and other transgressions, the pendulum swung away from active neglect and dissonance with respect to the ugly macho locker-room culture, which has tended to dominate professional, collegiate, and even high school football. Increasingly, there were calls for the sport to be banned, along with warnings that football might self-destruct under the weight of its successes and excesses.[31] As Jon Wertheim intoned in *Sports Illustrated*, "The same violence and intensity that . . . [makes football] so compelling to so many, will ultimately lead to its undoing."[32]

One of the most penetrating critics of the game in recent years has been Canadian journalist, widely read author, and provocateur Malcolm Gladwell, who opined that he was "quite confident . . . that we won't be watching football 20 years from now . . . . in large part because the sport is morally indefensible."[33] In covering the Michael Vick dogfighting scandal, Gladwell pointed out the "unbelievable hypocrisy . . . of people in football . . . getting up in arms about someone who chose to fight dogs." Gladwell concluded that it was difficult, if not impossible, to morally differentiate "dog fighting . . . from football."[34]

In 2012, *Washington Post* columnist Mike Wise opined that without a fundamental change in attitudes within the league, the NFL would "lose the [concussion] war." Wise was moved in part by the fact that one of the NFL's medical consultants, Robert Cantu, had determined that "kids under 14 years old shouldn't tackle each other with pads and helmets." Because of the bobblehead doll effect—big heads on weak necks— children are at "greater risk than . . . an adult."[35]

Those added risks to minors playing football have turned out to be profound. Reportedly there is "somewhere between a one-in-five and 1-in-20 chance of serious head injury over a four-month period,"[36] which normally is one season. Hence, even the NFL has moved to embrace flag football for youngsters—especially girls—and Dartmouth football uses and promotes an expensive tackling dummy known as a "Mobile Virtual Player . . . to reduce concussions."[37] In addition, Ivy League football has banned tackling during regular-season workouts.

For Wise the issue boiled down to this: "How do we reconcile celebrating a game so good for your soul but so bad for your body and brain?" A meaningful reconciliation of those two realities is unlikely to come soon. The profits to be made in America's favorite sport are too great and the sport too popular "to completely overhaul." Wise explained there is "something deep in the reptilian part of [our] brain . . . [that] is enraptured by big hits—the speed, force, sudden impact, the rawness of the moment."[38] This may well be true as far as it goes, but it raises the question why this particular "something" applies predominantly to American males. In addition to biology, it appears likely that sociological and cultural factors explain football's extreme popularity in the United States, but nowhere else.

George Will, the sometimes controversial but often insightful conservative columnist and devoted baseball fan, has reprised two compelling arguments about the "physical carnage, institutional derangement and moral seaminess [that is football.]" First, it is the only sport—other than boxing and newer types of sanctioned fighting—in which "long-term injury [is] the result, not of accidents, but of the game played properly."[39]

Second, and perhaps more tellingly, Will has noted—as others have done before him—that the labels on football helmets warn the equipment cannot "protect you from serious brain and/or neck injuries including paralysis or death." The best way "to avoid these risks [is not to] . . . engage in the sport of football."[40] To a large extent this is a lawyer-written liability waiver. At the same time, it also reflects common sense and reveals a fundamental flaw of the sport.

Media mogul billionaire, big systems thinker, and publicity magnet Mark Cuban, who also is the owner of the Dallas Mavericks, which competes with the NFL for market share, predicts a dim future for professional football. In 2014 he forecast that the NFL would "implode in 10 years." Cuban pointed to "the growing consciousness related to [football's] endemic health risks" and its "eventual oversaturation"[41] by scheduling too many nationally televised games, particularly those that compete with the NBA. Two years later, the ratings for NFL football games have begun to decline.

## FOOTBALL'S LONG-TERM VIABILITY

While Cuban's timeline probably is unrealistic, the view that sometime in this relatively new century football will no longer be America's favorite spectator sport appears to be persuasive, and may even understate the sport's current predicament. In 2014 the *Washington Post*'s education columnist, Jay Mathews, reported that sixty-seven of the one hundred top-ranked academic high schools in the nation no longer had football programs. In 1998, by comparison, almost all of the top academic high schools had teams.[42]

This burgeoning connection between high academic achievement and declining interest in football is significant in two respects. First is the popular notion, which fans can relate to, that generally "nerds" and "geeks" do not make good football players. As Bill Belichick can attest, however, many could and now do become innovative coaches and general managers. Second, and more importantly, strong supporters of academic achievement are more likely to discourage football as a sport for male children, especially their own.

This trend away from football can be seen in youth sports more generally. Soccer moms and dads have considerable influence over the athletic choices of their boys, as well as their girls. In addition, the quickly expanding notion that "good" parents are supposed to distance their children from playing football is already a part of our culture. This cultural shift is diluting football's reach and threatening its number one sport status, especially among upwardly mobile families and academic achievers.

It should not be forgotten that in the 1920s boxing was even more popular than baseball, and now it exists on the sports periphery. Cultural change can be almost immediate, as it was with the Beatles and the Internet, or, occur over many years, as it did with the risks of tobacco or climate change. The NFL is hoping—like the National Rifle Association with respect to guns—that it can deflect new policies from being implemented to address football's trail of injuries, violence, and bad behavior.

Ultimately, though, it is difficult to deny that what has been happening to football is culturally significant, and damaging to the game. As Steve Rushin opined in *Sports Illustrated*, "Football, played at its highest level, is catastrophic . . . grotesque and bookworthy. But the most insidious injuries . . . are invisible,"[43] oftentimes deliberately so. That image of football is becoming increasingly difficult to ignore or change.

Years from now tackling dummies may not be the only virtual human forms used in football. Games themselves may be contested at almost every position, except maybe quarterback and wide receiver, using mobile virtual players operated like drones, similar to how modern warfare has been evolving. In that future America, "Madden football" would become almost indistinguishable from the professional game.

# 16

# CHILDREN PLAYING FOOTBALL

## The NFL's Achilles Heel

Female athletes fought for years to update the rules and practices in various sports to allow them to be as aggressive and competitive as males. In certain ways, however, gender equality in athletics, which is legally and morally compelling, has traveled down the wrong path with female athletes emulating males to make their sports more dangerous. Yet, it is the male-dominated sport of football—due to its inherent violence, frequent lawlessness, and constant media scrutiny—that is likely to face curtailment first. Already many parents are either preventing their kids from playing this dangerous sport or encouraging them to engage in other sports or activities. This appears to be the primary reason why the NFL, led by Commissioner Goodell, has tried to create the misleading impression that tackle football is relatively safe to play, and becoming even safer than it once was.

Playing tackle football is not a safe activity for children or even older adolescents, and the prospects for making it so are discouraging. According to certain NFL coaches, a professor of kinesiology who has studied the problem, and two sports historians, tackle football is so dangerous, the best way to diminish on-the-field "premeditated mayhem"—other than banning the sport—would be to mandate that these young athletes play football without helmets, at least in practices, to help them learn how to modify their destructive behavior. [1]

That idea, however, smacks of desperation. It would be similar to teaching people to drive safely by not allowing anyone to use seat belts. It is conceivable that such a proposal could improve safety, marginally—although that seems very doubtful—but it also reveals for all to see that football is inherently dangerous. Being potentially a little safer is not the same thing as being reasonably safe.

## THE NFL HAS BEEN EMULATING BIG TOBACCO

Instead of confronting the safety issue, the NFL seems to have relied on the tobacco industry as a model to help formulate strategies of deception and denial. For the purposes of public perception, the NFL has tried to distance itself from Big Tobacco, which in a letter to the *New York Times* a league lawyer called "perhaps the most odious industry in American history." For years, however, "the two businesses shared lobbyists, lawyers and consultants." Giants co-owner Preston Tisch is credited with facilitating that working relationship. Tisch "partly owned a leading cigarette company . . . and was a board member of both the Tobacco Institute and the Council for Tobacco Research, two entities that played a central role in misusing science to hide the risks of cigarettes."[2]

Little has changed since with regard to the league's strategic game plan. Shortly before the 2016 Super Bowl, in his state of the NFL message, Commissioner Goodell tried to pretend that playing football was just one of many "risks in life. There are risks sitting on a couch," he argued earnestly. Like the town leaders in the movie *Jaws*, who sent their kids into the water to assure the tourists that it was safe, Goodell claimed that he would "want [his] son to play football."[3]

The insincerity of the commissioner's position did not escape attention. Sally Jenkins observed that Goodell had

> conflated the danger of brain trauma with the health benefits of exercise . . . as if discouraging kids from playing tackle football is tantamount to encouraging them to stay indoors and get diabetes. It was nonsense. Disingenuous, willfully deceptive nonsense, and he knows it.[4]

*Boston Globe* cartoonist Dan Wasserman brilliantly ridiculed the NFL's self-serving promotions for the league's fiftieth anniversary of the

Super Bowl. He created a mock advertisement underscoring the health risks of football-related concussions. The text of his editorial cartoon read: "This game [is] brought to you by CTE official brain disease of the NFL; by concussion: 'keep your head in the game'; and by brain trauma: get started on assisted living today!"

More significantly, George Lundberg, the pathologist who had been the editor of the *Journal of the American Medical Association* in 1983 when it recommended that boxing be banned, wrote a scathing op-ed piece in the *New York Times*. He warned that the "failure of the league to take effective actions to protect the brains of current players puts it into willful-negligence territory." Lundberg also condemned "the sports media [as] . . . mostly shills paid by the networks to entertain audiences and please the league, with little interest in using their pulpit for the cause of player safety."[5]

Two months later, despite such widespread criticism, the NFL again was caught trying to massage the truth. This time it involved the owners of its two Texas franchises after a league official at a congressional meeting had acknowledged "there is 'certainly' a connection between the brain disease and football." Apparently Bob McNair (Houston Texans) and Jerry Jones (Dallas Cowboys) became concerned about such an acknowledgment after some sports lawyers had opined that such an admission might cost the league money in the NFL's ongoing settlement with its former players.[6]

McNair asserted that the cause of CTE was still unknown, while Jones remarked that it was "'absurd' to think there's enough data to link CTE to football."[7] Chris Nowinski, a cofounder of the Concussion Legacy Foundation, called the NFL owners' remarks "woefully ill-informed."[8] Commissioner Goodell went in the opposite direction, however, implausibly claiming that the NFL's position about "a possible connection between CTE and football" had not changed "over the years."[9]

The impetus for the league's conflicting deceptions seems self-evident. Tackle football has an intractable problem. No safety measures have proven to be effective in substantially reducing, much less eliminating, most of the destructive impacts of the sport on brains, bones, ligaments, and other body parts. Nor can any of the incremental safety precautions alter the disturbing reality that minors who play tackle football are considerably more vulnerable to serious injuries than adults playing the sport. Not only are children's immature brains and skulls more susceptible to serious harm, scientific studies demonstrate "that players as young as 7 sustain hits to the head comparable in magnitude to . . . adult players."[10]

For many years, the NFL has employed myths, illusions, deceptions, and handsomely paid medical experts to mask or diminish the peril. As discussed in chapter 13, the deceptions began decades ago, but in recent years the effectiveness of such tactics began to fray. By 2009 the close connection between the NFL and the promotion of youth football had become a cause for national concern, especially with regard to concussions. By then tackle football for children had been declining. Nonetheless, high school football still attracted "more than 1.2 million teenagers" each year. Millions more played youth football. Yet, most of these younger players and their parents continued to be unenlightened about the "seriousness of brain injuries."[11]

In October 2009 the House Judiciary Committee held a well-publicized hearing that focused on brain injuries in the NFL and how that was affecting youth football. What was happening in the NFL also had major "trickle-down effects on high school and college players . . . [that could] be fatal," opined a Georgia congressman. Incredibly, the NFL's medical expert argued that league "practices [were] 'exactly what should be passed down to . . . youth football.'"[12]

That expert ignored—or was unaware—that a child's brain is substantially different from an adult's. Even then it was well known that younger brains, when they are injured, "require considerably more care and longer rest periods." Failure to recognize those essential differences invited youth fatalities and serious impairments. Researchers who had studied youth football found that nearly 16 percent of the time when these players lost consciousness on a play, they returned to the field that "same day." This was "considered particularly perilous."[13]

## THE LACK OF DATA ON CATASTROPHIC AND OTHER DEBILITATING FOOTBALL INJURIES

After this groundbreaking congressional hearing had concluded, virtually all football-related deaths or catastrophic injuries to young football players due to brain traumas became newsworthy to a national audience. Yet, the mechanisms to track such injuries remained relatively crude, which is true even today. For thirty years Fred Mueller had run the National Center for Catastrophic Sport Injury Research at the University of North Carolina. He was the only person who gathered information on the "more than 1,000 fatal, paralytic or otherwise ghastly injuries in sports from peewees to the pros."[14] Usually such incidents involved football, which is why Mueller had taken over the task from the American Football Coaches Association, which apparently wanted to distance itself from the carnage.

On average there have been about thirty-six catastrophic football injuries a year that Mueller was able to identify. How many he missed was unknown, particularly those conditions that develop more slowly. Tracking such debilitating and catastrophic injuries should have been a nationally coordinated public health mandate. Unfortunately there has been no centralized, comprehensive source of data about catastrophic and other debilitating injuries and conditions due to playing football. The lone exception has been certain information about injuries to professional football players, which is collected as part of the federal occupational safety requirements that NFL teams are obliged to follow.

Because of national concerns about brain trauma, in June 2016 the Centers for Disease Control and Prevention finally announced that, as recommended by the privately funded Institute of Medicine, it "plan[ned] to create and oversee a surveillance system to collect data on concussions across the entire country." How it would be designed, staffed, funded, and implemented remained unspecified, however. Moreover, as the *Washington Post* opined, "There's a long way to go on concussion control for children and adults alike. Better data collection will not solve problems of underdiagnosis or improper care."[15] It also would not track other types of potentially catastrophic and debilitating injuries and conditions that football players and other athletes, both young and old, sustain.

## THE NFL AND YOUTH FOOTBALL TRY TO MARGINALIZE THE SAFETY ISSUE

By 2012, the NFL and one relatively small segment of youth football had begun working in tandem to improve the perception of player safety. Both sides should have realized that without comprehensive data "to understand the problem, [it would be] hard to begin the work of prevention in an intelligent way."[16] Instead, the league put substantial money and other resources into trying to calm fears through public relations, while the cooperating youth league—Pop Warner football—continued to promote and enhance the character-building virtues of football.

The justification for this partnership had to do with mounting concerns about football that were "trickling down to the youth level," especially among parents. The primary concern was not the accumulating evidence of brain and other serious injuries, but rather reports indicating that from 2007 to 2011 there had been a 35 percent decline in kids aged six to twelve playing tackle football.[17] Before that downward trend became known, youth football had been perfectly content to ignore the accumulating negative health implications of the game for its players.

Roger Goodell and the NFL tried to position themselves as the knights in shining armor, but it was impossible to hide the badly tarnished metal, which was leeching toxins into youth football. The league pretended that its "motives for . . . safety measures [were] pure." The man who was paid so well for his public relations skills much of his adult life claimed: "I don't do things for public relations. . . . I do things because they're the right thing to do,"[18] such as marginalizing player violence against women (Ray Rice) and advocating for racially insensitive team names ("Redskins").

As the wife of a former NFL player who had CTE and then killed himself remarked, "They have to put on a show. . . . The pressure is on."[19] A *Washington Post* political survey revealed that the league's involvement was much more than just a show. In the 2008 and 2012 national elections alone, NFL "team owners and their families . . . contributed nearly $2 million to congressional campaigns"[20] in order to ensure the league's political influence would not wane.

Whatever the actual reasons were for Goodell's concerns—and it probably was a mixture of public relations, self-preservation, and, as he explained, his "love" of football—the league began to do everything possible to diminish the perceived risks. In addition to instituting relatively minor changes in the way the game was played, such as reducing the number of runbacks on kickoffs, the NFL implemented new rules to decrease "injuries by reducing wear and tear on players' bodies . . . in offseason programs." Organized team practices "were cut from 14 to 10." Furthermore, there would be "no hitting among players during the offseason."[21]

Beginning in 2013, NFL players were required to wear pads on their thighs and knees. For years that safety measure had been eschewed so players could increase their perceived speed and flexibility, and reinforce the ever-popular "play with pain" image. In addition, it was now "illegal for a ballcarrier to lower his head and use the crown of his helmet to initiate forcible contact with a defender." After that rule modification, Rich McKay, the chair of the NFL's Competition Committee, proclaimed that with regard to safety, "we feel pretty comfortable where the game is."[22]

The NFL also began working with Pop Warner football to promote certain safety measures for the nearly three hundred thousand kids who played in their leagues. The most publicized program was the "Heads Up" initiative to teach young players to tackle properly by leading with their shoulders rather than spearing opponents with their helmets, like so many NFL players, most notably defensive backs and linebackers, had been taught to do for decades. In addition, Pop Warner football decreed that tackling would be forbidden "for two-thirds of each practice" and there would no longer be "drills that involve[d] full-speed, head-on blocking and tackling." In particular the new rules banned a popular character-building drill "in which teammates encircle[d] a player and repeatedly rush[ed] him . . . knock[ing him] around like a pinball."[23]

Unfortunately, there were obvious limitations with these recommendations. In addition to the fact there were no formal mechanisms in place to enforce them and they did not go nearly far enough, the new guidelines bypassed the vast majority of minors who play organized tackle football. Over 3.2 million children were in leagues not affiliated with Pop Warner and frequently operated "with volunteer coaches, referees and doctors."[24] Furthermore, these safety restrictions did not apply to high schools, much less colleges.

## THE CRITICS OF FOOTBALL'S INCREMENTAL CHANGES STRONGLY DISAGREE

Even these incremental efforts to help make youth football somewhat safer had their strong critics on both sides of the issue. Many outside the football world, as well as certain skeptics inside, argued that making the game marginally safer to attract more kids to the sport—or more accurately, to lose fewer kids to other sports—was a Machiavellian sleight of hand. At the very least it was seen as a "NFL marketing move to increase youth participation, despite growing concerns over head injuries."[25] At its worst the effort was seen as a charade: "a PR Jedi mind trick," which ignored "a much bigger [health and safety] problem."[26]

Many former and current NFL players and coaches, on the other hand, worried that the game was being "water[ed] down" unnecessarily. This attitude remains prevalent at the high school level where many coaches have complained that the bad publicity has resulted in "football . . . not [being] as physical as it used to be,"[27] as if that were a bad thing. In addition, certain critics of the safety changes tried to argue that players were "more vulnerable to head hits in games if they take part in fewer contact drills during practices."[28]

This illogical argument skipped over the fact that from a health standpoint it does not matter whether a concussive impact occurs during a game or practice. In fact, most concussions happen during practices. Furthermore, a 2013 study in the *Annals of Biomedical Engineering* proved that what happens in "practice does not influence the number of head hits absorbed during games."[29] The medical literature strongly supports the commonsense observation that the more concussive impacts a player sustains, the greater the likelihood that brain damage will result. Thus, contact drills in practice can only make an already dangerous situation worse, not better.

Perhaps the most outlandish critics have been a small minority of doctors, like Steven Rothman, former Washington University pediatric neurologist, who have challenged medical ethics by urging "parents . . . [to] stop obsessing over concussions."[30] Similarly, football apologists have suggested that it is wrong to "extrapolate [medical] data from the NFL . . . to the youth level."[31] This reckless argument has a ring of truth to it because physiologically, children are different from adults.

Unfortunately, all the relevant medical evidence demonstrates that responsible parents should view tackle football as being more dangerous for children than adults. Immature brains are more vulnerable to trauma. Even young adults may be at heightened risk. In addition, kids "suffer more hits to the head in practices [than adults] . . . [each of which] can have similar force as those absorbed by adult players."[32] The longer a child plays competitive football, the more likely that these head traumas and other serious injuries are going to become problematic and potentially dangerous to the kid's health, both now and in the future.

## BANNING TACKLE FOOTBALL FOR CHILDREN UNDER FOURTEEN

Robert Cantu, one of the leading brain experts who frequently has consulted with the NFL, advocates banning tackle football until children turn fourteen. That guideline, however, raises the question as to why football should not be banned until a young adult's brain has fully matured, a process that often is not completed until age twenty-two or twenty-three. It would appear that this arbitrary age limit of fourteen was not based on sound physiological considerations, but because that is the age when children begin to play high school football, which is enormously popular. Trying to eliminate high school football as we know it would probably be politically disruptive.

Thus it is no surprise that, despite the recognized dangers, safety concerns seem to wane when these younger athletes begin to participate in high school football programs. In April 2014, for example, it was reported that no public secondary schools in the United States had yet adopted the NFL's Heads Up program. Maryland became the first to do so that year, but participation was only voluntary. [33]

Promoting safety probably was not the primary reason Maryland adopted that recommendation anyway. Making parents think the game was safe appeared to be more important. As one Maryland high school coach explained, "We need to . . . ease the minds of parents who are letting those kids play so we can keep growing our sport."

Fortunately, the idea of growing the sport through deception has become unpalatable to many educators and parents. Most medical experts have emphasized the need to make "honesty . . . [the] top priority"[34] in helping to make the decision whether kids should play football. Yet, such honesty by its nature can be scary and off putting.

*Washington Post* columnist Sally Jenkins employed that type of candor in describing what happens to a child's brain when the child is playing tackle football. Jenkins used the now familiar medical comparison of youngsters being like bobblehead dolls. "Watch the . . . neck whiplash back and forth. . . . [H]ear the toy rattle. . . . [I]magine your son's . . .

brain inside the shell." She concluded her public service message with sound parenting advice: "When your own little bobblehead . . . demands a helmet and shoulder pads . . . hand him a flag [instead]."[35]

Somewhat less eloquently, but to the point, former NFL linebacker Cato June conveyed a similar message. He warned an eager group of mostly African American boys in Washington, D.C., that "[tackle] football can be a dangerous game."[36] Actually, it is always dangerous. Some players are just luckier than others in avoiding serious injuries.

Despite new measures to improve safety and the NFL's concerted public relations push, there has continued to be bad publicity as tackle football appears to be "on the verge of a turning point." Doomsayers have argued that this will lead to a situation that eventually would place football "in pretty much the same place as boxing or ultimate fighting."[37]

Whatever happens, though, over time changing attitudes about football are likely to lead to significant losses of business for both the NFL and big-time college football. Even former and current NFL stars, including Terry Bradshaw, Howie Long, and Tom Brady, have publicly expressed the view that as parents they would not encourage—and perhaps even actively discourage—their sons from playing football. In addition, President Obama, who like any president is advised to avoid needless political controversies involving sports, told Americans "that he would think 'long and hard' before letting his son play football,"[38] if he had a son.

Such ominous warnings have come at a time when many former NFL players and their families have been suing the league over the severe brain and other impairments that they incurred while playing the game. Even based on NFL data, from 2004 through 2012 there was a substantial increase in football-related injuries, especially severe injuries. Furthermore, there was a steady increase in what were termed "mild traumatic brain injuries." This rate increase seemed to level off after the 2011 season when rule changes were implemented but began to rise again in 2015. The bottom line is that NFL players need "lifetime health care," given that "their injury rate is 100 percent and one-third [of them] will have to cope with brain disease."[39]

## THE NFL JOINS FORCES WITH GE AND THE MILITARY

Another way the NFL has responded to the awful news about brain trauma and other severe head and neck injuries to football players, both young and older, is by pouring more money and resources into masking and deflecting the danger. The league has attempted to provide hope for the future by changing some rules and training practices that were deemed to be especially problematic. Unfortunately, this self-serving exercise has been more about making people—especially parents—believe football is safe, than substantially improving safety. Kevin Guskiewicz, the founding director of the Sports-Related Traumatic Brain Injury Research Center at the University of North Carolina, put it succinctly: the NFL had "to protect their image. . . . [T]he headlines [were] not good."[40]

In March 2013 the NFL improved its public persona by launching a four-year, $50 million research partnership with General Electric (GE) to develop "imaging technology that would detect concussions and encourage the creation of materials to better protect the brain."[41] This search for a technological fix was on top of the NFL's funding of its controversial and flawed research studies. This additional money would try to shift the imaging technology focus away from establishing proof that those who play football are likely to sustain permanent brain damage. The objective was to identify brain damage early enough to mitigate permanent harm, or at least to create the impression that this was realistically possible someday in the near future.

The initial thrust was to "specializ[e] imaging equipment to detect head trauma." Not coincidentally, the NFL chose to partner with "G.E. a leader in diagnostic equipment like magnetic resonance imaging . . . [which] . . . ha[d] . . . not been honed for traumatic brain injuries like concussions." The CEO of GE was a former Dartmouth football player who said he wanted to promote head injury research as a business model. These advancements were intended to create "a potentially large and lucrative market," which would include not only athletes, but also "children and young adults around the world . . . [and] soldiers returning from combat."[42] This optimistic message was targeted at GE stockholders and the public, rather than neuroscientists who knew better.

The pot of gold at the end of the rainbow was the hope that such scanning devices would become sensitive enough to "forecast who might sustain concussions, and . . . show in real time the degree of brain injury and recovery."[43] The problem with that premise—as Nate Silver has demonstrated with many other types of forecasting—is that due to all of the various human and other variables involved in making such predictions, most of the time they are unreliable and unrealistic. This type of forecasting in particular is likely to be problematic whether the assigned task is to identify athletes who are most susceptible to brain impairments, are likely to sustain serious damage should they be concussed again, or will experience serious symptoms later in life. Even if a negative result could be used to "confirm that a patient does not have a [brain] disease, a positive [one] does not ensure he . . . has it, will develop it or will ever experience symptoms like memory loss or dementia."[44]

At best, imaging technology is many years away from being able to achieve reliable results that would allow for effective treatments of athletes with concussive symptoms. In the meantime, the carnage continues. Even what appears to be the most promising screening test, which has been developed by researchers at UCLA, is viewed as "experimental. [It] is perhaps years away from gaining federal approval."[45]

More importantly, effective treatments for CTE are unlikely because it is a "degenerative condition with no known cure." Robert Stern, who helped found the Center for the Study of Traumatic Encephalopathy at Boston University, observed that "this type of science moves slowly and must move very carefully." The danger is giving people at risk "false hope,"[46] which apparently is what the NFL is all about, in lieu of providing effective solutions.

Children and adults who play football continue to be brain injured on a regular basis. Even highly trained neurologists are left to guess when it might be safe for a concussed athlete to resume playing again. "Concussions are too idiosyncratic to be categorized neatly." As one of the authors of the American Academy of Neurology's concussion guidelines remarked, "There is no set timeline for safe return to play."[47]

These medical decisions must be carried out on a case-by-case basis, which inevitably leaves a great deal to chance. If luck is not on the player's side, then there can be potentially serious or devastating consequences. Deciding what to do is a very risky proposition that involves trying to properly weigh too many concussion unknowns to be reliable.

The second prong of the GE research targeted ways "to improve helmets and other protective devices."[48] That appeared to be a more readily achievable result. At the same time, given today's technology, the degree of protection that any head equipment can provide without incurring exorbitant costs is likely to be limited. Neurologists have concluded that currently there is "no clear evidence that one type of football helmet can better protect against concussions over another kind of helmet."[49] There would have to be a technological breakthrough in order to obtain the desired results at an affordable cost, even for the wealthy NFL, much less the rest of the football world, especially youth leagues and high schools.

Shortly after joining this research initiative with GE, the league also began collaborating with the military "to try to change attitudes of both athletes and troops toward brain injuries." The target audiences were "current players, active military personnel and future generations of athletes and servicemen." In addition to an awareness campaign, the two parties to the agreement said that it was possible that they would "share technology, medical information and marketing strategies."[50]

The common ground between the NFL and the military was somewhat strained from the start. It is one thing to prevent athletes from participating in football because of concussions; it is quite another to diminish troop strength based on similar concerns. Nonetheless, those issues apparently were conflated because the NFL and military share other common interests.

First, both institutions want to ensure that any negative publicity about brain injuries is well managed, as much as organizationally possible. Second, they both want to maximize participation levels—in combat and football—by minimizing the perception of risk. Third, they both want to limit their financial and/or legal liability for the many brain injuries that will continue to occur. One way of doing this is to place responsibility on the players and troops for not adequately identifying and managing their risks and have them pay for the long-term damage when injuries occur.

## FOOTBALL IS IN SERIOUS TROUBLE

Ultimately football, which remains "the most popular [sport] in the United States," is in trouble, despite all the smoke screens and collaborations with GE, the military, and youth football. Even in Texas where high school football reigns supreme, there are "widespread and growing concerns about the physical dangers of the sport."[51] The steadily increasing perception, supported by accumulating medical and scientific evidence, is that tackle football is unsafe.

That momentum will be difficult to reverse, even if it can be slowed. This will lead to an inevitable undermining of the sport. Yes, some parents, fans, and athletes will "remain unconvinced of the dangers, while others [will] view football as the best way to get to college." However, the most responsible view has been established: kids "don't need to play football,"[52] given the dangers it presents.

The ongoing dilemma that football faces was illustrated at a May 2014 conference that President Obama convened, which brought together "some of the country's top sports executives and researchers to . . . combat the nation's . . . concussion crisis." That meeting demonstrated "how quickly [concussions have become] . . . a mainstream cause and how uncomfortable" the NFL is in this national conversation. Although the NFL has spent millions of dollars on public relations and tightly controlled and manipulated concussion research—and plans to spend much more—there is an undeniable "paradox. . . . [T]he more the N.F.L. spends . . . the more it is highlighting those problems [and] . . . worrying the audience that it is trying to assure."[53]

Fortunately for the NFL a politically astute president "stayed far away from proposing any new regulations . . . on cherished sports programs in schools and in communities." Instead, in part he gave the NFL and its supporters a forum where they could continue to promote "programs that attempt 'to convince parents that football can be made safer.'" Nonetheless, parents were learning from experts that "there is no empirical evidence that tackling procedures can reduce the rate or severity of concussions,"[54] much less make the sport reasonably safe for kids to play.

Even if safety could be improved by changing the nature of the game and taking certain precautions, this would fall well short of demonstrating that football could—or would—be played in a reasonably safe manner. At its core football is aggressive and violent, and most of those who play, coach, make money from, and/or faithfully watch the sport embrace the aggression and violence as being manly, entertaining, and strategically necessary. The Case Keenum incident in November 2015 (see chapter 2), only a couple of years after what had happened to Robert Griffin (see chapter 3), was a clear indication that player safety remains a secondary concern, which tends to be outweighed by money, winning, and perpetuating the football character-building mythology.

What happens in the NFL with regard to concussions is still guided by smoke and mirrors intended to reduce owner and league liability and maintain escalating profits. Adam Kilgore of the *Washington Post* astutely observed that the Case Keenum fiasco would provide the "truth about player safety, and [its] consequences." Either the league would acknowledge that it is management's responsibility to ensure safety "by holding teams to the same standard as players. Or it [would] expose the league's concussion protocol as a toothless suggestion, merely a public relations shield."[55]

The NFL chose to try to limit its liability by placing the responsibility for player safety on the players themselves. They are the ones who must "pay the fines and face potential suspension" for playing the game unsafely. Yet, when the St. Louis Rams' coaching staff obviously screwed up on national television by deliberately placing Keenum in danger of further injury, "the league declined to penalize anyone," calling the sad episode a "learning experience."[56]

If this was a teachable moment, it appears that the league failed to learn anything of lasting value. Less than a year later another situation involving an NFL referee screwup threatened the mental health of All-Pro quarterback Cam Newton. More importantly, unfairly saddling players with the primary responsibility of protecting themselves is likely to backfire.

Sooner or later lawyers for former and current players, along with parents of children who might someday have been prospective NFL players, are likely to deflate the NFL's football. This outcome will be inevitable, unless the ever-expanding bad press can be contained, which is becoming increasingly doubtful. Perhaps that is why Goodell and the NFL, like Big Tobacco, are so committed to developing viable markets overseas. Globalization continues to be a priority, even though it poses serious scheduling and transportation problems, it loses money, and the overall foreign fan interest beyond London has not been encouraging.

Even more discouraging is the evolving science regarding brain traumas caused by football. The latest evidence suggests that multiple concussions are not the only grave concern. Repeated hits to the head—an integral part of the game no matter how it is sugarcoated—create subconcussive impacts, which may well exceed the overall health danger contributed by concussions.[57] These nonapparent impacts occur throughout games and practices. While this type of brain science may still be evolving, what is known now is alarming. The prudent course of action, when exposing kids and young adults to such dangers, would be to insist upon caution by respecting the available medical and scientific evidence.

Not surprisingly, more and more NFL players are deciding to shorten their careers, even if it means losing out on millions of dollars in salaries, out of concerns for their health.[58] In addition, NFL and college players are more apt to state publicly, or at least imply, that tackle football may not be something that kids should play. More importantly, as Bennet Omalu, the chief medical examiner and pathologist upon whom the movie *Concussion* was based, has warned, we have a "moral duty" not to allow children to play football, at least until they have "reached the age of consent."[59] Apparently parents are listening. According to a 2016 *New York Times* editorial, over the past six years youth football for children aged 6 to 14 has decreased from 3 million to 2.2 million. In addition, the Pop Warner league—the NFL's stepchild—has become the plaintiff in a class-action lawsuit filed by parents whose sons have been diagnosed with CTE-like symptoms after playing youth football as kids.[60]

With all the popular sports to choose from, there is no compelling reason why minors should play tackle football, or box or fight competitively, for that matter, at least until it can be demonstrated that doing so has become reasonably safe. Hockey, wrestling, rugby, lacrosse, and other aggressive contact sports, along with heading in soccer, should be more closely scrutinized and monitored as well. With football, however, the dangers have become apparent and undeniable. Thus, the burden should be on those who want kids to play tackle football to show that the risks are manageable and worth taking. In the meantime, children—including older adolescents—should be strongly discouraged from taking those risks.

## 17

# FOLLOWING SUIT

## Concussions in the NHL and NCAA Football

$P$laintiffs' lawyers understand that American law operates with legal precedents that can expand to cover new but analogous situations. The hundreds of lawsuits filed on behalf of former NFL players, which were alleged to have been proximately caused by concussions and other brain traumas, became viable as precedents once the NFL agreed to a lucrative settlement. Like the NFL itself, these lawsuits are driven primarily by money.

Without attorneys' fees there would be very little civil justice. Thus, it is hardly surprising that this type of personal injury litigation, if successful, would be expanded to target other major sports enterprises that have ignored or marginalized their athletes' concussions and other brain traumas. In recent years former athletes with concussion-like symptoms have also sued the NHL and NCAA football.

## BRAIN INJURIES IN HOCKEY

Physical and mental impairments that arise in North American hockey are not as widespread as in football, but they may not be any less harmful to the damaged athletes involved. Hockey violence tends to be more bloody, theatrical, and discrete. Concussive impacts generally occur when skulls collide with the ice, the boards, Plexiglas, or the elbows or sticks of opponents. Like football, these collisions can be incidental, accidental, or deliberate.

Unlike football where the concussive hits are delivered on every play in many different places all over the field, hockey blows to the head, while common, are not as ubiquitous. In addition, much of the permanent damage inflicted in hockey tends to be cosmetic, involving broken and missing teeth and scars on the face. As with football, though, the dividing line between delivering punishing blows to help one's team win and trying to deliberately injure an opponent can be thin.

In North American professional hockey, much of what happens on the ice has been needlessly violent. This is particularly true when it has involved staged fighting to entertain the raucous fans in big arenas, or management-instigated thuggery to intimidate or protect a valued scorer. While the fighting may be manufactured, a punch to the head can be potentially even more damaging than in boxing because the hockey contestants drop their gloves. One need only compare Olympic, college, and women's hockey with the NHL, AHL, and the Canadian minor and junior leagues to realize that many, and arguably most, of these serious head injuries could be eliminated with relatively modest rule changes that would adequately constrain fighting and physical assaults on the ice.

Despite all of the sport's calculated violence, concussion litigation in the NHL followed football lawsuits for two good reasons. First, professional football draws considerably more media scrutiny and generates more money than hockey overall, although probably not in Canada where hockey is "sacred." However, Canadian laws are much more resistant to this type of litigation, which is an American specialty. Second, football-caused concussions and concussive impacts are considerably more frequent than in hockey where the damage tends to be more isolated, often targeting players—usually one to a team—designated as enforcers, who tend to dominate the fighting.

Nonetheless, once American personal injury lawyers started making real headway with football-related brain injury litigation, their attentions naturally turned to hockey where the parallels are striking, if not always perfectly analogous. Not surprisingly from a legal perspective, deliberate fighting has taken center stage in the lawsuits against the NHL.

## HOCKEY CONCUSSIONS BECOME A PUBLIC CONCERN

The first concussion-based hockey litigation to gain national attention in the United States and Canada involved the designated enforcer, Derek Boogaard, who died of a drug overdose in 2011 while recuperating from a hockey-related concussion. His family sued in 2013, alleging his death was due to substance abuse and addiction, which physicians employed by the two NHL teams Boogaard had played for—the Minnesota Wild and the New York Rangers—had facilitated. Submerged in those initial claims, though, was an allegation that Boogaard sustained brain damage as a result of being a designated fighter. The implication was "that the league and the union knew that its fighters faced . . . a risk . . . [of] degenerative brain disease linked to repeated head trauma"[1] but did little or nothing to intervene.

After the initial lawsuit was dismissed for certain procedural defects, Boogaard's family filed a new wrongful death action against the NHL. In this subsequent litigation the plaintiffs alleged that the league was "responsible for the physical trauma and brain damage that Boogaard sustained . . . as one of the league's top enforcers." The new law firm representing Boogaard's family previously had sued professional football "on behalf of Dave Duerson, a former Chicago Bear . . . who [had] committed suicide . . . and was found to have CTE."[2]

Boston University researchers found that when Boogaard died he also had the same brain disease,[3] as did a number of other designated NHL enforcers. In 2010, researchers concluded that the brain of "Bob Probert, a well-known [designated] fighter for the Detroit Red Wings . . . [had] chronic traumatic encephalopathy."[4] As "former hockey enforcer" Bob Ray predicted, it appeared inevitable that "a more ambitious suit" involving many former hockey fighters would follow. In addition to Boogaard and Probert, the list of deceased hockey enforcers with CTE included Rick Rypien, Wade Belak, Steve Montador, and Todd Ewen, all of whom had passed away before turning fifty.[5]

It was not just the designated fighters in hockey who were being concussed. By 2013, the media was reporting on a wave of concussions throughout the NHL. One of the major catalysts for those reports involved serious head injuries to several of the game's most visible stars, including Pittsburgh Penguins league MVPs Sidney Crosby and Evgeni

Malkin. At the time, Crosby was the game's most popular—and arguably its best—player.

Crosby had to sit out sixty games due to a hit in the head that he sustained during the 2011 Winter Classic, which had been played outdoors on a substandard ice surface. When combined with the off-season Crosby would endure a "14 month concussion saga."[6] It was reminiscent of what had happened some fifteen years earlier to Eric Lindros, another of the game's stars who was incapacitated, repeatedly, from concussions in what should have been the prime of his athletic career.[7] Slowed by those injuries, Lindros never reached his full potential as a superstar hockey player. The same type of diminished output has impaired Crosby's greatness, although by the 2015–2016 season he had recovered enough of his skills to make the All-Star team and be voted Most Valuable Player in the 2016 Stanley Cup Finals. Yet he still was not even the best player on his own team.

Crosby was one of many hockey players to be sidelined by brain trauma. The Canadian Broadcasting Corporation estimated that for the 2011–2012 season alone, approximately ninety NHL players (13 percent) had missed games because of concussions. Whether this represented a substantial increase in the number of concussions or merely better reporting was difficult to discern. Regardless, beginning in the fall of 2012 "concussions and hits to the head [became] frequent talking points in the N.H.L."[8] These types of hockey injuries were no longer viewed as isolated incidents.

One of the most tragic NHL concussion-related stories involved future Hall of Fame defenseman Chris Pronger. In 2011 he suffered "a severe eye injury and head injury . . . three weeks apart," which derailed his brilliant career. Pronger experienced repeated migraine headaches triggered by the slightest sensory overload, had a "shrinking field of vision" that substantially diminished his hockey abilities, and, not surprisingly, was driven into a "black hole of depression," which suggested emerging symptoms of CTE.[9]

Ironically, over his illustrious eighteen-year career Pronger had a reputation for "always deliver[ing] more punishment than he received." He played the game to win, not to make friends. Thus, Pronger accepted what had happened to him without voicing any recriminations. He would have viewed himself as a "hypocrite to ask for sympathy now."[10]

Nonetheless, even Pronger conceded that the game had to change. He believed that the players should "look out for themselves by talking about symptoms and protecting themselves on the ice." This was a perspective that he shared with NHL owners and management. It also reflected a hockey culture in which young players from Canada are taught to glorify the game as a Canadian "way of life," which epitomizes "speed, skill, and toughness."[11]

## BRAIN SCIENCE IMPACTS HOCKEY

By September 2013, concussions in hockey had become enough of a concern that the Mayo Clinic in Rochester, Minnesota, held its second conference devoted exclusively to that narrow topic. The takeaway message from leading medical researchers at "Summit II" was that hockey "causes too much brain trauma, and it must change fundamentally." The attendees recommended "significant modifications in body checking and an end to fighting," not only in professional hockey, but in the juniors as well.[12]

Around the same time, a Toronto neurosurgeon who had closely studied concussions in male hockey players published his findings, which focused on the types of male hockey players who were most likely to be negatively impacted by these brain traumas. Those most at risk, he concluded, tended to be "short . . . defensemen or those who take a lot of penalties." In addition, he found that young players appeared to be "more susceptible, as well as players with a concussion history."[13]

Apparently, there was a substantial, widespread risk of concussions among many different types of male hockey players. Only taller, older athletes who played forward, did not get penalized frequently, and had never sustained a concussion before were not especially "susceptible." Among hockey players that seems to be a relatively small unsusceptible universe.

Arguably the CTE-related health risks posed to professional hockey players in North America come close to rivaling athletes in the NFL. According to prominent NHL agent Allan Walsh, of those players who have had their brains examined after they died, "over 90 percent have CTE. CTE is basically melting their brains." This is comparable to what is being found with deceased NFL players. Former NHL players complained that in addition to providing "inadequate oversight and care to treat brain injuries," teams were "promot[ing] the game's violence, including bare-knuckle bouts on the ice." Moreover, they contend that the NHL is well "behind the NFL in dealing with concussions and returning players to the playing surface." Despite creating a "concussion work group in 1997," as of 2016 it still did "not have a neurologist on the panel."[14]

## CLASS ACTIONS ARE FILED AGAINST THE NHL

In November 2013, ten former players filed the first potential concussion-based class action against the NHL. In addition to alleging "negligence and fraud," the plaintiffs contended that the league "should have done more to address head injuries." They also asserted that the NHL "celebrated . . . a culture of speed and violence," which greatly increased the risk of brain damage. In particular, the league has "continue[d] to glorify and empower players known as 'enforcers' . . . [whose] singular intention [is] injuring the opposing team."[15]

Cultivating its own culture of denial, the NHL responded by claiming that it was "completely satisfied with the responsible manner in which the league and the players . . . have managed player safety." Unlike the NFL, however, the NHL had initiated modest steps to protect its players. The NHL did not have sound concussion protocols for responding to players injured on the ice, but with regard to the appearance of safety, the league was "evolving."[16]

The NHL had created a Department of Player Safety to review games and help ensure that player penalties were "far more stringent than . . . a decade ago." Commissioner Gary Bettman promised that any player who "blatantly flouts the rules in a manner that causes a head injury . . . should expect to be severely disciplined."[17] Like Goodell and the NFL, however, Bettman was placing most of the responsibility for safety on the players themselves. Bettman did very little to suppress staged fighting, which so many North American fans still believed was the lifeblood of the sport, or to ensure that when players were concussed, they received immediate diagnoses and proper treatment.

In 2014, nine more former professional hockey players filed a second lawsuit against the NHL, alleging that the league "'intentionally created, fostered and promoted a culture of extreme violence' for profit." The NHL, through its deputy commissioner, did not refute the merits of the allegations. Instead it responded that the complaint provided no "valid basis for liability or damages as against the National Hockey League."[18]

The NHL offered the same response in February 2015 when twenty-nine more former players filed another action against the league. Shortly thereafter the NHL's reputation suffered another blow when former hockey enforcer Stephen Peat, who had reported having "memory loss and headaches—often associated with C.T.E."—almost died after, accidentally or deliberately, setting fire to his father's house.[19]

NHL lawyers responded to the lawsuits by arguing that all of the concussion cases against the league should be dismissed. A federal judge denied all those motions as being "premature."[20] In the process, she also rejected the argument that these claims should be precluded based on the collective bargaining agreement between the league and its players. She pointed out that the plaintiffs were "retired and no longer subject to any CBA."[21]

As a result of her rulings, the federal judge placed the NHL in a legal "'quandary' [that] [n]o other league has faced." While the NFL's lawsuits were about to be settled, those against the NHL remained viable. Nonetheless, in order to prevail, the former hockey players would still have to prove "that the league hid information about the dangers of fighting" and that the resulting injuries that they sustained while playing in the NHL "led to their current ailments."[22] Initially this appeared to be a high legal hurdle, unless the former players could somehow demonstrate that league officials had actually known about these dangers.

In March 2016, though, the litigation calculus changed substantially after the contents of damning e-mails between "Commissioner Gary Bettman and his top lieutenants" became public. Nearly five years earlier the "N.H.L.'s top officials . . . [had] privately acknowledged that fighting could lead to concussions and long-term health problems, including depression, and that so-called enforcers frequently use pills to ease pain." Brendan Shanahan, a former player who was now a senior vice president for the league, stated in one of his e-mails that "fighters used to aspire to become regular players. . . . Now they train and practice becoming more fearsome fighters. They used to take alcohol and cocaine to cope. . . . Now they take pills . . . to sleep . . . to wake up . . . to ease the pain . . . to amp up." In addition, another league official had e-mailed that "fighting raises the incidence of head injuries/concussions, which raises the incidence of depression, which raises the incidence of personal tragedies."[23]

These types of admissions are a personal injury lawyer's dream scenario. They made it much more likely that the former hockey player plaintiffs would ultimately prevail, either through continued litigation or a generous settlement. If there was a settlement, however, the lessons learned from the NFL agreement—which clearly favored team owners—would prove instructive to the plaintiffs' lawyers. Moreover, a congressional committee demanded information from the NHL about what it has been doing to prevent and treat concussions, noting that hockey appeared to be lagging behind other professional sports, including the NFL.[24]

## THE NCAA LITIGATION

The NCAA was first sued over concussions in 2011, well before the initial class action against the NHL had been filed. Much of the early NCAA litigation was framed in the context of the woeful neglect of the health needs of college football players and other athletes in NCAA-managed sports. It was alleged that coaches were failing to teach players how to tackle properly, medical staffs were failing to identify and respond to head traumas appropriately, and teams were shirking their responsibility for concussions by expecting their athletes to report their injuries, rather than instituting specific team protocols for doing so.[25]

Several years later in a press release, the NCAA announced that it was agreeing to settle "several consolidated concussion-related class actions" for $70 million. This appeared to be a very small cost of doing business. Without admitting any liability, the NCAA promised to provide "concussion testing and diagnosis of current and former NCAA student athletes," which it should have been doing years ago. In addition, the NCAA agreed to provide for "baseline concussion testing of NCAA student-athletes" and ensure that medical personnel would be "present" at all games and "available" for all practices.[26]

The NCAA refused to pay for the type of "bodily injury claims" and resulting impairments that were the focus of the concussion litigation against the NFL. Furthermore, the agreement's "return-to-play guideline" for concussed athletes proved to be very disappointing. The NCAA recommended—but failed to require—that colleges ensure "student-athletes with a diagnosed concussion . . . not be allowed to return to play or practice on the same day."[27]

This favorable settlement for the NCAA continued to languish awaiting "approval by a[n Illinois] federal judge."[28] In 2016, before the settlement was finally approved, lawyers representing other former college football players filed six new lawsuits against the NCAA, various football conferences, and a number of universities.[29] Each of these actions focused on the critical issue of bodily injuries to players. A few weeks later four more such lawsuits were filed, including one by the brother of Heisman Trophy winner Archie Griffin against the NCAA and Big Ten. One "Chicago-based law firm" was responsible for all of these legal actions and promised to file several more in the weeks to come.[30]

The common contention in all these claims was that the university and college defendants, including the NCAA, had "kept their players and the public in the dark about an epidemic that was slowly killing their athletes," which "severely increased their risks of long-term brain injuries."[31] The key issue to be decided involved the legal concept known as assumption of risk: whether these former young athletes knew what could happen to them brain injury–wise, if they continued to play football.

Until recently, though, high school and college football players and their parents did not know much about concussions, concussive impacts, CTE, and other long-term impairments that football can cause, although they probably were aware that playing football was likely to lead to a variety of short-term physical injuries. It is important to emphasize that almost all of these former athletes had made the decision to play college football while they were still adolescents in high school. Furthermore, the fact that the NCAA and its members considered football players to be student-athletes, rather than pseudoprofessionals, heightened the duty on those "educational" institutions and athletic programs to protect these still-young players from known harms.

As a law professor explained in *Forbes*, "Sooner or later, [one of these] case[s] will go to trial and the depositions, interrogatories and testimony will reveal . . . just how much was known by those who administer the sport [of football] and when they knew it."[32] Based on the class action settlement that the NCAA tentatively agreed to, even as recently as 2014 many of these college football programs did not have concussion protocols in place. Not surprisingly, most of these lawsuits were filed against high-profile schools such as Auburn, Oregon, Penn State, Georgia, Utah, and Vanderbilt. The athletic departments at those universities have deep pockets and normally spend large sums of money on football, except when it comes to providing safe and healthy environments and outcomes for their football playing student-athletes.

# 18

# CONCUSSION CONCERNS FOR FEMALE ATHLETES

**W**hile football—and, to a lesser extent, ice hockey—for men have received much of the media's attention in covering sports-related concussions, and deservedly so, concern about brain injuries is becoming less male dominant. Media coverage of the issue has been expanded to include several sports that female athletes play. The third leading cause of sports-related concussions in American high schools is girls' soccer.[1] Except for football and boy's hockey, it "ranks at the top . . . in terms of concussion rate."[2] When one includes all sports, girls' basketball and lacrosse rank fifth and sixth, respectively, just behind boys' lacrosse.

Yet, despite the growing recognition that various sports are dangerous for female athletes, there has been a dearth of medical and related research studies on brain injuries where women are the subjects. "It is clear that concussion and brain injury of women has been sorely overlooked," one brain trauma expert explained to Amie Just of the *Washington Post*.[3] Similarly, Anne McKee, a neuropathologist and the director of Boston University's CTE Center, has opined that "we currently know so little about how gender influences outcome after trauma."[4]

As of March 2016, of the 307 brains that had been obtained by the Concussion Legacy Foundation on behalf of CTE research, only four belonged to women. Most of the relevant information on female athletes and brain trauma has been anecdotal, as reported in the media, focused mostly on soccer and ice hockey. What we do know, statistically, however, is "that women and girls suffer concussions 1.4 times more often than [men and boys] in comparable sports. And, often, the women and girls have a longer recovery period."[5]

## SOCCER

The most publicized concussion concerns involving female athletes have focused on soccer, in part because of the sport's popularity and in part because studies indicate females incur these injuries more easily than males. The leading problem is the impact on nonadult female players' brains when they use their heads to score or to advance or control the ball. In addition to concussions, "heading poses the risk of . . . sub-concussive hits . . . that [don't] yield any symptoms but can nevertheless be damaging [over time as] . . . the blows accumulate."[6]

As a result, a number of soccer programs around the country have placed restrictions on heading for players of both sexes before they enter high school. Yet, there is little reason to conclude that the risk subsides once those kids turn fourteen. At the same time, while heading appears to be the most frequent single cause of head trauma for female soccer players, the other types of concussive impacts when measured collectively cause most of the brain damage to girls and boys.

As in any sport, the practical questions about how to deal with this risk typically come down to whether player safety is worth changing the nature of soccer, in this instance by making it a serious infraction of the rules to head the ball. The answer for the immediate future is that safety likely will lose out most of the time, except for the very youngest competitors. Given sexist attitudes in sports, though, it probably is easier to promote concussion safety for girls and women than for boys and men. Thus, girls' soccer is probably more open to accepting safety restrictions, as long as the game remains largely the same for both sexes.

Girls and their parents seem to take these head injuries more seriously, and, along with their coaches, tend to be somewhat more cautious in deciding when to resume playing contact sports after such an injury occurs. Despite its sexist origins, this caution is a good thing. The culture of playing hurt, which infested male sports many years ago and continues today, has not penetrated female team sports quite as deeply, including in soccer. In part this is because there still tends to be a residual perception that female athletes are more fragile than their male counterparts. Nevertheless, as Briana Scurry, the former starting goalie on the U.S women's national team, recounted, "In the mid-[19]90s, you get your head hit, you get your bell rung, you shake it off . . . [u]nless you're knocked out. Even [then] . . . once you recover you get up and you keep going."[7] At her elite level, the "play with pain and injuries" culture was more similar to that of the men.

The prevailing explanations for why girls and women incur concussions at higher rates in soccer than boys and men have focused on differences in physiology, rather than culture and environment. Based on numerous studies, "girls are more susceptible to concussions across all sports played by both genders."[8] This is true even though girls' sports, especially lacrosse and hockey, have specific rules aimed to diminish contact. Nonetheless, subtle—and not so subtle—cultural factors may play a significant role in contributing to this gender dichotomy with respect to soccer concussion rates.

Regardless, it is important to remember that boys' football is still number one in terms of concussion rates by a wide margin, followed by boys' ice hockey. Also, comparing the number of concussions reported in any high school sport by gender does not account for reporting differences between boys and girls, or the severity of the blows to the head that the athletes in various sports receive. Football and hockey played by males appear to regularly deliver impacts that tend to be greater and more frequent than what occurs in any other popular sport, including girls' soccer, girls' basketball, girls' lacrosse, or girls' ice hockey.

This does not mean that female athletes do not suffer career-ending brain injuries or are immune from CTE. Although the public reports to date of such injuries have been relatively rare as compared to male athletes, a "growing body of research suggests . . . female athletes suffer relatively more concussions . . . with more dramatic symptoms." Based on a study in the *American Journal of Sports Medicine*, which focused on high school sports that have similar rules for boys and girls, girls get concussed at twice the rate. In college sports it appears that "among all . . . athletes, female soccer players had the highest overall concussion rates."[9]

This last statistic suggests that the willingness of female college soccer players to self-report concussion symptoms, and their coaches to promote safety more readily, may account for much of that higher rate. It would be shocking to learn that female collegiate soccer players actually have a higher concussion rate than males who play collegiate football or hockey. It also would raise questions as to why in high school the opposite seems to have been true. Nonetheless, it seems clear that female college soccer players incur a substantial, serious risk of concussions no matter what comparisons are being made.

Lauren Long, a former college soccer player, claims "she suffered 10 concussions and continues to deal with emotional and cognitive consequences [years later]." She cofounded Concussion Connection, but emphasizes that "not all players who suffer concussions experience the same consequences." She also believes that the primary concern should not be whether an athlete in a sport is going to be concussed, but rather when it does occur, what is going to happen to ensure that the athlete is safe?[10]

Former American World Cup champion goalkeeper Briana Scurry may be the most well-known female athlete trying to overcome a life-altering concussion. In April 2010, Scurry's brain was concussed when a forward slammed into her while she was attempting to make a save. Shortly thereafter she retired from soccer, failed in her "short-lived gig with ESPN and . . . [was] push[ed] . . . into depression."[11]

She could not understand what had happened to her and why she was not getting better. Scurry experienced "persistent pain" due to migraines and other chronic headaches. In addition, she had imbalance, memory loss, and being "spacey, anxious and depressed," which proved to be the most disturbing symptoms of her concussion. Whether all of those devastating symptoms were due to this one concussion, accumulated concussions, or some significant part of what she had experienced in her quick descent from the top of the female soccer world, remains unclear.

What proved to be undeniable, however, was that Scurry's life changed dramatically for the worse after being concussed. This is a status she has shared with numerous elite athletes of both sexes, including Cindy Parlow Cone, Scurry's teammate, who retired from soccer in 2006 due to post-concussion syndrome.[12] For nearly three and a half years "Scurry's day-to-day activities resembled nothing close to the life she flourished in before the hit" that appears to have set off her symptoms.[13]

It was not until she had "bilateral occipital nerve surgery at Georgetown University" that she recovered enough from her symptoms to become an advocate for women's brain health. Scurry thinks the most important thing anyone can do if they are concussed, especially athletes, is to "be honest to everyone . . . including loved ones, doctors, coaches, family members and everyone associated with the [recovery] process."[14] Yet, honesty may not be enough should her symptoms return or new ones develop due to the brain traumas she endured playing her sport.

## ICE HOCKEY

Ice hockey appears to be one of the most dangerous sports for women, even though—unlike the men—it "penalizes body checking and does not have a history of fighting." While "there is a dearth of information focused on concussions in women's hockey," there are strong indications that the concussion rates are high. An eight-year study of women's hockey conducted by the International Hockey Federation found that "at the world championships and the Olympics . . . concussions were the third-most-common injury (15.5 percent)." That is consistent with self-reported injuries among NCAA student-athletes, which found that more than 20 percent of women hockey players "had experienced at least one concussion." In addition, a "small study of two Canadian college teams . . . found that female hockey players sustained concussions almost twice as frequently as [the] men did." [15]

This evidence suggests that, along with soccer, there has been a substantial increase in the reported incidence of concussions by female athletes playing ice hockey. Whether increases are because female athletes are stronger, fitter, faster, and more aggressive, and/or due to better reporting and greater awareness is difficult to determine. Regardless, concussions have become a serious problem for girls and women in a number of sports, and ice hockey is near the top of the list. It remains somewhat hidden, however, because not very many female athletes play ice hockey as compared to soccer and other sports.

Several high-profile female Olympic ice hockey players have reported having life-altering concussion symptoms, which has helped to publicize the problem. Amanda Kessel, America's leading scorer at the Sochi Games and the 2013 College Player of the Year, almost "end[ed] her career . . . at 23 because of . . . symptoms from a concussion sustained before the Olympics."[16] Nearly two years passed until she was able to return to college hockey at the University of Minnesota. Kessel's "teammate Josephine Pucci retired . . . at 24, cognizant of her [repeated] concussion[s]." Similarly, Canada's hockey Olympian, Haley Irwin, was unable to play in the Olympic tournament until the semifinals due to a concussion, while another one in January 2015 "kept her from playing professionally."[17]

As Briana Scurry has observed, for women who play contact sports at an Olympic or professional level there is a tendency for head injuries to be underreported and ignored, much like what happens with the men. Money changes the nature of these sports and the athletes who play them. One longtime women's ice hockey coach explained that when elite female athletes "compete for higher stakes . . . , [they develop] this inability to care about the [health] consequences of playing the sport."[18] At the same time, that tunnel vision, which encourages athletes to ignore serious health issues, probably is diminished somewhat by the realization that the "stakes" for women athletes almost always lag behind the men.

# 19

# BRAIN AND OTHER SEVERE INJURIES IN BASEBALL

Brain and other severe injuries to baseball players appear to be less prevalent than in many other contact sports. More common, though, are serious injuries to largely unaware fans struck by hard-hit line drives, bats, and bat shards, which are propelled at high velocity into the stands. Baseball is not a dangerous sport like football or hockey, but it does create circumstantial dangers that could and should be mitigated more than they are now.

## SEVERE PLAYER INJURIES

Stories, articles, reports, and investigations about the threats of brain traumas and other devastating injuries are more likely to focus on the most popular spectator sports. Thus, those types of injuries to players in baseball have generated significant media attention, even though they seem to be considerably less common than in football, hockey, or many other sports. At the high school level, for instance, the concussion rate for baseball is less than girls' volleyball, which means that there are twelve scholastic sports that pose a greater concussion risk.[1]

It was not until December 2013 that the first former major-league player was found to have CTE postmortem. Ryan Freel, who had suffered numerous baseball-related brain injuries, died in 2012 "at [age] 36 of a self-inflicted shotgun wound."[2] Freel had retired in 2010 after sustaining "nine or 10 concussions," along with other injuries, which had shortened his career, and quite possibly his life. He experienced a similar progression to what has been reported with a growing number of former football and hockey players who have been repeatedly concussed.

In 2006 Freel told the *Dayton Daily News* that "he had an imaginary friend . . . 'who lives in my head who talks to me and I talk to him.'" This was presumed to be a symptom of a mental disorder related to his multiple concussions, which were thought to have contributed to his suicide. Yet, he also might have been trying to make light of the cognitive distress that he had been experiencing. Whatever the explanation, Freel missed thirty games in 2007 after being concussed in a collision with a teammate.[3]

In baseball, there are a number of circumstances that appear to substantially increase the risk of brain and other severe injuries to players: pitchers either deliberately or unintentionally throwing at or near a batter's head; fielders running into a wall or fence trying to make a difficult or spectacular catch; collisions between runners and catchers at home plate; and runners trying to break up double plays at second base.

With one notable exception, Major League Baseball (MLB) has addressed the first two dangers by having umpires aggressively enforce game-removal sanctions against pitchers who appear to be throwing at a batter's head, while teams have placed protective cushioning on the outfield fences. The exception has been the many managers and coaches, who still instruct, encourage, and/or permit their pitchers to intentionally throw at the opposing batter. Most of the time this is done because either the opposing team threw at one of their players or someone on the other team violated one of the absurd, unwritten rules of baseball that define "appropriate" on-the-field decorum for players. Fortunately, in today's game most of the time—but not always—pitchers target an offending player's body below the head. Unfortunately, sometimes they miscalculate or lose control of their pitches.

## TAKE-OUT SLIDES

Until recently, MLB largely ignored the other two especially dangerous situations, which involved runners hurtling into catchers or infielders to avoid an out. The first of those two situations was addressed by changing the existing rules in 2014, while the rationale for ignoring the other circumstance diminished quickly in the glare of public opinion.

Throughout baseball's history, runners mowing down catchers who were trying to tag them out at home plate, or ripping into them with their spikes, had been a violent staple of the game. Even after Ray Fosse's career had been curtailed when Pete Rose recklessly slammed into him during the 1970 All-Star Game, the irresponsible attitude of MLB was to say that catchers assumed the risk of runners doing what was necessary to win. Rose actually won acclaim for his toughness and the overly aggressive way he played the game.

Attitudes shifted somewhat, however, after the San Francisco Giants superlative catcher Buster Posey, at the beginning of the 2011 season, almost lost his career to an awful-looking leg injury as a result of a home plate collision. Following considerable debate, discussion, and dissenting views, MLB decided to make a major rule change. This was done not so much to promote safety per se, but to protect baseball's business interests by avoiding injuries to valuable players and dampening widespread criticism from fans and the media alike.

For the 2014 season, MLB initiated what was termed an "experiment" to prohibit runners from crashing into catchers at home plate. This prohibition, which a year later became permanent, applies only if the catcher positions himself just outside the base path, near enough to make a tag but not directly in the runner's way. Otherwise, should the catcher block the plate, the runner may collide with him, potentially causing an injury, as long as the runner does not "deviate from his direct pathway . . . to initiate contact."[4]

The number of years it took before this rule change was promulgated, along with its timing, made a number of commentators wonder whether liability concerns due to the concussion litigation in football may have spurred this action as much as Posey's injury itself. According to those commentators, MLB did not want to follow in the footsteps of the NFL, which had been "slow in responding to the concussion problem . . . denying it for years, at great cost . . . to the league's reputation."[5] Baseball was still recovering from all the bad publicity that had been generated because it had ignored steroids and other performance-enhancing substances for such a long time (see chapter 6).

Inexplicably, this new rule did not cover the closely analogous situation of take-out slides at second base. This suggested that regardless of any litigation concerns, MLB was not going to act against its perceived financial interests in satisfying its fans, until there was a sustained public outcry. During the 2015 baseball playoffs, the issue of reckless slides into second base, which MLB had continued to ignore, became national news. Chase Utley of the Los Angeles Dodgers slid dangerously hard into Ruben Tejada of the New York Mets in game two of the National League Division Series, breaking Tejada's leg while the Mets shortstop was trying to execute a double play.[6] Utley received a two-game suspension for going out of the base path, while Tejada would not be able to play for several months, including the rest of the playoffs and the World Series.

Questions arose immediately whether the short suspension was sufficient punishment and the existing baseball rule on slides was enough to prevent this type of awful result from happening again. Statements by Utley's representative and Joe Torre, the executive vice president for operations, on behalf of MLB highlighted the ambiguity of the existing rule and its applications. Utley's agent pointed out that take-out slides at second base have been a routine part of the game almost since its inception and had not resulted in suspensions. Torre responded that while he did not believe there had been any intent to injure, the "slide was in violation of Official Baseball Rule 5.09(a)(13), which [was] designed to protect fielders from precisely this type of rolling block that occurs away from the base."[7]

Utley's intent, which was obvious to most baseball fans watching, was to do what was physically necessary to impede the fielder, even if it resulted in a serious injury. Ultimately, though, whether the player making a slide is in or out of the base path is a judgment call by the umpires, meaning considerable ambiguity still remains. Instant replay may only be used to determine whether the vulnerable fielder touched the base, not whether the runner remained in the imaginary base path.

Like the collision at home plate, serious injuries can also occur when the runner remains within the base path and collides with a vulnerable fielder who is trying to make the double play. In fact, this danger had been so apparent to most umpires that for years they tended to look the other way when a shortstop did not actually touch second base trying to make a double play. This "so-called neighborhood play [has been] an unwritten rule going back decades that allows infielders to protect themselves by getting out of the way of hard-charging runners."[8] In many ways, the umpires' solution was a better way to protect players from injuries than the current written rule.

That unwritten accommodation began to fray, though, once the advent of instant replays began to reveal for all to see—especially baseball purists—that umpires were not enforcing the written rules on those types of neighborhood plays. Thus, strict enforcement came in conflict with a tradition that protected players but still allowed for the occasional collision to entertain the fans and feed into the macho-athlete mystique. Not surprisingly, MLB and the players union worked out a compromise that improved player safety somewhat, but probably did not ameliorate the danger as well as strict adherence to the neighborhood play would have.

The revised rule added unnecessary ambiguity, which has made close calls more difficult. Under the new policy, slides to break up double plays "will have to include a bona fide attempt to reach and remain on the base. Contact with the fielder is permissible, but the runner cannot change his path to initiate contact or engage in a 'roll block.'"9

## FANS IN THE STANDS

Prioritizing safety over baseball traditions and maximizing revenues for owners also have been obstacles to protecting fans from potentially devastating injuries, if they have purchased seats in the highly valued lower decks closest to the field of play. Fans in those seats are especially vulnerable to vicious line drives unintentionally directed at their heads, as well as from bats—or sharp pieces of bats—that are launched into the stands. To guard against such injuries MLB has advised fans to wear baseball gloves and remain alert throughout the game. But relatively few do. An overwhelming percentage of fans are at risk, especially youngsters, people who are not athletic, and people who have watched very few baseball games in the past.

In the NHL a similar danger existed from fans being hit by pucks. That changed after a thirteen-year-old girl was killed in 2002. The league directed teams to put in protective netting and Plexiglas barriers to ensure that another potentially devastating fan injury did not happen. Nearly thirteen years later, following a couple of well-publicized incidents of fans being severely injured by foul balls and flying bats, MLB finally instituted a new fan protection policy. Yet, compared to what the NHL had done to protect against flying pucks, MLB's changes were too little, too late.

The difference in attitude appeared to be based on legal liability and how it was perceived by American courts. For many decades baseball has enjoyed special legal protections, which not only extend to antitrust matters, but also liability. What is known as the "baseball rule" has allowed professional teams to effectively avoid liability for fan injuries by including a warning on every ticket. It states that fans assume the risk of being injured when they attend a ball game.

According to Joe Nocera of the *New York Times*, the liability calculus began to change, however, "during the third inning of a game between the Yankees and Oakland Athletics at Yankee Stadium on . . . Aug. 25, 2011." A "Manhattan real estate executive named Andy Zlotnick . . . [was struck by] a scorching foul ball . . . [which] completely destroyed the bones around [his] left eye socket, fractured his sinus and upper jaw, and did extensive damage to the left side of his face." Reportedly treatment of those injuries cost over $100,000, of which "about $25,000 [was] out of pocket."[10] The Yankees either reneged on a verbal promise to cover the out-of-pocket expenses or never had intended to do so. Up until then fans had almost no chance of recovering legal damages if they were injured at a baseball game.

From a judicial perspective what had happened to Zlotnick was significantly different from a typical baseball fan injury case. Yet that difference seemed slight. When Zlotnick's face was smashed, it had been raining. His view of the batter and ball had been obstructed by a fan holding an open umbrella. Thus, after Zlotnick sued, his claim was not automatically dismissed. The judge found that by "allowing open umbrellas during the game, the Yankees . . . negligently increased the danger posed by the game of baseball."[11]

Elsewhere there were other judicial rumblings that baseball's liability exemption for fan injuries was no longer impenetrable. In 2014, "appeals courts in Georgia and Idaho . . . refused on technical grounds to adopt [the] long-standing legal principle . . . that shields teams and stadium owners from liability as long as a screen protects spectators in the most dangerous seats—those behind home plate."[12] More importantly, in 2015 an Ohio appeals court reversed a lower court, which had granted summary judgment to the Cleveland Indians in a case that was closely analogous to Zlotnick's.

In Ohio, the plaintiff had sued for damages after being injured by a ball that struck him when he had moved in the late innings. His lawyer alleged that all fans in that seating area had been asked to vacate to make way for a fireworks display after the game. As in Zlotnick's case, this particular plaintiff was allowed to sue, despite baseball's assumption of the risk protections, because of "attendant circumstances" that were not normally present.[13] A meaningful legal distinction had been drawn, which provided the court with grounds for concluding that the general precedent of the "baseball rule" did not apply.

Two other developments, around the same time, contributed to a perception that fan injuries were a growing problem for MLB and its new commissioner, Rob Manfred. First, there was a startling *Bloomberg News* investigation, which in 2015 had documented the large number of injuries caused mostly by foul balls "at major league games." Those investigators concluded that about "1,750 spectators get hurt each year . . . [which is] more often than a batter is hit by a pitch." Among those unintended injuries were a few extremely disturbing head and skull traumas to children, as well as to adults like Zlotnick. The article noted that unlike the NHL, "which mandated netting behind the goal line and higher Plexiglas above the side boards . . . , Major League Baseball [had] done little to reduce the risk."[14]

Second, based on shifting attitudes about fan safety and the cracks in baseball's assumption of risk legal armor, two law firms filed a "class action lawsuit on behalf of all season ticket holders against Major League Baseball and Commissioner Rob Manfred." It alleged that "Manfred . . . 'failed to uphold his duties to enact safety measures against the danger of foul balls and broken bats through a pattern of negligence [and] misrepresentation.'"[15]

With great fanfare, MLB's commissioner recommended that every team "erect protective netting in front of the most exposed field-level seats from one dugout to the other."[16] Unfortunately, what Manfred was proposing did not adequately protect the fans at risk. In large part this was because MLB was still trying to juggle competing concerns: safety, legal liability for acknowledging a known danger, and the loss of revenue if netting made premium seats less attractive to ticket holders.

The most obvious deficiency was that Manfred's proposal did not cover exposed field-level seats beyond the dugout where a lot of the hard-hit balls land. Furthermore, the new policy was only a recommendation.

Teams and businesses that own the baseball stadiums could still choose to protect—or not to protect—their fans how they pleased.

Not surprisingly, teams have continued to rely on baseball's assumption of the risk rule to protect them from liability. Their position remains that "it is up to the fans to pay attention. . . . [W]hen they come to the ballpark, they do so knowing that they . . . might be hurt."[17] Making matters worse, the new policy does not provide for compensation to injured fans to pay for their medical bills, long-term impairments, and loss of time at work. Much like players who can no longer perform, injured fans typically are on their own.

By making these changes, though, baseball acknowledged—at least implicitly—that there is a basic standard of care that teams should exercise. This recognition may well provide plaintiffs' lawyers with enough legal ammunition to convince courts that the assumption of risk protections accorded baseball are no longer absolute. Someday the baseball rule may be overturned in many or most jurisdictions. Moreover, should a team fail to follow MLB's recommendations, or do so incompletely, that team could be opening itself up to liability if, as a result of not providing enough protection, a fan is injured.

Over time, what is deemed legally acceptable for baseball teams to do with respect to protecting their fans is likely to evolve. That will create greater liability risks for teams and better opportunities for injured fans to receive appropriate compensation. All MLB teams have made some effort to comply with the new commissioner's recommendation, "though in some cases, teams really didn't do much beyond widening the netting behind home plate a few feet in either direction."[18]

The Minnesota Twins and a few other clubs may have complicated legal matters for the league by "extending their netting to the far ends of the dugouts, protecting seats usually sold to season-ticket holders." While this is the more prudent course of action for every team to take, it could impose liability on all the teams that continue to do less when "trying to balance intimacy [of the baseball experience] with safety."[19]

Ultimately, as Joe Nocera pointed out, "safety needs to come before intimacy,"[20] and someday it probably will. The dangers to fans have become too apparent to continue to be ignored or marginalized. Yet, it remains likely that with regard to these new safety measures, most teams will only do what is perceived as necessary to avoid liabilities that could eat into their profits. Thus, despite a number of new serious fan injuries from foul balls and broken bats in 2016, including one during game 7 of the World Series, MLB did nothing more than say that it would be "'evaluating and reviewing the data' during the off-season."[21]

# Part IV

# Why Elite Athletes Sacrifice Their Health

# 20

# PERFORMANCE-RISK REWARDS
# UNDERMINE HEALTH

## THE ACCELERATED HEALTH RISKS OF BEING AN
## ELITE ATHLETE

Playing with pain, taking drugs to suppress pain or enhance athletic performance, and enduring brain trauma, broken and shattered bones, torn and shredded ligaments, and other serious and potentially catastrophic impairments continue to be prominent health risks for athletes in America's most popular spectator sports. Football, whose popularity in the United States is unsurpassed, poses the greatest risks to its players. The strong linkage between increased health risks and popularity is not a coincidence.

At the same time, in the sports world there is a resigned, almost casual acceptance of the physical and mental impairments and addictions that these athletes endure. This raises the question of what the leagues and organizations responsible for operating and benefiting from these sports do to minimize those risks and care for their prized athletes' welfare when they become impaired. The answer tends to be what is necessary to fully exploit an athlete's talents—and too often considerably less than that.

Health neglect continues to exist for elite athletes at all levels of competition, especially when they are no longer able to compete. Even at the top of the athletic food chain, American collegiate, Olympic, and professional athletes often receive poor health care, and very little in the way of aftercare, rehabilitation, and disability benefits when their impairments and addictions become permanent and debilitating. In addition, when impairments involve mental disabilities and cognitive deficiencies, stigma and social stereotypes, which are heightened in the sports world, encourage athletes to keep their conditions secret.

In many ways, health care for elite athletes tends to be exploitation stacked in favor of those who organize, manage, and benefit from, but do not play, these sports. For professional, college, and Olympic athletes health care is inadequate with respect to both prevention and long-term care. The situation is even worse for the vast majority of American athletes who are hoping to become elite. This power imbalance also has created serious privacy and confidentiality gaps. Typically it is the teams paying for the limited health care their athletes receive that are the real clients, regardless of the medical ethics involved.

And for those elite American athletes who have stopped playing their sports due to physical and mental impairments, or develop serious and sometimes grave health conditions later in life as a result of having played professional, Olympic, or collegiate sports, few programs exist to care for their needs. Mostly, the athletes are on their own, regardless of the circumstances or the need. If former athletes lack the resources or wherewithal to care for their costly long-term physical or mental impairments and/or addictions, the results can be debilitating, devastating, and occasionally catastrophic. This is true even though it has become abundantly clear that in our most popular spectator sports, being—or trying to be—an elite athlete presents greatly accelerated health risks.

## PERFORMANCE-RISK REWARDS DIMINISH ATHLETES' HEALTH

The United States has not been known for its inclusive and comprehensive health care practices for anyone who cannot pay. Affordable care is provided grudgingly, if at all. Thus, it is hardly surprising that with regard to our most popular spectator sports, any type of health care and prevention tends to be distorted by performance-risk rewards, especially the generation of revenues.

Elite athletes are viewed as moneymaking commodities and perceive themselves as supermales or superfemales who have remarkable powers of recovery and special abilities to endure pain. Overwhelmingly these athletes—and athletes-to-be—favor short-term fitness to play well now over long-term well-being—much like American politicians and voters give far more weight to what happens today or is about to happen tomorrow than what may happen in the more unknowable future.

Elite athletes—and those who manage and benefit from those athletes' talents and skills—tend to view health care from a narrow prism of attaining the fitness and pain endurance that are necessary to perform at or near peak levels for as long as possible. Normally this athletic catharsis lasts for a few years, or more rarely a decade or conceivably two. Almost everything that is done to improve health and fitness of athletes in sports is guided by perceived performance measures, outcomes, and rewards.

Athletes are constantly motivated to resort to various types of risky—and frequently improper or illegal—means to boost their competitive performance, which often compromise, or even devastate, their long-term health. Particularly in contact sports, wear and tear on the body is expected and various means are employed to minimize the negative effects on performance, to speed recovery, or to delay the inevitable. When drugs and other potentially toxic and addictive substances are added to the training, nutrition, treatment, and rehabilitation mix, long-term—and even short-term—negative health outcomes become less predictable, less beneficial, and more harmful.

British sports scholar P. David Howe has concluded that "the acceptance of risk [is] an inevitable consequence of professional participation in sport."[1] It also is a likely consequence for those hoping to become professionals or pseudoprofessionals competing in Olympic or collegiate sports. As the potential athletic rewards increase, so do the motivations for athletes to take greater risks with their bodies and their minds. Too often they are encouraged and pushed on by their teams, handlers, supporters, and families, who are invested in the most positive athletic and financial outcomes possible.

Unfortunately, there are relatively few words of caution, certainly as compared to the many prescriptions to go for broke, which is what the best athletes are supposed to do, regardless of the consequences. Potential scholarships to private high schools and colleges and usually unrealistic possibilities of lucrative careers as professionals, not to mention the pride and glory of being an elite athlete, are more than enough motivation for most of them to risk their physical and mental health. This is particularly true for those who appear to have—or believe they have—few other comparable opportunities. Since the second half of the nineteenth century sports have provided a perceived—but often unrealistic—opportunity to scale the social and economic ladder.

Generally coaches of elite, potentially elite, or perceived to be elite athletes are not primarily educators who teach their charges the benefits of morality and the valuable lessons of life, as various sanguine sports myths would suggest. This is why the very few coaches who even appear to be educators stand out, or are made to stand out, at least until their own transgressions are revealed. Typically, though, if they are viewed as being really good at what they are being paid to do, coaches are not moral beacons. Instead they inculcate the skills, intensity, commitment to team, dedication, and shared values that are necessary to win and succeed, athletically, without cheating too much, or at least in less obvious ways than their opponents. The Dean Smiths and Pat Summits of the coaching world are extremely rare, which is why they are celebrated so much and placed in protective cocoons so their complete legacies do not upset the myths.

Not surprisingly, this tunnel vision and lack of candor tend to be inimical to effective preventive and rehabilitative health care strategies for elite athletes and athletes-to-be. Too often in our throwaway society we exploit all that we can enjoy today and in the near future, ignoring, dismissing, or postponing the day of reckoning that will surely come later. All the empty, unused stadiums and related leftover rubble in major metropolitan areas of the United States symbolize this attitude. On the human side, athletes ravaged by CTE, substance abuse, and other debilitating physical and mental impairments punctuate such reckless abandon.

There is little doubt that elite athletes "have better medical provisions than were available to competitors of yesteryear." Throughout this century, the potential for improved health care has increased in many different ways. Among other things, it has provided us with improved medical treatments, including sophisticated surgeries, genetic manipulations, and other interventions. Unfortunately, in the sports world improved health care is primarily available in order to boost athletic performance, rather than to maximize long-term physical and mental health.

As Howe intones, athletes' health is seriously jeopardized by rampant and uncontrolled "commercialism . . . and the importance of pain, injury and risk in the contemporary sporting world." On too many occasions, "sports medicine is . . . a tool used by sports administrators and club officials to fast-track elite sporting performers . . . back into competition." This leaves the athletes with the primary responsibility to look out for their own health and well-being. Too often such neglect produces poor, tragic, or even catastrophic results in order to feed a sports culture in which "the ultimate goal is to have . . . [athletes perform] . . . so that they can earn their 'keep.'"

Unhealthy practices and long-term health problems are found in all of America's most popular spectator sports, as has been documented throughout this book. Nevertheless, four types of glaring health risks illustrate, in compelling ways, how elite athletes have been exploited for their immediate performance capabilities at the expense of their overall well-being:

- baseball pitchers who risk their arms by throwing too hard and too often, particularly at a young age
- the acceptance of serious physical and mental injuries to athletes who play professional football
- the absence of proper health care and disability benefits for collegiate athletes, especially those who play in the major sports programs that generate the largest revenue streams for their universities and colleges
- the failure to adequately address stigma and stereotypes that negatively affect and often devastate athletes who have or are likely to have mental impairments or addictions as a result of playing their sports

# 21

# ARM INJURIES TO ELITE YOUNG PITCHERS IN BASEBALL

**D**ecades ago, but still in the modern era, professional pitchers would routinely throw for many more innings than they do now, both in single games and during a season, apparently with far less risk of incurring the types of arm injuries that have been called an epidemic today.[1] Sandy Koufax's arm burnout was the exception, not the general rule. Given the velocity he generated and the torque on his curveball, however, he might have been foreshadowing what has happened to today's pitchers.

## THROWING HARD YOUNGER, MORE OFTEN, WITH MORE TORQUE

Today's pitchers tend to be bigger, stronger, and in many ways fitter than ever before. Good pitchers, like good quarterbacks, tend to be the best athletes in their sports communities. Thus, the increasing prevalence of arm injuries appears to be due, at least in part, to the early age in which pitchers begin throwing hard, often year-round, especially if they want to be viewed as being elite at the next level of competition. Sandy Koufax was pitching in the major leagues when he was nineteen years old.

In recent years the average velocity of pitches has been increasing, along with the torques on pitchers' arms because of the variety of curves and sliders that they throw. So many young pitchers with notable talent try to throw like Nolan Ryan, who somehow defied normal physiology.

Medical researchers at the American Sports Medicine Institute have concluded that forty pounds of biomechanical force is the point at which the
normal human arm breaks apart.[2]

Today, that amount of force is what the typical major-league pitcher
experiences on a regular basis before and after he makes it to the big
leagues. Therefore, it seems reasonable to surmise that the hardest throw-
ers endure a considerably greater impact than that. For young pitchers
with immature arms using less sophisticated training methods, the potential injury point is significantly less. That alone could explain the rash of
arm injuries to so many young, hard-throwing pitching stars like Stephen
Strasburg, Matt Harvey, Dylan Bundy, Jameson Taillon, and Jose Fernandez. Even though their pitch counts as professionals have been tightly
controlled, all of them have "blown out their elbow[s]," temporarily or
forever.

Arm injuries also occur with greater frequency to "elite high school
[pitchers who] throw in the upper 90s." *Sports Illustrated*'s Tom Verducci found that of the "top 30 [pitcher draft] picks from 2010–2012 . . . 38
percent [had] . . . Tommy John [elbow] surgery before age 22."[3] These
arm problems are not a particularly new phenomenon, although they have
been becoming more frequent it seems. Back in 2006, *USA Today* ran a
feature, which concluded that "increasingly ace 11- and 12-year old hurl-
ers [were] developing overuse injuries—most noticeably . . . in their . . .
shoulder[s and elbows]."[4] As a result of growing concerns about such
injuries, many youth leagues—but certainly not all of them—began enforcing pitch counts and mandatory rest periods between pitching out-
ings, particularly for starting pitchers.

That change, like reducing contact during practices in some football
youth leagues, was as much a smoke screen as an effective solution. What
youth leagues did not do was limit the number of months in the year that
these young pitchers throw. Too often the accumulated strains on Little
League pitching arms require surgeries years later, assuming these young
athletes continue to pitch in high school, college, and/or as professionals.
Not only do the many assaults on their arms accumulate over time, as
players age into adulthood their tendons and ligaments become less flex-
ible and more subject to tearing.

Whatever the biomechanical explanations may be as to why youngsters are placing more strain on their arms—which is producing more
injuries, particularly later on in their careers—the primary motivation for

assuming this risk appears to be money and fame. The rewards that go to collegians and professionals who pitch extremely well, even for a few years, pushes these special and not so special kids, encouraged by their parents and coaches, to establish pitching dominance at an early age. Young elite pitchers do this by using pitches that immature arms are not well adapted to throw without creating substantial elbow and shoulder problems. The kinds of throws that make elite pitchers extraordinary appear to be high risk over the course of a player's career, but especially when pitchers are adolescents or young adults trying to make an impression on scouts and other talent evaluators.

## TOMMY JOHN SURGERY AND TEARING ARMS TO SHREDS

One of the most popular medical procedures for those whose arms become damaged or are likely to become damaged is Tommy John surgery, named after the first pitcher to successfully undergo the operation in 1974. It is used now not only to repair long-term damage, but also to attempt to repair and restore pitchers' arms after years of abuse at a young age so they can potentially throw harder than they did before their injuries manifested themselves. This assumes, though, that those players are diligent during the many months of rehabilitation that is required to maximize their recoveries and there are no setbacks. Otherwise, this risk taking can fail miserably, leaving prospects with broken arms and broken dreams.

For many of those pitchers, Tommy John surgery and the intense recovery process afterward are viewed as performance enhancing, at least in the short term. In that skewed sense, the operation can be perceived as an opportunity to enhance their careers. If the pitchers already have signed lucrative contracts and are being paid well while they rehab with good doctors and skilled trainers, their long layoffs may seem less oppressive and even necessary in order to continue receiving extraordinary monetary rewards.

Not surprisingly, the number of Tommy John and other invasive arm surgeries has skyrocketed as the hype surrounding them has intensified. In the major leagues where these arm operations are tracked, there were just seventeen Tommy John surgeries in the twenty years after the first one was performed.[5] In the next twenty years, however, there were 655, with 456 of them being performed during the ten-year period from 2004 through 2013. By the end of April 2014, there already had been thirty-one of these complex elbow operations, threatening to break the annual record of sixty-eight, which was set in 2012.

As *Washington Post* baseball writer Dave Sheinin has noted, two aspects of this substantial increase in arm injuries and surgeries appear to be not only remarkable, but disturbing. First, today's pitchers, when they begin their major-league careers, "have more overall mound experience . . . [and] are . . . more fundamentally sound in their pitching motions"[6] than any previous generation. These players tend to throw harder as measured by the biomechanical impact on their arms. This suggests that pitchers' arms are being overused in different ways than in the past. Nonetheless, baseball insiders continue to complain that pitchers are being babied both in the minor and major leagues. This suggests that carefully managing pitch counts has not solved the problem. One major problem with that approach seems to be the physiology involved. Once a pitcher attains a certain maximum velocity, each additional mile an hour the pitcher adds increases the impact on his arm "by multiples . . . like the Richter scale [for earthquakes]."[7]

In other words, the closer pitchers come to consistently throwing their fastballs and sliders in the high nineties—much less the low hundreds—the more likely their arms will be "torn to shreds."[8] Being able to throw that hard, consistently, has become a requirement for many pitchers who do not have the control and variation that allows them to be successful with less velocity. Today major-league hitters generally have the skills to take advantage of fastballs that are neither deceptive nor exceedingly fast. Thus, being fundamentally sound in one's pitching motion is far different from being able to pitch well in terms of location and utilizing change of speeds and a variety of pitches and motions.

## THE ART OF PITCHING WITHOUT THROWING TOO HARD

In the long run, a pitcher may well be better off health- and career-wise throwing his fastball at ninety to ninety-four miles an hour or slower, rather than ninety-five to one hundred.[9] The ability to throw that hard for six or more innings on a consistent basis and completely recover on only four or five days' rest has created a credible suspicion that many of the pitchers who are able to do this, like Roger Clemens once did, are using various performance- and recovery-enhancing measures, both legal and illegal. From that perspective, a sound training policy would be to encourage pitchers to learn the art of pitching, so that they do not have to depend so much on throwing hard. Unfortunately, with regard to learning these more nuanced skills, it appears that today's young professional pitchers—and wannabes—are less prepared than their predecessors.

Hall of Fame pitcher Greg Maddux achieved the pinnacle of baseball success by using this nuanced approach, averaging less than ninety miles per hour on his fastball. At the same time, the perception has been created that registering at least a strikeout an inning by throwing as hard as possible much of the time is what the most celebrated pitchers do. In addition, they are rewarded for doing this by various pitching analytics. Greg Maddux, who retired in 2008, was arguably among the two or three most exceptional pitchers of his era, but never came close to attaining the celebrity of pitchers like Roger Clemens and Randy Johnson, who threw harder and struck out many more batters per inning. It was only later in his career, and after he retired, that Maddux's greatness was more fully appreciated.

Nolan Ryan remains a legend because he was the hardest thrower of his day, setting season and career records for strikeouts and no-hitters. By other measures, though, he was often very good, but only occasionally great. Tim Lincecum in 2008 and 2009 won consecutive Cy Young Awards with the San Francisco Giants and a huge payday before his career was derailed by arm fatigue and other injuries.

In his prime, Lincecum was known for his violent pitching motion, low earned run average, meager hits per inning, and high strikeout totals. Yet, even in his best seasons, Lincecum never won more than eighteen games. Given his relatively small physical stature and the fact that his father was a biomechanical engineer, Lincecum was celebrated as a pitching marvel. Once he lost several miles an hour on his fastball and slider, however, he became a mediocre major-league starting pitcher at best, who as of 2016 had yet to master the art of pitching well without high velocity. He was cut by the Giants and was given a second chance by the pitching-depleted Los Angeles Angels, but was released before the season ended. He has never come close to reprising his greatness.

On the other hand, there is the remarkable story of longtime pitching star Mark Buehrle, who registered more than two hundred wins and fourteen straight seasons of two hundred innings or more without ever being seriously injured. He has been a consummate pitcher, yet a consistently soft thrower and underappreciated performer. His "average fastball velocity . . . [is] a tick over 83 mph," which is the second slowest in the majors. Unfortunately, he also is viewed as being "so far removed from anybody else, his example only applies to him."[10]

Regardless, Buehrle has been a testament to the advantages of not overthrowing and learning how to pitch to locations and to use change of speeds instead. He has been the turtle who won the race against most of the fastest hares. The fact that his style—like that of Greg Maddux—is rarely followed does not prove that this approach cannot be adapted for many or even most other pitchers. Youngsters should learn the basics of arm conservation, and the value of doing so needs to be promoted more aggressively. Of those pitchers who can throw ninety-five miles an hour, there are relatively few who have successful major-league careers, in substantial part because the injury rates are so high and the complementary pitching techniques so poorly taught and learned.

## YOUNG PITCHERS ARE PITCHING TOO MUCH

A second major problem for elite pitchers is that while they may be throwing less frequently at the minor- and major-league levels than ever before, as adolescents they are pitching more, when they should be pitching less. As with other major sports in the United States today, many elite athletes play one sport almost all year round, so that they can specialize and further develop their exceptional talents. Unfortunately, the American Sports Medicine Institute, which studied young pitchers, "found that kids who pitched competitively for more than eight months of the year were five times as likely to undergo arm surgery." Not surprising, kids who pitch in "warm-weather climates [have] . . . a higher incidence of Tommy John surgery."[11]

Even if pitchers take a break from baseball, they still may be overusing their shoulders and arms by playing other sports that place additional stress on the joints, tendons, and muscles in their dominant arm. This happens frequently with star pitchers, who often are great athletes in other arm-dependent sports, especially being quarterbacks in football, but also as basketball, hockey, or tennis players.

The far from universally followed Little League rules to limit the number of pitches kids can throw in a game certainly helps control the potential arm damage, if those rules are strictly enforced. Unfortunately, too often pitch restrictions by themselves fail to ameliorate the damage because so many of these kids never get a chance to properly rest their arms. Journalist and author David Epstein, citing a recent "longitudinal study . . . at Loyola University in Chicago" on youth sports, concluded that there is an "epidemic of hyperspecialization . . . , [which] is both dangerous and counterproductive." That study found young athletes "who were highly specialized had a 36 percent increased risk of suffering a serious overuse injury."[12]

Such overuse can occur when athletes rely on the same muscle groups in several sports. Thus, while it makes sense to encourage kids to try a variety of sports, it makes more sense to encourage them to participate in sports that utilize different muscle groups so those body parts actually get a respite. Thus, kids who play baseball seriously should rest their arms by playing soccer or running track, or even better by playing chess, being on student council, or participating in drama.

In addition, the types of pitches that youngsters are encouraged to throw place excessive strains on their arms. Like professionals, their elbows and shoulders also can be literally "torn to shreds." Playing baseball year-round can be a substantial risk, even for young players who do not pitch. One study indicated that nearly 50 percent of youth baseball players who sustained serious lesions on their elbows were not pitchers.[13] Somewhat counterintuitively, catchers had the highest risk of such injuries, accounting for about 25 percent of them, even though they are far outnumbered by pitchers.

Yet, it is the elite pitchers who are more likely to sustain career-ending or debilitating arm injuries. Moderation and common sense, which could prevent many of these arm problems in these prized young athletes, tend to be jettisoned in the pursuit of scholarships, professional contracts, and personal glory. As detailed by Jeff Passan in both *Sports Illustrated* and his book on the subject, one of the most insidious influences on the arms of young pitchers who want to be viewed as elite are "showcases and tournaments run by companies," which invent competitions, in addition to baseball games and practices, to determine who can throw the hardest.

One company called Perfect Game "posts national player rankings for every age group starting with freshmen in high school. Kids obsess over the rankings,"[14] along with the college and professional scouts.

The irony is that the closer most elite pitchers come to attaining their baseball dreams, the greater the risk seems to be that their arms will break down. Whether and how to assume that risk are not the types of decisions that most young minds make well. Someone needs to be looking after their best interests, which clearly is not happening much of the time.

# 22

# FOOTBALL INJURIES IN THE NFL AND COLLEGE

**W**hile long-term concussion risks of playing football have received most of the media's attention—particularly those linked to CTE—the frequency of injuries during games and full-contact practices should be alarming as well. That is why many commentators believe injuries—or their relative absence—are the single most important factor in determining which professional and college football teams are successful, especially in the NFL where there is significant parity among the teams. Injuries in the NFL, as well as in major collegiate football programs, have become a cottage industry for those who want to provide the latest player and team information to owners of fantasy football teams, gamblers, and other fans.

Today, it is very easy to find that type of NFL and NCAA superconference football injury information, which affects the outcome of games. It is far more difficult, though, to obtain annual totals in the NFL, much less broken down by the types of injuries. It is even more difficult to find meaningful statistics on football-related injuries for athletes who play in college. The NCAA's last published compilation covered 2004–2009. It measured injuries based on something called "athlete exposures," which allowed these collegiate programs to claim the football injury rate was ridiculously low: only "8.1 per 1,000 athletes." Thereafter, the NCAA turned over data collection to an affiliated nonprofit called the Datalys Center For Sports Injury Research and Prevention, which apparently maintains secrecy by only providing statistics on request to athletic programs of NCAA members.[1]

Nonetheless, despite the lack of comprehensive public information, it should be apparent that in professional, collegiate, and high school football, injuries are rampant. In the NFL, according to the league's own statistics, the number of injuries in a year approaches three-quarters of the number of total players. There are about thirteen hundred injuries per year[2] and about seventeen hundred players. Even kickers and punters— who generally avoid contact, are specially protected by the rules, and are used for only a very few plays each game—are injured frequently. While there are significant differences in injury rates based on the positions these athletes play, the carnage is spread all over the field, every single game, on every play.

Furthermore, the overall injury rates, as measured by the NFL, have remained high, especially concussions, which in 2015 actually substantially increased[3] despite the rule changes. Making matters worse, these injury compilations do not include drug addictions and other long-term physical and mental impairments that compel players to retire from professional and collegiate football, or present serious symptoms years or decades later. The current compilations only estimate the more immediate damage to players.

## THE *PITTSBURGH TRIBUNE-REVIEW* STUDY OF THE NFL

Much of the carnage in competitive football is obscured because meaningful statistics are hard to come by. During the summer of 2005, the *Pittsburgh Tribune-Review* published the results of the most comprehensive investigative study—before or since—about what has been happening with regard to injuries week to week during the NFL's regular season. The *Tribune-Review* published its results toward the end of the Paul Tagliabue era just as concussion concerns were gaining momentum. Since then, the injury problem has grown worse—or at least has been identified more readily, which would make the problem appear to be worse.

For the Pittsburgh study, a team of investigative reporters gathered all the weekly injury reports in the NFL from 2001 through 2004, "tallying the who, what, when, where, and why of 6,558 injuries over [those] four years." The reporters supplemented their statistical research with NFL injury reports for the past sixty years and interviewed "hundreds of current and former players, coaches, league officials, trainers, . . . sports physicians and university statisticians." The intent was to ensure that the study's conclusions reflected the opinions of the "gridiron expert[s]" they had consulted.[4]

The findings were stunning. They also quantified NFL injuries in a number of different ways. The results appear to have provided much of the impetus for the players union and former players to take actions against the league, including litigation. At a bare minimum, that study provided compelling data to those who, for different reasons, were most concerned about such injuries and their implications: players, former players, the NFL, various lawyers, and the sports media.

During the four-year period that the study had examined, approximately "half of the NFL's players [were] hurt every season." Not surprisingly, players on defense sustained more injuries than those on offense. A defensive back had "a 30 percent greater risk . . . than a quarterback . . . [who] touches the ball on every offensive play." Two-thirds of all defensive backs were injured each season; half of them were hurt a second time with an "unrelated injury."[5]

A major reason for this high rate of injuries at that particular position is physics. While all the other players had increased their body mass by "25 percent . . . over the past six decades . . . , the average cornerback or safety [had] barely changed [in size]." Since defensive backs have to regularly tackle receivers, tight ends, running backs, and quarterbacks head-on, this growing size differential has made these smaller players especially vulnerable "to routine spine, head and bone injuries." Similarly, placekickers and punters, who were thought to be largely immune from "the violence,"[6] had a 20 and 14 percent risk, respectively, of being injured each year, even though they are called on to play only a few downs in each game.

Furthermore, the study found that overall "half of NFL players [would] leave football because of a debilitating injury." Twenty-five percent were known to "suffer lifelong degenerative bone and joint conditions or mental illness." In addition, "more than a third of all linemen [suffered] from obstructive sleep apnea, not to mention . . . high blood pressure, fatigue and heart problems." Despite the high rates of long-term physical and mental impairment, the study confirmed what was already well known by then: that "impoverished"[7] former players, of which there continue to be many, did not receive adequate long-term health care after their NFL careers were over.

The players union, which according to the collective bargaining agreement was responsible for paying for such care out of the many millions of dollars active players had received from the league, was defaulting on its responsibilities. Annually there were "more than 500 new claims . . . from impoverished veterans, but the union ha[d set aside] only enough cash to help a fraction of them,"[8] and never supplemented that amount to address the growing need for better health care and related benefits. Moreover, it was likely that many legitimate claims were never filed because otherwise entitled players believed it would be fruitless to do so.

The investigators involved in the *Tribune-Review* study concluded that the steady increase in injuries was not only due to the fact that players were becoming larger, faster, and stronger—pushed on, no doubt, by the widespread use of performance-enhancing substances. In addition, over the years the game had grown more violent due to "blitzing behemoths and high-velocity collisions . . . between receivers and men hurtling to crush them." Linemen on both sides of the ball had learned a variety of new aggressive physical techniques to combat their opponents. Nevertheless, as the "league shifted the rules to spur offensive production there was a disproportionate increase in injuries to defenders." The myth that professional football used to be more violent than it is today cannot be reconciled with the physical and biomedical realities. The pre-1978 game with its "weekly scrum of lumbering linemen and pounding rushers . . . 'killed you slowly.'" Today's game "'[kills] you quickly' with punishing high impact, high-velocity body blows."[9]

Moreover, reliance on rewards for defensive players, either in the form of praise or money, to encourage them to deliberately injure opponents, and the use of chop blocks and other techniques by offensive players to incapacitate defensive players through their legs, have demonstrated all too graphically how the game has devolved. Football has become ritualized combat in which almost anything that can be done without the referees calling a penalty will be tolerated, and often encouraged. There is very little perceived value in playing by the rules or avoiding situations in which opponents are more likely to be seriously injured. Football is not a sport that produces healthy competition. It is survival of the fittest and luckiest, which, in that skewed sense, makes football players like the gladiators of Rome.

# 23

# THE NCAA PROVIDES SHAMEFULLY INADEQUATE HEALTH CARE FOR ITS STUDENT-ATHLETES

**W**hen it comes to the health of its athletes, perhaps no organizational structure governing major American spectator sports is more irresponsible and uncaring than the NCAA and its members, especially the universities and colleges with major football and basketball programs. Despite burgeoning revenues generated from athletics, health care for college athletes remains an unconscionable mess. In most respects it is even worse than health care in the NFL, which is an important reason why the call to unionize college athletes resonated so loudly.

The overriding issue for college athletes, beyond being paid for their athletic contributions, is gaining rights and entitlements so they can obtain health benefits and better control their college lives.[1] This includes obtaining assurances that "the next generation of athletes diagnosed with concussions and other medical ailments . . . [will] be taken care of."[2] NCAA president Mark Emmert's position has been vague at best. In lieu of unionization, which he says would be "'inappropriate . . . , long-term medical coverage . . . [should be the subject of] a good debate. . . . The devil is in the details,"[3] he has proclaimed with little urgency or conviction.

Emmert has acknowledged that there is a need for "legitimate, good, high quality [health] coverage going forward." Unfortunately, he said, there would be difficulties getting the necessary approvals from the NCAA's "membership." If the past is a key indicator, after a time-con-

suming, self-congratulatory debate it is likely that the NCAA will continue to do little or nothing to protect its indentured student-athletes. Traditionally, the NCAA has almost always valued making more money for
member schools more than providing for the health of its athletes. Little
has happened to change that reality. Three examples illustrate the depth
of the health care abuses and dysfunctions that have characterized
NCAA-governed athletic programs in recent years.

## LITTLE HELP FOR DEBILITATING INJURIES

The first incident originated some forty years ago. Yet, it was written
about again during the movement to unionize college athletes because
after all that time little has changed for the better. Fred Rensing became
quadriplegic during a football practice at Indiana State University in 1976
when he tackled a teammate who was returning a punt.[4] That catastrophic
accident left him without the use of most of his body, although his mind
was fully intact.

Ironically, how Rensing chose to respond to his university's refusal to
provide him with compensation helped shape the law that now strongly
favors the NCAA and its member schools. His ordeal demonstrated the
vulnerability of all collegiate athletes when they sustain severe physical
and/or mental impairments while playing for their universities and colleges. Indiana State's insurance only covered "initial expenses" for hospi-
talization and treatment, which is typical of what happens now as well.
The rest of Rensing's treatment, rehabilitation, and long-term care Indiana State left him to cover, as a remembrance of his career-shortened
contributions to its athletic program.

After his injury, health-related payments initially were quilted together from several sources: his family's insurance policy, money from his
parents directly, and "community . . . fund-raisers to help offset the initial
costs."[5] When he was finally released after months of rehabilitation,
Rensing returned home to his parents' garage, which they had transformed into a wheelchair-accessible bedroom. He was better off than
many collegiate athletes would have been in that situation because he had
parents with some financial resources to help him out.

Nevertheless, Rensing realized that for the rest of his life there would
be large medical and related expenses for him to pay regularly, his being

employed was highly unlikely, and he "would always need caretakers to dress him, feed him and help him out of bed."[6] In 1977, after Indiana State refused to cover any of his long-term expenses, he decided to apply for workers' compensation benefits to help pay for his care. That program, among other things, was created to provide a regular stipend to employees who were injured on the job. The greater the injury and medical expenses are, the greater the award. The cost is split between the employer and the applicable state.

When his administrative claim for benefits, which the university opposed, was summarily dismissed, Rensing appealed. His turned out to be a "novel" lawsuit in Indiana, which had the potential to create an important legal precedent governing whether college athletes in Indiana—and elsewhere—were employees as defined under state law. Rensing's claim was vigorously challenged by "Indiana State . . . , the N.C.A.A., as well as nearby [Indiana] universities."[7] For financial reasons, all of these educational institutions opposed providing workers' compensation benefits to athletes who are permanently impaired playing collegiate sports.

The legal outcome hinged on two factors: whether Rensing's scholarship was considered a "contract for hire"; and whether collegiate athletes are pseudoprofessionals, or student-athletes "governed by 'strict' rules 'designed to protect [their] amateur status.'" It took six years for the case to be resolved. In 1982, a divided state appeals court ruled in Rensing's favor. The scholarship he had received was deemed to be a "contract for hire . . . [which] created an employer-employee relationship."[8] A year later, however, a divided Indiana Supreme Court reversed. A majority of those justices concluded that Rensing had not been paid as a professional employee. Rather, he was considered to be a nonprofessional student-athlete—as conveniently defined by the NCAA—who had received benefits that were strictly limited because of his amateur status.

The state high court's rationale was based largely on a myth. The NCAA had created the mythology in the mid-1960s after two different courts in other states had concluded "scholarship students killed in the course of their athletic duties were . . . university 'employees' due workers' compensation." Under the leadership of its executive director at the time, Walter Byers, the NCAA "coin[ed] the well-worn phrase 'student-athlete' to describe college athletes." According to Byers, he had invented the phrase as an Orwellian deception to be "embedded in all NCAA rules and interpretations as a mandated substitute for such words as players and athletes."[9]

That self-serving legal fiction has insulated universities and colleges from their financial responsibilities to athletes, not the least of which is providing adequate health care and disability benefits to those who are severely injured playing their sports, even when they are generating profits for their schools. The NCAA has had the audacity to use Byers's distorted concept of amateurism to deliberately limit the health care universities and colleges were permitted to provide to their student-athletes.[10] Under the NCAA's twisted logic, which regrettably courts have accepted, providing most types of health care and disability benefits to college athletes would make these student-athletes professionals. Even with the impaired athletes' consent, colleges would violate the presumed sanctity of the student-athletes' protection by providing them with essential health-related services.

In 2013 the NCAA relented, but only incrementally. Universities and colleges were given "more freedom to provide [health] care for athletes." In other words, there no longer was a prohibition, but, then again there was no actual health care mandate. Schools have to "certify that players have a primary health insurance policy . . . , [which] the universities do not have to pay for," unless they want to. In the event of a "catastrophic injury," a new NCAA program "kicks in when expenses exceed $90,000."[11] That means that most student-athletes are responsible for the first $90,000 needed to care for any sports-related injuries. Furthermore, if the symptoms of a sports-related health impairment should occur after an athlete has left—or been dumped from—the program, there is no coverage at all.

## DUMPING STUDENT-ATHLETES WHO CAN NO LONGER PERFORM DUE TO INJURIES

Even with those minor health care concessions, some of the most unconscionable health care abuses against college athletes have been allowed to continue. Not only may universities and colleges choose not to pay for health insurance and health care, even for injuries that occur on the playing field, after an injury they retain the right to revoke a student-athlete's scholarship. The stated rationale justifying such heartless revocations is entirely self-serving. Apparently once athletes become impaired enough that they are no longer cash cows able to fulfill the terms of their scholarships, the agreement between the athlete and the university or college may be voided.

Legally, the situation is treated as if the athletic program had purchased damaged goods and thus deserves some sort of rebate. More disturbingly, it is the university or college that determines whether an athlete's impairment is sufficient to cancel the scholarship. This distasteful state of affairs provides the context for another story, which exemplifies NCAA-facilitated health care abuses.

Kyle Hardrick came to the University of Oklahoma in 2009 as a prized basketball recruit. That first fall during practice, he injured his knee but was told he did not need physical therapy. His pain and dysfunction, though, continued not only for that season, but the next as well. Finally, in January 2011 his mother paid for him to have an MRI, which revealed that Hardrick had been trying to play with a torn meniscus.

Nevertheless, after challenging the family orthopedist's findings, the university refused to authorize and pay for the surgery. Instead, Hardrick had to use his family's insurance policy. Afterward questions remained about the health of his knee and his continuing ability to perform at the elite level necessary to play in a major college program. As a result, the Oklahoma basketball program deemed Hardrick's collegiate athletic career to be over, along with any hopes he had of playing professionally, and revoked his scholarship. This meant he was responsible for all the future medical costs associated with his damaged knee, as well as the cost of tuition and expenses if he chose to stay at Oklahoma.

## A GRUESOME INJURY DRAWS CONCERN, BUT LITTLE ELSE

Another example of the dumping of a high-profile damaged college athlete by a university involved a big-time basketball player. During the 2013 NCAA Tournament, Louisville's Kevin Ware sustained a gruesome injury on network television, which was replayed numerous times to a national audience. At the time, college athletes were being strongly encouraged to unionize, in large part so they could obtain improved health care benefits. Thus, Ware's severe injury became part of the national conversation about inadequate health insurance for college athletes, particularly for star players who "help generate hundreds of millions of dollars for their universities."[12]

For most of the 2012–2013 season Ware had been Louisville's starting point guard and heralded as a likely future NBA player. That was the year in which Louisville won the national championship. Because of his injury, Ware had to be hospitalized for "surgery to repair compound fractures to his tibia." Who would be paying the cost of any extended rehabilitation was unclear since the university only had "a secondary [health insurance] policy on its varsity athletes." Thus, it appeared likely that once Ware left the program, he would be "personally responsible for any health care expenses related to the injury,"[13] including any lingering impairments or nonapparent conditions that developed later.

These revelations produced a great deal of rancor toward the NCAA and big-time college basketball, even among ardent fans. Before that incident most fans did not understand or appreciate how much these university and college athletic programs were shortchanging their athletes. They assumed that these cash-rich programs were providing comprehensive health care to those players. The executive director of the National College Players Association observed that with all the money being generated by major collegiate sports, particularly basketball and football, "there are plentiful financial resources available . . . to ensure that all injured athletes—at all levels and not just at the biggest schools [are covered]."[14]

It turned out that the media's concerns about Ware's welfare were justified as his situation only grew worse. A year later, shortly after Louisville had lost during the 2014 NCAA Tournament, Ware was strongly encouraged—or told—to transfer, since it was likely that he would be losing his Louisville scholarship due to the lingering damage that his injury had caused. Before that season had begun, Louisville's coach, Rick Pitino, had remarked that the point guard's "limp in practice was concerning . . . and . . . declared [Ware] out for the season."[15] Apparently there had been sufficient funds available from alumni to hire paid escorts for recruits, which led Louisville to suspend itself for the 2016 NCAA Tournament, but no money was available to support a once-prized athlete whose talent had diminished because he had been injured playing for the university.

While attempts to unionize student-athletes under the auspices of the National Labor Relations Board ultimately failed on legal grounds, this unionization effort publicized the fact that the NCAA and its member universities and colleges badly neglect health care for their athletes. That neglect has been most apparent when serious impairments are involved. The primary concern has been to ensure that these athletes are able to perform at the highest level possible on game day in order to maximize wins and revenues. If these modern-day gladiators can no longer perform well, or their health care appears to be too costly and/or their athletic potential has been diminished as a result of an injury, these universities and colleges, through their athletic departments, typically abandon them. Health care for student-athletes only exists as long as these students can continue to perform as elite athletes, not a moment longer.

# 24

# STIGMA, STEREOTYPES, AND SECRECY UNDERMINE ATHLETES' MENTAL HEALTH

**M**any of the worst stereotypes and prejudices in America's most popular spectator sports involve mental impairments. An ironic twist has been added to this type of stigma and discrimination with revelations that concussions and subconcussive impacts to athletes playing many of those sports can cause severe mental disorders. These mental conditions may manifest themselves over years, as they have with many former football players, or almost immediately.

Specialists in neurology and psychiatry "say the days, weeks and months that . . . follow a traumatic brain injury can be crippling, particularly for young people."[1] Suicides by high school, college, and professional football players and other athletes who have experienced these head traumas are no longer viewed as extraordinary. Young adulthood and concussive impacts can be a lethal combination.

Tragically, treating athletes with mental disorders badly has been deeply ingrained in the American sports world. It is typically accentuated by a veil of secrecy, until tragedy strikes and media coverage becomes mandatory. Professional, collegiate, and Olympic teams concoct elaborate ruses in order to hide the fact that a player has a mental condition.

Adding to their distress, athletes who are unable to get on the playing field due to such an impairment are viewed as "'head case[s]' . . . one of the most damning labels in the front office"[2] and in locker rooms. They tend to be disparaged, and to disparage themselves, because even though they have no serious physical injuries, they are unable to play or practice with their teams. Their mental disorders are viewed as a lack of character, rather than an illness or disease. The sports environment often helps to prolong their conditions and makes them worse.

As compared to athletes with physical injuries—or even substance abuse problems—having a "mental illness remains largely stigmatized . . . and . . . largely undiagnosed."[3] In 1998, Robert Lipsyte wrote in the *New York Times* that "the discussion of any kind of mental illness [in sports] . . . had not progressed much beyond the 1950's Jimmy ("Fear Strikes Out") Piersall story."[4] Nearly "half a century [later] . . . the sports world . . . [has] remained largely in the dark on matters of mental health."[5]

Surprisingly this lack of enlightenment has continued, even though it is becoming increasingly apparent that due to the extreme stresses of competition, childhood athletic traumas, CTE, and unhealthy lifestyles, athletes "might be more prone to mental illness than the population at large." Certainly many elite athletes, due to their dedication and tunnel vision, are likely to experience stress, brain traumas, and other circumstances that hasten, worsen, or even cause mental disorders. At the same time, because of this heightened stigma of mental disabilities, athletes have been extremely reluctant to disclose (much less discuss and address) their conditions or problems. For many years only a few stories about elite athletes with mental disorders emerged, but usually only after the individuals had quit playing or because they had no other choice.

Terry Bradshaw, the CBS commentator who quarterbacked the Pittsburgh Steelers to four Super Bowls and was the NFL's MVP in 1978, revealed that he had episodes of depression throughout his career. After a game "he would hemorrhage sweat and dissolve into tears." Bradshaw admitted that even though he knew his non-football "life was going to hell in a hand-basket," he did not seek professional help. Instead, he and the people around him pretended that he was fine.

Vin Baker, who played professional basketball from 1993 to 2006, was frequently incapacitated by depression, the symptoms of which were difficult for him to hide. His unpredictable episodes led him to be perceived as unreliable and unmotivated. As one of his more sympathetic, but unenlightened, coaches told him, "Don't let the blues get you down!" Just "run it off,"[6] as if such advice would overcome a mental illness.

Former New York Mets pitcher Pete Harnisch was one of the few athletes to publicly acknowledge having a mental illness while he was still a player. Harnisch admitted to having a "depressive episode" that began Opening Day in 1997 and lasted most of that season. Yet, Harnisch "recoil[ed] at being a poster boy for depression," so he claimed unconvincingly "that his body chemistry [had been] destabilized when he abruptly quit a 13-year chewing tobacco habit."[7] Reportedly, his manager, Bobby Valentine, was so angry at Harnisch for his long bout with depression that at a team meeting he called his player "gutless," and soon after, Harnisch was traded.[8]

Professional hockey player Shayne Corson played fifteen distinguished NHL seasons, including winning a Stanley Cup and being selected to play for Team Canada. Corson admitted that throughout his career he would wake up "in the middle of the night panicking—'my heart pounding, tears in my eyes . . . I wouldn't know what to do.'"[9] During the 2002 playoffs, as a member of the Toronto Maple Leafs, Corson's anxiety became so debilitating and painful that he left the team. Instead of being sympathetic, "members of the press unleashed their daggers,"[10] accusing Corson of walking out on his team, and worse. And unlike what would have happened to him if his injury were physical, Corson forfeited millions of dollars that remained on his contract.

Unfortunately, due to stigma, stereotypes, and the ignorance of others, elite American athletes still feel the need to hide their mental disorders when symptoms arise; those who do not, often experience hate, a lack of empathy, and/or recriminations after their impairments are publicized. There have been numerous stories of professional athletes, coaches, and even referees who have had extreme difficulty trying to cope with their mental disorders in the sports world. These examples are in addition to the growing legions of former athletes who have been trying to cope with the symptoms of CTE and other degenerative cognitive impairments.

## PROFESSIONAL AND COLLEGIATE BASKETBALL

### Chamique Holdsclaw and the WNBA

One of the best women college basketball players of all time, Chamique Holdsclaw, experienced emotional problems sometime after joining the

WNBA's Washington Mystics in 1999. In 2002 and 2003 she had out-standing seasons, but thereafter symptoms of severe depression emerged, brought on in part by the death of the grandmother who had raised her. Reportedly, the basketball prodigy would miss practices, "sitting alone in the dark. . . ." She also "started drinking."[11]

Few knew what was troubling Holdsclaw because like most athletes she kept her mental problems a secret. When she finally opened up, Holdsclaw said that she was "labeled . . . a quitter . . . an enigma . . . or a 'problem.'"[12] Her illness was widely perceived as a character flaw, which was incompatible with being a good person, much less a great profession-al basketball player.

In July 2004, she went on an extended leave of absence for what was described as "an unspecified medical condition."[13] She missed the rest of the season. Neither she nor her team felt comfortable revealing the true nature of her situation. That October when reportedly she asked to be traded, her condition was revealed, not out of empathy, but as a justifica-tion for the Mystics giving up on one of the greatest players of all time. Holdsclaw thought "a fresh start 3,000 miles away would help, even though . . . she didn't want to play basketball."[14]

Not surprisingly, the move did not cure her illness. In 2006, which was her second season with the Los Angeles Sparks, she capped a "year-long battle with depression . . . [by] tak[ing] an entire vial of her once-daily antidepressant." This resulted in her being confined in a "psychiat-ric ward, rattled by hallucinations."[15] She retired from professional bas-ketball the next year but returned as a role player with the Atlanta Dream. Her last WNBA game was in 2010.

In 2012 Holdsclaw published her autobiography, which focused on her "mortal struggle with despair."[16] She, like former soccer star Briana Scurry and former San Francisco 49ers linebacker Chris Borland—who both apparently suffered their mental traumas due to concussions—tried to redefine herself as a "mental health advocate." Yet, within a few months, she would be "arrested and charged with aggravated assault for allegedly smashing the windows in the car of . . . [her] . . . former teammate [and] ex-girlfriend."[17]

Being a gay athlete with a mental illness placed her in an especially vulnerable position in terms of having to endure two stigmas. Making matters much worse, she was charged with committing a violent felony. It was first reported incorrectly that she had doused her ex-girlfriend's car in gasoline and "may have been trying to ignite it." What actually happened, according to police, was not much better: Holdsclaw had fired a bullet into that vehicle.[18] Based on her mental condition and perhaps her former sports celebrity status, Holdsclaw was allowed to plead guilty to felony assault without going to jail.[19] Unlike what normally happens to defendants with mental disabilities,[20] the American legal system helped ensure Holdsclaw received the empathy and treatment that had been lacking in the WNBA.

## Royce White and the NBA

Another major story involving a professional basketball player's battle with mental health issues occurred in the NBA, which is normally known as a player's league. Royce White was All-Big Ten, an honorable mention All-American, and one of the most physically talented athletes in the 2012 draft. Still, his draft stock was placed in limbo after he revealed he had an anxiety disorder, which included "a severe fear of flying" and "obsessive compulsive tendencies."[21] The key considerations in drafting him became: "How much risk are [NBA] teams willing to accept?"[22] And what changes would front offices be willing to make to reasonably accommodate this talented player?

Unlike most athletes with mental impairments who hide their conditions, White early on had bravely decided to be guided by "transparency," which led him to announce that flying around the country made him "scared as hell." *PTI* (*Pardon the Interruption*) sports commentator, podcast host, and former *Washington Post* and *New York Times* sports reporter and columnist Tony Kornheiser apparently has a similar anxiety disorder, which was a contributing factor in his leaving a much sought-after position as a broadcaster on *Monday Night Football*. John Madden apparently had a similar disorder. Both Kornheiser and Madden were given luxurious buses to use—with drivers—to accommodate their fear of flying so they could continue to broadcast these nationally televised games. Unfortunately, athletes with mental disorders tend to be treated with far less empathy than sports media personalities.

Although at one point White was viewed as a potential lottery choice, he dropped down to the Houston Rockets, who had the sixteenth pick in the first round. Despite his disappointment, Royce expressed gratitude that Houston was willing to take "a chance on me. They didn't have to."[23] At first his appeared to be a feel-good story.

Soon, however, a rift developed over the proper way to deal with his mental health issues, especially the provision of reasonable accommodations that would allow him to maximize his talent. The Rockets, the NBA, and most of the basketball media thought the team's front office should be allowed to make the decision as they pleased without having to adhere to any league or professional guidance.[24] Rockets management would decide each accommodation dispute when it arose without establishing a coordinated plan.

White, mental health professionals, and disability experts understood that planning for the players' accommodations involved complex questions, which required specific medical and legal expertise.[25] Thus, White insisted on an accommodations plan, which the Rockets refused to develop or implement. Neither White nor the Rockets budged from their positions, creating an impasse.[26] In the sports world this was viewed as White overstepping his bounds. Despite his basketball skills and talent, he was sent to the developmental league, which was unheard of for a player of his caliber.

As Phil Taylor explained to White in a patronizing and paternalistic open letter in *Sports Illustrated*, professional sports "will always be hazardous for someone with your anxiety condition. . . . 'Basketball might not be what is best for you.'"[27] Taylor's sentiment was similar to the somewhat more sympathetic journalistic advice Jonathan Martin received from the *New York Times'* William Rhoden, who wrote that Martin might want to quit professional football if, due to his emotional difficulties, he was not tough enough to withstand bullying from other players.[28] The clear implication from both journalists was that in the macho world of sports there is no place for athletes like White and Martin who need to be treated differently because of their mental health needs.

White, even before he was discriminated against, had become "an outspoken . . . advocate for mental health." He criticized the "disconnect between physical health and mental health" in athletics and insisted on a "protocol that would spell out in writing how his mental illness would be addressed," which, under the Americans with Disabilities Act (ADA), is supposed to happen with most employees who have a disability. The Rockets dug in their heels by arguing that providing an accommodation for White was "a potential violation of the collective bargaining agreement."[29]

While the team's lawyers had asserted a legitimate potential defense in refusing to properly accommodate White under the CBA, Rockets management certainly was not abiding by the spirit of the ADA. One of the main purposes of requiring reasonable accommodations is to provide a reliable structure so that both the employee with a disability and the employer know what to expect when situations like this arise. Nonetheless, the cooperation and flexibility needed for these accommodation agreements to work well for both parties appear to be anathema to the inflexible and often tyrannical organizational structures of professional and collegiate team sports. If it failed so miserably in the NBA, it had little chance of succeeding in other professional leagues.

By the fall of 2013, White had been traded to the Philadelphia 76ers, who "waived him from their roster . . . before he had played a single non-exhibition game, leaving him to sit out the final days of his $1.7 million contract." This so-called trade appeared to be a face-saving gesture for the NBA because the 76ers never did anything that indicated any intent to allow White to play by accommodating his special needs. One of the major bones of contention continued to be White's fear of flying. All he said he wanted was for his team to "let him travel by bus when possible," rather than making him fly all the time. He hoped—unrealistically as it turned out—to be traded to "a team that . . . [took] mental health seriously enough to put some effort into it . . . because it is the right thing to do."[30]

It took many months for him to be even signed by another team, this time the Sacramento Kings. Not surprisingly, it was under a temporary ten-day contract at a minimal salary, meaning that he was starting over again as a professional player and the odds were seriously stacked against him. The next season he was completely out of the league, which always seems to happen to professional players when they complain that they are being discriminated against because they have a mental disorder or are gay. NBA insiders blamed White's predicament on his failure to "break down barriers . . . coping with [his] mental health." In that biased sports narrative, White's inability to overcome his illness without accommodations made him "the worst first-round pick ever."[31]

In the NBA where star players receive special considerations all the time, even with respect to enforcing the rules of the game, and the home team generally is called for fewer fouls than the road team, it is abhorrent to think that a player's disability cannot be accommodated in reasonable ways. Think of what would have been lost if the brilliance and eccentricities of Stephen Hawking had not been accommodated by his employers. In smaller but still similar ways, professional sports teams lose out whenever they fail to take steps to reasonably accommodate skilled athletes who are different. Moreover, such intransigence is a prominent example of how teams and leagues fail to address the health of their athletes.

## Collegiate Coach Chris Craig

A third disturbing story involving mental illness and a basketball figure concerns Chris Craig, who a few years ago was poised to become a highly successful collegiate basketball coach after finishing third at the National Junior College Athletic Association Championship in 2010. His fall from grace was as unexpected as the onset of his schizophrenia. According to George Dohrmann in *Sports Illustrated*, Craig's condition "distanced him from his family and robbed him of the game he loved."[32]

More accurately, though, Craig's family and basketball colleagues gave up on him when Craig quit coaching and began acting bizarrely, apparently unable to separate his religious delusions from reality. Those close to him initially expressed the sentiment that he deserved forgiveness for what his illness had caused him to do, but only if he was able to get better. As is typical, his mental impairment was viewed more as a character flaw than a disease. Yet, at first, his basketball status allowed Craig's religious rants and other abnormal actions to be treated less harshly in the communities in which he still was recognized, but only as long as those delusions were viewed as Christian rather than "Islamic." Once he crossed that religious line, however, he was viewed as being dangerous.

Soon Craig began to disappear from public view, trying to negotiate a very lonely and troubled existence. His wife established the grounds for his ostracism from their family and community by publicly announcing that his behavior had caused their child to suffer. Slowly but surely, his narrative was transformed from a coach who was once a pillar of the community to a forgotten and dangerous man. "Chris is still a great person inside," said his wife. Yet no one, including his former college basketball employer, wanted anything to do with the man Chris Craig had become, leaving it all up to him to return "to being the Chris we knew."[33]

# PROFESSIONAL AND COLLEGIATE FOOTBALL

## Erik Ainge and the NFL

It is not just professional and collegiate basketball that have demonstrated a lack of understanding and commitment in dealing with athletes and other people connected to the game when they become impaired by a mental disorder. In many ways basketball is more open to diversity and health issues than other sports, especially football and hockey. One of the more compelling football examples is former Jets backup quarterback Erik Ainge, the nephew of Boston Celtics general manager Danny Ainge.

The former Jets quarterback had a long history of addictions combined with what subsequently was diagnosed as bipolar disorder. At age twelve, he began alternately self-medicating and feeding his mental condition, first with marijuana and later with Adderall, heroin, cocaine, and alcohol. Like many football players, during his senior year at the University of Tennessee he also became "addicted to painkillers . . . downing them by the handful." Because of his bipolar disorder–fed "self-destructive lifestyle that included multiple overdoses, drunk driving, extended stays in rehab and relapses,"[34] his college athletic exploits were marginalized and eventually his professional football career was ruined.

Even though it should have been apparent based on his college history, from the start of the Jets' training camp in 2008 the team either did not know, wanted to ignore, and/or did not care about his condition or his history of mental disturbances. In the NFL, like most other professional team sports, almost all that counts is what a player does on the field of play. Players who cannot suit up are quickly forgotten, no matter what the reason for their absence might be. It becomes much worse, however, when there is no apparent physical injury that can explain their absence.

In November the NFL suspended him four games for taking steroids,[35] but taking performance-enhancing drugs or powerful painkillers is something many players do. Taking recreational drugs, however, is an entirely different matter, but only if doing so negatively affects a player's performance on the field or casts the team in a bad light. Early in 2009, things became so bad that Ainge had to enter a drug detoxification center and was compelled to tell Jets management what was happening to him, breaking the familiar code of secrecy. It was around this time he was first diagnosed with bipolar disorder, which it turned out, not surprisingly, that he had had "for a long time."[36]

Often what is viewed as a drug problem masks an underlying mental disorder that has been kept under wraps through denial and/or falsehoods. In the world of athletics it is far more acceptable to be compromised by drugs or alcohol than to be flawed by a mental illness. Normally, teams view mental disorders as something for the athletes to deal with and keep to themselves, rather than setting up support systems to help the players cope with their conditions.

Upon his release from detoxification, Ainge kept away from drugs for a time but did not take medication for his mental illness, becoming a self-described "hard-core alcoholic." He was "driving under the influence almost every night," and there was nobody associated with the Jets or the league trying to stop him. Alcoholism was a convenient alternative to taking drugs, now that the NFL during the season was testing him for drugs "three or four times a week"[37] because he had been identified as a chronic abuser.

During the end of the next off-season, however, in July 2010 just before training camps were to begin, Ainge "relapsed with hard drugs . . . [during] a two-week bender."[38] When he went back into rehabilitation, he was given medication to treat his bipolar disorder. Although still under a contract with the Jets, Ainge was encouraged to retire in June 2011. Both he and the Jets cited so-called injuries, rather than his mental disorder and addictions, as the reason.[39] Since he has been out of the NFL and relieved of the pressures to win and succeed as a quarterback, Ainge seems to have turned his life around. Although he has been arrested once on drunk driving charges, for several years now he has hosted a popular local Tennessee sports radio show.[40]

## Daniel Olson and Norbert College

The saga of Daniel Olson, an all-state quarterback for a Michigan high school team coached by his father, underscores the unnatural pressures of trying to be an elite athlete. According to Jeff Olson, Daniel's father and coach, his son had battled "severe anxiety and depression for years," but it was football that placed him in a "dark hole." The last stage of Daniel's disease seems to have been triggered after he had led his high school team to the state finals in 2010, but lost. Even though Daniel was directly responsible for his team scoring four touchdowns and was viewed as "the best player on the field . . . , he focused on the few mistakes he made."[41]

Instead of embracing his momentary stardom and being accepted at St. Norbert College where he would play defensive back as a freshman, "for weeks . . . Daniel woke up with night sweats, thinking about the loss." These obsessions continued during his first season of college football in 2011. He managed to perform more than adequately until "his panic attacks became unbearable."[42] A few months later he quit college altogether because he was being overwhelmed by anxiety and nothing worked to reduce his pain. He took his life a little more than a year later.

People in his town were shocked. While Daniel's bouts of depression were common knowledge, he was viewed as a tough kid and he hid his worst symptoms very well. This lack of awareness by others, including family members, is common with suicides. Jeff Olson's team won the state championship that same year. Daniel's father attributed their great season in part to his players being able to "feel Daniel's presence." When he was alive, though, no one could sense the depth of his pain, not even his father who also was his coach.

## Lance Easley, NFL Referee

Lance Easley, who for a short time was an NFL referee, experienced mental illness of a different sort, with a reckless assist from football fans and the sports media. In 2012, Easley worked as a replacement official during an infamous *Monday Night Football* game between Green Bay and Seattle.[43] Due to hysterical media criticism of the officiating by replacement referees in that contest, the NFL would be compelled to sign a new agreement with the regular officials. The league had locked them out after their union had asked for higher salaries and better benefits consistent with the NFL's escalating revenues.

In that pivotal game Easley ruled, on the final play, that Golden Tate caught the game-winning touchdown pass, after another referee had signaled "a touchback, meaning he thought it was an interception." As Easley pointed out, it was one of those "hard decisions . . . [that] are gray; they're not black and white."[44] There was an honest difference of opinion between two replacement officials as to what had actually occurred. This was something that happens frequently in NFL and college games no matter who is officiating.

Nevertheless, many fans and the sports media had been criticizing the NFL for the lockout, citing poor decision making by replacement officials as the major reason why the unpopular lockout should end. Thus, what should have been accepted as a tough decision for any official to make turned into a popular referendum on what was perceived to be a "bad call," which in the skewed minds of football fans was representative of the ineptitude of the replacement officials. Easley was personally attacked and vilified in the media, repeatedly, which greatly worsened his ongoing "struggle[s] with depression." According to Easley, this incident also brought on "post-traumatic stress disorder . . . , panic attacks . . . and even suicidal thoughts." He compared it to "los[ing] . . . a loved one."[45] After the sports media onslaught, he became an emotionally battered man who had great difficulty dealing with his football-inspired demons.

## "THE YIPS" IN PROFESSIONAL BASEBALL

In professional baseball a small number of players experience a particular type of mental disorder that is inflamed by the game itself. It is the extreme anxiety that can attach to the routine play of throwing a baseball accurately. Occasionally even the best college and minor- and major-league players make throwing errors, but these normally are aberrations that are supposed to occur very rarely. Yet, for a few players, what used to be the routine of pitching to a batter, throwing an opponent out at a base, or a catcher throwing a ball back to the pitcher becomes a nightmare. This has happened to otherwise superlative MLB players in the past, including Steve Blass, Steve Sax, Mackey Sasser, and Rick Ankiel.

The nickname for this condition is "the yips."[46] It also is a condition that affects the ability of golfers and basketball players to perform routine athletic tasks, such as making short putts or shooting free throws. Sometimes it is temporary; other times it can destroy an athlete's career. It is one reason why sports psychologists have become so popular.

How this psychological phenomenon occurs in professionally trained athletes is described well in a 2014 *Washington Post* article by Adam Kilgore about Aaron Barrett, who at the time was a Nationals pitching prospect. As a ninth-round pick in the 2010 MLB Draft, Barrett was sent to the team's minor-league affiliate to work on his fundamentals so that someday he might become a starting pitcher in the big leagues. Suddenly, without any other tangible signs of a mental disturbance, the mechanics Barrett was there to improve began to deteriorate, which brought on a loss of confidence. His control all but disappeared as he "threw nine wild pitches and walked 22 hitters in [just] 21 innings."[47]

At that rate, his bout of the "yips" would drive him out of professional baseball sooner rather than later. Fortunately, he had a pitching coach who understood the benefits of addressing this type of anxiety patiently through successive approximation, rather than applying all-or-nothing solutions. The coach "conceived a series of drills . . . [in which Barrett] turned double plays . . . so he could feel what it was like to make a different kind of throw without thinking." Barrett was repeating mechanics that were similar to throwing a pitch, but clearly different enough to reduce his anxiety. Barrett turned double plays until he felt comfortable enough to resume pitching. By the beginning of the 2011 season, he was able to return to minor-league competition, but with one front office initiated compromise. He was turned into a reliever since they did not trust him to start, at least not those who controlled his contract.

Even though Barrett seemed to be back to normal pitching-wise, his bout with the yips had made him mentally damaged goods. The Nationals' front office decision to make him a reliever appeared to be based on a stereotype rather than an assessment of Barrett's pitching skills or his previous problem with the yips. In most ways, being a relief pitcher is considerably more stressful than starting. A good reliever is expected to come into a game with a brief warm-up in pressure situations in which runners are likely to be on base. To be successful, relievers must be able to deal with that pressure by throwing strikes and otherwise demonstrating enhanced control of their pitches. Mistakes are much more costly when runners are in scoring position.

Nevertheless, despite the front office's lack of trust of a player with a mental disorder, Barrett proved to be psychologically resilient. Unlike many baseball players who have experienced the yips, he recovered fully and has been on the Nationals' big-league team since the 2014 season, although he missed much of 2016 recovering from Tommy John surgery. Unlike many players who have overcome this particular affliction and believe they should "refuse to discuss it, lest they tempt a return [of the yips]," Barrett has "embrace[d] the blip that threatened his career" with a more nuanced and healthy mantra: "If you can't talk about it . . . you're not over it."

## GOLF AND TENNIS: THE PGA AND WTA

Golf is another sport in which different types of panic attacks, including the yips, can undermine a golfer's performance. As they age, professional golfers appear to be more likely to get the yips while putting. Thus, the advantages they have accumulated in terms of knowing how to play the game are substantially diminished—and often more than negated—by an inability to control their nerves in pressure situations. The inability to deal with this anxiety seems to be a natural part of the aging process for many professional golfers.

What happened to PGA golfer Charlie Beljan, however, when he became psychologically paralyzed by extreme panic attacks in the prime of his career was abnormal. Through his struggles, Beljan was able "to put a human face on the issue of debilitating anxiety."[48] He became a human interest story—a player conquering steep odds—just as he was about to be jettisoned from the PGA Tour for not winning enough money to remain eligible.

The competition to retain one's tour card is extremely intense, especially when a golfer is on the borderline facing a demotion to the minor-league tour. The golfer's athletic career and livelihood are at stake. In this pressure-cooker environment Beljan "play[ed] through a series of televised panic attacks"—that millions of people painfully watched—and somehow managed to win his first tour event. His was no ordinary case of athlete anxiety. After Beljan had played the second of four rounds, he had to spend the night in a local hospital to be sure that he had not been experiencing a heart attack.[49]

Winning his first PGA tournament did not end Beljan's mental health struggles, although it did make him relatively famous for a short while as "the face of anxiety."[50] It also allowed him to continue to compete on the tour. Before he became a professional golfer he was viewed as "quirky" and even "infamous" because of the peculiar routines he employed to deal with his condition. Obsessive-compulsive behavior often accompany extreme anxiety. Keegan Bradley, who won the 2011 PGA Championship, is another golfer who is described as having "jittery nerves"[51] and a preswing routine that appears to be very odd. What helped Beljan cope was his willingness to remove the veil of secrecy from his mental illness. As a result, the media and his competitors viewed him as "a genuine, caring, social person"[52] open to talking about his condition.

In terms of being accepted by his peers, the fans, and the media, he was much more fortunate than former professional tennis player Rebecca Marino, whose depression has received very little sympathy. At one time she was a very promising Canadian champion who as a teenager was ranked as high as thirty-eighth in the world, which was unusual for so young a player. By the time she was twenty-two in 2013, however, she chose to give up the game and her professional career. She attributed her crash to unpleasant publicity and vicious comments she received through social media, which fed her depression in destructive ways.[53] She was being verbally bullied by her fans and critics.

Before Marino announced her retirement, "she deleted her Twitter and Facebook accounts because she knew what was coming." She explained that social media had made her depression much worse. In particular, "she was berated for her weight [and by] gamblers who lost when she lost." Marino had come to realize that it would be better to change her tennis "world than herself."[54] She did not want to lose who she was to a lack of empathy for, and even hostility toward, athletes who have mental disorders.

Many athletes participating in professional, Olympic, or college sports—or competing for the opportunity to do so—can place their mental health in jeopardy. When that happens, those in the sports world do little to help. Frequently they make matters worse, sometimes intentionally, but usually due to ignorance or lack of understanding. At the same time, there are many former athletes with emerging or imminent symptoms of CTE and other forms of brain damage who will need special care. Many, as exemplified by football great Sam Huff, run the substantial risk of becoming cognitively impaired to such an extent that they can no longer care for themselves. When that happens, unless they are one of the few former athletes to have made life plans that specify how they should be cared for should they be deemed mentally incompetent, they will have their lives governed by someone else. Too often this can lead to exploitation, especially if the former athlete has substantial assets.

# CONCLUSION

## Protecting Athletes' Health in Cartel-Governed Sports

### ECONOMIC INTERESTS THAT JEOPARDIZE ATHLETES' HEALTH

The benefits to elite athletes of performing well in our most popular spectator sports are readily apparent, if measured by inflated salaries, endorsements, college scholarships, glory, and self-esteem. It is around money, publicity, and fame where the tunnel vision of athletes, teams, management, owners, organizers, universities, and the cartels that manipulate these sports for their own purposes are mostly united, even when largely selfish disputes arise about the sharing of revenues. Those common interests, however, only extend to health in limited, self-interested ways in order to ensure that these athletes

- perform well
- play through pain and injuries
- recover from their performance-depleting injuries and other impairments as quickly as possible

These common interests that too often compromise the overall health of athletes in our most popular sports are motivated mostly by the desires of all the involved parties to generate more revenue. This even includes the drug testing carried out by WADA and the U.S. Anti-Doping Agency, which is a big business in and of itself,[1] and the management of youth sports where "embezzlement" has become a common practice.[2] In this greedy environment, addictive painkillers, performance-enhancing drugs, and the underreporting, marginalizing, and even ignoring of potentially serious physical and mental impairments too often become substitutes for medically appropriate health care for elite athletes.

In addition, team doctors, owners, athletic directors, coaches, and management frequently violate athletes' treatment-related rights to privacy and confidentiality. Medical and other professional ethics may be diluted or dispensed with altogether because the doctors and other medical and training staff members who treat these athletes are hired and paid for by the teams.

Moreover, if these once-prized athletes can no longer compete well, retire, or are cut from the team, anything more than pretenses of caring for those players' health quickly disappear, at least on the management side. Residual and long-term physical and mental impairments, including drug addiction and substance abuse, which have resulted from being prepared—often illicitly or illegally—to compete at the highest levels possible become the athletes' problems. Beyond winning and making money, the health of these athletes—even for themselves—is a low priority, and awful examples for youngsters who hope one day to become elite.

So much of what is done to keep elite athletes fit enough to participate in their sports is at cross-purposes with keeping athletes healthy in life. Too often what happens in locker rooms and other nonpublic places in preparing athletes to complete is secretive and pathological, encompassing unhealthy or self-destructive practices that frequently involve cheating and breaking the law. Furthermore, the gaudy aspirations of athletes to serve as positive role models for America's youth more often than not work in reverse, as kids are taught how to be like their supposed heroes who sacrifice their health in order to be successful. Similarly, those who operate youth sports emulate the cartels that run professional, collegiate, and Olympic sports by allowing selfishness and corruption to be normal business practices. To borrow the words of the *Washington Post*'s Norman Chad, these role models and pillars of youth sports operate in "a world with no moral compass; they get a bully pulpit because, in a society with skewed values, they are celebrated for having all the wrong ones."[3]

Obviously the athletes share much responsibility for giving life to and participating in these self-destructive locker-room cultures that are part of our most popular spectator sports. Football in the NFL and big-time college programs may be the exemplars of these unhealthy behaviors and practices of athletes in America, but they exist in some form throughout our professional, intercollegiate, and Olympic sports world. Coaches, trainers, team management, and organizers in America's most popular sports actively support and sometimes facilitate these unhealthy and pathogenic behaviors. They provide the settings, lack of oversight, lack of transparency, and behind-the-scenes encouragement and incentives in which these practices flourish. Afterward, the individuals and entities that are supposed to protect the athletes mostly look the other way to avoid responsibility as these destructive practices continue to occur.

This environment is especially damaging for younger athletes aspiring to be elite, who typically lack the maturity and insight to properly assess the dangers of unhealthy living and pathogenic behavior. They are constantly being tempted by the immediate rewards that taking these risks can provide them with, including fame, college scholarships, Olympic medals, or pro careers. These temptations are particularly difficult to resist when their sports heroes and competitors appear to be engaging in the same self-destructive behavior, and their coaches and young teammates are imploring them to do whatever it takes to be more competitive and athletically successful. The good sportsmanship and healthy values displayed on television during the Little League World Series are well-orchestrated deceptions that bear little resemblance to what goes on in these elite youth sports the rest of the time.

## SPORTS CARTELS ARE ULTIMATELY RESPONSIBLE

The ultimate responsibility for the abuses and corruption that jeopardize elite athletes' health lies with those self-governing entities that control our most popular spectator sports at the highest levels of competition. These largely autonomous sports leagues, federations, and organizations normally are beholden to those who make the most money in those sports: the owners and organizers. Thus, the individuals who control the sports cartels look out for the athletes, coaches, and the public primarily when it is in their business or organizational interest to do so. At best, their loyalties are selective and typically tied to public relations and monetary considerations. They are the "Godfathers" of our most popular sports.

For the most part, these powerful, self-interested sports cartels are allowed to govern themselves without having to obey state and federal laws. They are treated more like public charters than business enterprises. This form of self-governance provides the ideal incubating ground for unhealthy, self-destructive, illicit, and illegal behavior and conditions to be passed down to youth sports as well. The incentives governing athletes' behavior are tied to generating more revenues and publicity. Thus, the penalties to deal with unhealthy behavior and cheating only tend to occur once the transgressions are publicly revealed and those revelations seriously threaten corporate sponsors or other revenue streams.

By then, most or much of the damage already has been done and normally few mechanisms exist or are put into place to ensure that similar transgressions will not be repeated, reprised, or reformulated in the future after the public scandal has subsided. Furthermore, the penalties are almost always targeted at the athletes. Teams, coaches, management, and organizations are rarely penalized, while owners or organizers who control the cartels never are held accountable, unless they flagrantly violate federal criminal laws, and the Justice Department chooses to act, which rarely happens—and then only against internationally based sports organizations, or the Russian government.

Whether it is the NFL, NCAA, IOC, WADA, FIFA, MLB, NBA, NHL, MLS, IAAF, or ITF, or various affiliates, to a greater or lesser extent they all facilitate unhealthy behavior and practices by American athletes who participate in our most popular spectator sports. These sports leagues and organizations tend to be selfishly selective in their enforcement policies guided mostly by internal business and other organizational considerations. Rarely do they adopt and rigorously enforce rule changes that would curb athletes' unhealthy practices, substantially reduce their long-term physical and mental impairments, or meaningfully address the use of illicit and illegal performance-enhancing substances, unless doing so is in the cartel's business interests, or viewed as a necessary cost of doing business. When the most powerful anti-doping authority in the world—WADA—was asked by U.S. lawmakers why there had been a multiyear "delay in investigating Russian sports," rather than acknowledging that it was due to organizational conflicts of interest, WADA's president claimed that "there was no clear authority vested in us to undertake investigations."[4]

More often than not, these mega sports entities have the audacity, spurred on by strong economic incentives, to directly or indirectly participate in the obscuration and cover-ups of obvious health-related improprieties or offenses. Certain leaders of a number of international sports cartels, including the IOC, IAAF, and FIFA, have profited handsomely from shoddy enforcement, taking bribes, and even establishing extortion schemes. Moreover, none of these sports leagues or organizations take aggressive actions to promote healthy or safe conditions for their athletes, unless and until the offending sport's revenue streams are put at risk, or when governmental authorities threaten to enact regulations or conduct prosecutions, which is rare.

When these sports enterprises finally do act, it tends to be in arbitrary ways, which too often violate the due process rights of the relatively small percentage of athletes who are designated for, or unlucky enough to receive, punishments. In addition, owners, teams, coaches, and/or management are almost never sanctioned for their direct or indirect involvement in jeopardizing the health of these athletes. What happens enforcement-wise is mostly for show in order to prevent governments and courts from becoming directly involved, and to ensure that revenues continue to grow unburdened by public condemnation due to these scandals.

The much-publicized banning of Russian athletes from the 2016 Summer Olympics appears to have been a reluctant overreaction to criticism of the IAAF. In the end it only resulted in the punishment of track-and-field athletes representing a country that by consensus has attained least favored nation status among the Western media and journalists. Doping throughout the rest of the sports world has continued to go on as usual, including during the Olympics in Rio where once again the competence of the host nation's testing facilities was called into question.[5]

In sports commerce, as in other global businesses, managing crises, public relations, and plausible deniability substitutes for acting to promote healthy values. This self-interested camouflage and denial of responsibility greatly diminish the possibility that our elite athletes—and those younger athletes who are trying to become elite—lead healthy lives, are protected by reasonable safety precautions, and receive essential health care and disability benefits if they become physically or mentally impaired or addicted.

The U.S. Department of Justice may launch a high-profile investigation on rare occasions when the political climate is just right. However, this very occasional enforcement approach, without a great deal more, is a terrible way to ensure that most elite American athletes, and those younger athletes who are trying to become elite, remain relatively healthy, especially later in their lives. A variety of systemic health dysfunctions exist while these athletes are competing and learning how to compete, and afterward when, as former athletes, they must lick their wounds and hope they will not succumb to various physical and mental impairments. Too often these accumulating impairments become debilitating, devastating, and occasionally catastrophic.

Virtually all the powerful sports cartels and their various affiliates, to a greater or lesser extent, have reneged on their responsibilities to protect the health of their athletes. Time and time again, these leagues and sports organizations have demonstrated that when the choice is between economic self-interest and doing what is best for athletes' health, the athletes' well-being will be shortchanged. The only cartel that seems to be trying to function in ways that protect the health of its athletes, at least much of the time, is the NBA, especially since Adam Silver took over as commissioner. The other cartels have been consistently deficient.

## COLLECTIVE BARGAINING TO PROMOTE ATHLETES' HEALTH, WITH TWO PROVISOS

Given what has happened over many years to jeopardize American athletes' health in our most popular spectator sports, it seems evident that some form of government intervention and regulation—well short of prohibitions—is necessary to clean up the mess and ensure that it does not return after attention spans wane. None of the existing organizational structures in sports have proved to be capable of meaningfully addressing this public health problem on their own. Collective bargaining between unionized American athletes and our major sports leagues has been a successful way to deal with sports management's lack of accountability for many types of improprieties or transgressions, including a few that have been health related. Unfortunately, as documented in part by the Harvard Law School's "The Football Players Health Study," those collective bargaining agreements (CBAs) as presently constituted have left most professional, Olympic, and collegiate athletes in America largely or entirely unprotected when it comes to their health needs.

To begin with, only male athletes who play in the NFL, MLB, NBA, NHL, and MLS are covered by relatively effective CBAs. Second, none of these agreements protect former players, other than incidentally. Third, even those athletes who are members of strong unions still tend to be at considerable risk with respect to their health. Concussions and other severe injuries in football, as well as performance-enhancing drugs in baseball, illustrate—along with many other well-publicized transgressions covered in this book—how easily and often elite athletes' health can be corrupted, taken for granted, and/or abused.

Fourth, American athletes participating in collegiate, Olympic, or other international sports, as well as most female athletes and all former professional and collegiate athletes, are not covered by effective CBAs. Lastly, collective bargaining has minimal influence on health-related transgressions committed by owners, coaches, management, and Olympic organizers, except if their actions violate specific terms of a governing CBA, assuming one exists. Thus, owners, coaches, management, and Olympic organizers are rarely—if ever—held accountable in any major spectator sport for their health-related transgressions.

Government regulation of health matters in American sports, if it were to mirror regulation of other corporate entities doing business in the United States, would very likely encounter overwhelming political opposition, and still leave major loopholes uncovered. Thus, it makes much more sense to actively pursue legislation that strongly encourages the adoption of effective CBAs throughout the American sports world, not only for active athletes, but former athletes as well. This result could best be achieved by adopting some version of the existing CBA structures found in our four major sports. At the same time, improvements in the care and treatment of athletes should be removed from the normal collective bargaining process to avoid making the health of players a contentious subject of negotiations. In addition, there should be federal legislation enacted to create governmental authorities to provide regulatory and judicial oversight and guidance to fill in the gaps that are unlikely to be covered by CBAs alone. The United States already is funding anti-doping agencies[6] and other aspects of sports health for tens of millions of dollars and receiving very little in return, other than the appearance of successful monitoring and enforcement.

## A National Commission on Sports Health

Congress should establish an independent national commission composed primarily of health providers and health educators, with no financial or other tangible ties or links to the governing sports cartels, including the NCAA, to promote and protect the health of athletes at all levels of competition. This commission would promulgate federal health standards for all our major spectator sports. In addition, the commission would provide regulatory guidance for youth athletic programs and high schools, which should be adopted by state and local governments with certain variations to account for jurisdictional differences. One emphasis at all levels of competition should be standards and guidance to provide athletes with transparent, appropriate, medically approved, and physician prescribed examinations, treatments, and services by certified health providers, even if doing so might enhance an athlete's performance, and thus be viewed as creating a competitive advantage. Health of the athletes should be paramount.

At the same time, however, part of the commission's mandate would be to establish standards for determining whether regularly prescribed treatments and services that provide perceived competitive advantages should be viewed as medically unnecessary, and thus inappropriate. This should be a transparent process, rather than one that remains secret until Russian hackers reveal it for the world to see. In addition, as recommended in chapter 11, the commission should create a list of performance-enhancing substances that should be banned because they jeopardize the health of athletes that use them. Moreover, any new substance or alterations in the formulas of existing substances should be temporarily banned, unless and until it can be medically certified as being safe for athletes to use in specified dosages. The burden should be on the athletes to demonstrate that any performance-enhancing substance is medically necessary and being prescribed and used appropriately.

This national commission should be authorized to establish rules governing health in all professional, Olympic, and intercollegiate sports that hold competitions in the United States, with penalties for noncompliance. These rules and penalties should apply whether or not a sport has a CBA, although more latitude in self-regulation should be shown to sports that have CBAs that have been federally certified as meeting minimum health standards. The national commission also should establish standards to certify those CBAs, as well as guidelines for youth programs and high schools, that states—within certain specified parameters—should be financially encouraged to adapt or modify to suit their particular jurisdictional needs.

## A Federal Magistrate Court for Health Standards in Sports

In addition, Congress should create a new court, which would be presided over by special federal magistrates, to hear cases and issue penalties in health-related matters involving professional, Olympic, and collegiate sports in America, most notably implementation of the national commission's health standards. This magistrate court's original jurisdiction would include: leagues, universities and colleges, teams, management, owners, and organizers, which violate commission-mandated health standards that fall outside the agreed upon administrative jurisdiction of a governing CBA. In addition, this court would have jurisdiction whenever either side has reasonable grounds to appeal a CBA-governed arbitration ruling.

If a sport has no authorized CBA, the federal magistrate court should have original jurisdiction over that sport's health issues until a CBA has been certified. In such a circumstance, the court should be charged with holding hearings to determine whether health-related rule violations have been committed and to administer mandated penalties once federal attorneys issue a charge. As with all other federal magistrate courts, a decision on any matter within its jurisdiction could be appealed by either party to a federal district court assigned to hear those appeals. The existing rules and precedents, which already govern such magistrate proceedings and appeals, should apply in these health-related sports cases as well.

# NOTES

## PREFACE

1. Ian Dishart Suttie, *The Origins of Love and Hate* (London: Kegan Paul, Trench, Trubner, 1935).

2. See D. K. Hall-Flavin, "Borderline Personality Disorder: A Clinical Perspective," BPDFamily.com, March 8, 2012, www.bpdfamily.com.

## INTRODUCTION

1. Mike Wise, "Lance, Manti and Modern Mythmaking," *Washington Post*, January 19, 2013.

2. David Kindred, "Fantasy League," *Washington Post*, January 20, 2013.

3. "They Said It," *Sports Illustrated*, July 22, 1968.

4. Wise, "Modern Mythmaking."

5. Kindred, "Fantasy League."

6. Tom Brokaw, *The Greatest Generation* (New York: Random House, 1998).

7. David Halberstam, *The Best and the Brightest* (New York: Random House, 1969).

8. Bill Pennington, "The Trusted Grown-Ups Who Steal Millions from Youth Sports," *New York Times*, July 7, 2016.

# 1. REAL MEN PLAY HURT

1. William C. Rhoden, "Sports of the Times—George Atkinson's Old-School Values," *New York Times*, December 8, 2009 (accessed December 8, 2012), www.nytimes.com/2009/12/08/sports/football/08rhoden.html ?r=1&ref= sports .

2. Mike Jones, "Old School Player, New Reality," *Washington Post*, August 23, 2013.

3. Adam Kilgore, "Wilson's Dangerous Concussion Claim," *Washington Post*, August 28, 2015.

4. Marc Tracy, "Concussions Ended His Football Dreams. Now He Helps Others Achieve Theirs," *New York Times*, November 20, 2015.

5. S. L. Price, "It Would Hurt More Not to Play," *Sports Illustrated*, December 7, 2015, 58.

6. Price, "It Would Hurt More," 58.

7. Brian Cazeneuve, "You Gotta Play Hurt," *Sports Illustrated*, May 3, 2014, 53–59.

8. Cazeneuve, "You Gotta Play Hurt," 53–59.

9. Cazeneuve, "You Gotta Play Hurt," 59.

10. Cazeneuve, "You Gotta Play Hurt," 59.

11. William C. Rhoden, "When Players Put Team First, They Put Themselves at Risk," *New York Times*, October 25, 2015.

12. Nathan A. Heflick, "Man Up Roethlisberger, It Was Only a Concussion," *Psychology Today*, November 30, 2009.

13. Rhoden, "Players Put Team First."

# 2. TEAMMATES, COACHES, FANS, AND OTHER UNHEALTHY INFLUENCES

1. William C. Rhoden, "Sports of the Times—George Atkinson's Old-School Values," *New York Times*, December 8, 2009 (accessed December 8, 2012), www.nytimes.com/2009/12/08/sports/football/08rhoden.html ?r=1&ref= sports .

2. Alan Schwarz, "Rules Trickle Down; Cash Won't," *New York Times*, August 30, 2013.

3. Dashiell Bennett, "The Jay Cutler Criticism Is the Reason Why the NFL's Concussion Problem Is Not Going Away," *Business Insider*, January 24, 2011 (last visited May 27, 2014), www.businessinder.com.

4. Jeff Z. Klein, "Coaches Defy Doctors after Players' Concussions, Study Finds," *New York Times*, November 20, 2012.

5. Brendan Prunty, "Anyone Have a Lozenge?" *New York Times*, November 22, 2015.

6. Andrew Das, "Chelsea Manager May Allow Doctor Back on the Bench," *New York Times*, August 15, 2015.

7. Ken Belson, "A Player Concussed, and a Policy Questioned," *New York Times*, November 23, 2013.

8. Sally Jenkins, "For NFL, Protocol Reveals a Disconnect," *Washington Post*, December 5, 2015.

9. Mike Wise, "Rose's Call to Sit Out Is Right One," *Washington Post*, May 8, 2013.

10. John Feinstein, "Strasburg Decision Is Still Haunting," *Washington Post*, September 24, 2013.

## 3. RG3'S PAINFUL STAY IN WASHINGTON

1. Mark Maske, "Redskins Fined $20,000 for Robert Griffin Concussion Announcement," *Washington Post*, October 19, 2012.

2. Maske, "Redskins Fined $20,000."

3. Kent Babb, "Threat of Head Injuries Constant," *Washington Post*, October 10, 2012.

4. Babb, "Threat of Head Injuries."

5. Babb, "Threat of Head Injuries."

6. Associated Press, "Urlacher Would Hide Injury," *New York Times*, November 16, 2012.

7. Tracee Hamilton, "If RGIII Gets the Green Light, Fans Should Buckle Up," *Washington Post*, December 12, 2012.

8. Mike Jones, "Shanahan: Robert Griffin III Has 'Mild LCL' Sprain," *Washington Post*, December 10, 2012, http://www.washingtonpost.com/blogs/football-insider/wp/2012/12/10/shanahan-robert-griffin-iii-has-mild-lcl-sprain/.

9. Sally Jenkins and Rick Maese, "Do No Harm: Medical Care in the NFL Plays to a Different Standard, Often Yielding Troubling Results," *Washington Post*, March 17, 2013.

10. Jenkins and Maese, "Do No Harm."

11. See Mike Jones, "As Griffin Recovers, Who's Responsible Going Forward?" *Washington Post*, March 29, 2013.

12. Tracee Hamilton, "Redskins Fail to Learn from RGIII Injury," *Washington Post*, March 22, 2013.

## 4. THE PITFALLS OF TEAM-DIRECTED MEDICAL CARE

1. Rick Maese, "Report: NFL Should Overhaul Player Care," *Washington Post*, November 17, 2016. See Harvard University's Football Players Health Study, "Protecting and Promoting the Health of NFL Players: Legal and Ethical Analysis and Recommendations," fooballplayershealth.harvardedu, November 17, 2016). (Note the study was carried out by Harvard Law School.)

2. Sally Jenkins and Rick Maese, "Do No Harm: Medical Care in the NFL Plays to a Different Standard, Often Yielding Troubling Results," *Washington Post*, March 17, 2013.

3. Jenkins and Maese, "Do No Harm."

4. Jenkins and Maese, "Do No Harm."

5. Rick Maese, "Survey: Players Distrust Team Medical Staff," *Washington Post*, February 1, 2013.

6. Rick Maese, "Ex-players: NFL Pushed Risky Drug Use," *Washington Post*, May 21, 2014.

7. Jenkins and Maese, "Do No Harm."

8. Sally Jenkins and Rick Maese, "In the NFL Culture, Pain and Drugs Are the Norm," *Washington Post*, April 14, 2013.

9. Jenkins and Maese, "Pain and Drugs."

10. Jeff Z. Klein, "Coaches Defy Doctors after Players' Concussions, Study Finds," *New York Times*, November 20, 2012.

11. Jeff Z. Klein, "Boogaard Lawsuit May Shake Up Hockey," *New York Times*, September 26, 2012.

12. John Branch, "In Suit over Death, Boogaard's Family Blames the N.H.L.," *New York Times*, May 12, 2013.

13. Ken Belson and Mary Pilon, "Concern Raised over Athletes' Use of Pain-killer before Games," *New York Times*, April 12, 2012.

14. Belson and Pilon, "Concern Raised."

15. Tyler Kepner, "A Slugger Fights for the Yankees, but Mostly against Them," *New York Times*, August 18, 2013.

16. Seth Davis, "The Demons of Rex Chapman," *Sports Illustrated*, July 27, 2015, 47.

## 5. PERFORMANCE-ENHANCING MEASURES

1. See Ruth Padawer, "Too Fast to Be Female," *New York Times Magazine*, July 3, 2016, MM32.

2. Peter Lattman and Natasha Singer, "Learning the Hard Way about a Banned Ingredient," *New York Times*, March 17, 2013.

3. Ross Tucker and Jonathan Dugas, "How to Fight Doping in Sports," *New York Times*, August 1, 2015.

4. Juliet Macur, "Anti-doping Lab's Flaws Put Olympics in Bind," *New York Times*, November 16, 2013.

5. Peter Keating, "Who's Cheating Who?" *ESPN the Magazine*, September 2, 2013, 14.

6. Keating, "Who's Cheating Who?," 4.

7. See Associated Press, "Study Claims Imaging Tests Show Larger Rubber Core," January 3, 2007, http://sports.espn.go.com/mlb/news/story?id=2719191 .

8. Alan M. Nathan, Lloyd V. Smith, Warren L. Faber, and Daniel A. Russell, "Corked Bats, Juiced Balls, and Humidors: The Physics of Cheating in Baseball," *American Journal of Physics* 79, no. 6 (June 2011): 575–80.

9. Mary Pilon and Gina Kolata, "New to Most Fans, IGF-1 Has Long Been Banned as a Performance Enhancer," *New York Times*, January 29, 2013.

10. David Epstein and George Dohrmann, "The Zany Story of Two Self Ordained Sports Science Entrepreneurs," *Sports Illustrated*, February 4, 2013, 58–66.

11. Ken Belson, "To the N.F.L., 40 Winks Is as Vital as the 40-Yard Dash," *New York Times*, October 1, 2016.

12. Isabelle Khurshudyan, "Capitals' Diet Now Includes More Than Just Winning," *Washington Post*, December 10, 2015.

13. "Testing Makes Perfect," *Bloomberg Businessweek*, April 4, 2016, 20.

14. See Andy Miah, *Genetically Modified Athletes* (New York: Routledge, 2004).

15. George Mitchell, "Drugs in Sports an Ongoing Menace," *Washington Post*, January 10, 2014.

16. "Testing Times," *Economist*, July 20, 2013, 12.

17. See Geoffrey Rapp, "Blue Sky Steroids," *Journal of Criminal Law & Criminology* 99, no. 3 (2009): 599.

## 6. BASEBALL'S TARNISHED LEGACY

1. George Mitchell, "Drugs in Sports an Ongoing Menace," *Washington Post*, January 10, 2014.

2. Buster Olney, "Just Say Yes," *ESPN the Magazine*, December 24, 2012, 60–61.

3. Harvey Araton, "It's Time to Reconsider Barry Bonds for the Hall of Fame," *New York Times*, July 24, 2015.

4. Mitchell, "Drugs in Sports."

5. Barry Svrluga, "Gordon's Suspension Alters Marlins' Plans," *Washington Post*, April 30, 2016.

6. Tom Verducci, "Here We Go Again," *Sports Illustrated*, November 19, 2012, 22.

7. Ken Belson and Jere Longman, "Baseball Dopers' New Drug Is an Old One Used by East Germany," *International New York Times*, May 6, 2016.

8. Svrluga, "Gordon's Suspension."

9. Svrluga, "Gordon's Suspension."

10. Associated Press, "Mets' Mejia Banned for Life," February 12, 2016 (last visited February 19, 2016), www.timesunion.com.

11. Svrluga, "Gordon's Suspension."

12. Lynn Zinser, "To Baseball's Chagrin, Steroid Era Goes On," *New York Times*, August 24, 2012.

13. Araton, "It's Time."

14. Michael Powell, "Jake Arrieta Shows He's Human, despite Accusations to the Contrary," *New York Times*, April 29, 2016.

15. Michael Powell, "Rose's Ban, a Product of His Flaws, Highlights Others' Faults," *New York Times*, December 20, 2015.

16. See Jon Wertheim, "Why Men Cheat," *Sports Illustrated*, August 19, 2013, 17–18.

17. Wertheim, "Why Men Cheat," 17–18.

18. Tracee Hamilton, "Athletes Continue to Prove That They Need a Boost in Supplementary Education," *Washington Post*, July 30, 2013.

19. Hamilton, "Athletes Continue to Prove."

20. Zinser, "To Baseball's Chagrin."

21. Howard Bryant, "Spring Thaw," *ESPN the Magazine*, March 31, 2014, 8.

22. Powell, "Rose's Ban."

## 7. FOOTBALL'S BRAZEN LACK OF COMPLIANCE

1. Tom Verducci, "Swampland Chronicles," *Sports Illustrated*, February 11, 2013, 16.

2. Barry Svrluga and Mark Maske, "NFL, MLB to Probe Allegations in Report," *Washington Post*, December 28, 2015.

3. *Wikipedia*, s.v., "List of Suspensions in the National Football League" (last visited February 24, 2014), http://en.wikipedia.org/wiki/List_of_players_and_coaches_suspended_by_the_NFL .

4. Verducci, "Swampland Chronicles," 16–17.

5. NFL, "Report: Adderall Remains Drug of Choice for Many NFL Players" (last visited February 24, 2014), www.nfl.com/news/story/Oap1000000242017/article/report-adderall-remains-drug-of-choice-for-many-nfl-players; see also Judy Battista, "Drug of Focus Is at Center of Suspensions," *New York Times*, December 2, 2012.

6. Mark Maske and Mike Jones, "Adderall Use Said to Be behind the Suspension of C. Griffin," *Washington Post*, December 6, 2012.

7. Tracee Hamilton, "Athletes Continue to Prove That They Need a Boost in Supplementary Education," *Washington Post*, July 30, 2013.

8. Mary Pilon and Gina Kolata, "New to Most Fans, IGF-1 Has Long Been Banned as a Performance Enhancer," *New York Times*, January 29, 2013.

9. David Epstein, "Moving the Needle," *Sports Illustrated*, October 29, 2012, 18.

10. Tom Pelissero, "Players to Be Blood-Tested in Camp for HGH Study," *USA Today*, July 22, 2013.

11. Brent Schrotenboer, "First Year of HGH Testing in NFL Catches No One," *USA Today*, February 2, 2015 (last visited December 17, 2015), www.usatoday.com .

12. NCAA, "Understanding the NCAA's Drug Testing Policies" (last visited February 26, 2014), www.ncas.org/health-and-safety/policy/drug-testing.

13. Verducci, "Swampland Chronicles," 16–17.

14. Chris Jones, "Crime and Punishment," *ESPN the Magazine*, June 10, 2013, 124.

15. Jones, "Crime and Punishment," 124.

## 8. CYCLING, OLYMPIC SPORTS, AND WADA

1. Brad Wieners, "Liestrong," *Bloomberg Businessweek*, October 17, 2012, 86.

2. David Epstein, "Moving the Needle," *Sports Illustrated*, October 29, 2012, 17.

3. Dan Turner, "Armstrong: Nobody's Buying the Witch-Hunt Line, Lance," *Los Angeles Times*, August 24, 2012.

4. Howard Bryant, "The Not-So-Fine Line," *ESPN the Magazine*, September 17, 2012, 10.

5. Sally Jenkins, "USADA's Campaign Is Far from Fair," *Washington Post*, August 25, 2012.

6. Bryant, "Not-So-Fine Line," 10.

7. Juliet Macur, "Armstrong Faces New Doping Charges," *New York Times*, June 13, 2012.

8. Amanda Coletta, "Speedskater Poised to Upend Rule of Sports' Highest Court," *New York Times*, February 11, 2016.

9. Rebecca R. Ruiz, "Sports Arbitration Court Ruling against German Speedskater Claudia Pechstein Is Upheld," *New York Times*, June 7, 2016.

10. Ian Austen, "Report Describes How Armstrong Mastered Undermining Antidoping Tests," *New York Times*, October 12, 2012.

11. Austen, "Report Describes."

12. Jenkins, "USADA's Campaign."

13. Juliet Macur, "Anti-doping Agency Exposed Armstrong, but What about the Others?" *New York Times*, October 21, 2013.

14. Ian Austen, "British Cyclist Releases Test Results but Does Little to Silence His Critics," *New York Times*, December 4, 2015.

15. Crouse, "Shadow of Doping."

16. Karen Crouse, "Shadow of Doping Is Never Far from Pool," *New York Times*, August 2, 2015.

17. Rebecca R. Ruiz, "Drugs Pervade Sport in Russia, World Anti-Doping Agency Report Finds," *New York Times*, November 9, 2015.

18. Juliet Macur, "A Second Chance for Sebastian Coe to Clean Up His Sport," *New York Times*, January 14, 2016.

19. Steve Eder, "M.L.B. Seeks Records on Rodriguez Doctor," *New York Times*, October 15, 2013.

20. Associated Press, "Tiger Woods Doctor in Doping Probe," *Richmond Times-Dispatch*, December 15, 2009.

21. Amy Shipley, "Growing Old Gracefully," *Washington Post*, May 20, 2012.

22. Shipley, "Growing Old Gracefully."

23. Shipley, "Growing Old Gracefully."

24. S. L. Price, "Judge Ye Not," *Sports Illustrated*, August 13, 2012, 76.

25. Maxwell J. Mehlman, *The Price of Perfection: Individualism and Society in the Era of Biomedical Enhancement* (Baltimore: Johns Hopkins University Press, 2009), 134.

26. Price, "Judge Ye Not," 76.

27. Amy Shipley, "A Shadow of Doubt," *Washington Post*, July 5, 2012.

28. Epstein, "Moving the Needle," 17.

29. Scorecard, "The Race Goes On," *Sports Illustrated*, August 31, 2015, 16.

30. Eddie Pells and Pat Graham, "Tyson Gay Tests Positive for Banned Substances: 2 Other Track Stars Fail Drug Tests," Associated Press, July 14, 2013.

31. Pat Graham, "Track Stars Tyson Gay, Asafa Powell, Sherone Simpson All Fail Drug Tests," Associated Press, July 14, 2013.

32. Tim Rohan, "Antidoping Agency Delays Publication of Research," *New York Times*, August 22, 2013.

33. Rohan, "Antidoping Agency Delays Publication."

34. Juliet Macur, "Doping Rules Are Tougher Only If Applied," *New York Times*, November 12, 2013.

35. Macur, "Doping Rules."

36. Macur, "Doping Rules."

37. Macur, "Doping Rules."

38. Rebecca R. Ruiz, "Rio Doping Lab Suspended as Games Near," *New York Times*, June 25, 2016.

39. Macur, "Doping Rules."

40. Idil Abshir, "Kenya's Gold Medal for Corruption," *New York Times*, August 23, 2016, Opinion Pages.

41. Michael Powell, "Winter Sports Athletes Ask for the Doping Spotlight," *New York Times*, March 29, 2016.

42. Sam Dolnick, "Russian Biathlon Coach Had Suspicions, Too," *New York Times*, February 7, 2014.

43. Juliet Macur, "There's a Dark Cloud over Our Sport," *New York Times*, February 7, 2014.

44. Macur, "Dark Cloud over Our Sport."

45. "Go Figure," *Sports Illustrated*, March 3, 2014, 16.

46. Katie Carrera, "Backstrom Will Get Silver Medal; IOC Says Ban 'Fully Justified,'" *Washington Post*, March 15, 2014.

47. Katie Carrera and Dave Sheinin, "Caps' Backstrom Fails IOC Drug Test," *Washington Post*, February 24, 2014.

48. Carrera and Sheinin, "Caps' Backstrom."

49. Scott Burnside, "Backstrom Victim of Testing Debacle," ESPN.com, February 23, 2014.

50. Carrera and Sheinin, "Caps' Backstrom."

51. Ken Belson, "Nicklas Backstrom Misses Final after Failed Drug Test," *New York Times*, February 23, 2014.

52. Carrera, "Backstrom Will Get Silver Medal."

## 9. THE LAISSEZ-FAIRE APPROACH TO DOPING IN TENNIS

1. Christopher Clarey, "Tennis's Watchdog Seems to Operate in the Dark," *New York Times*, January 18, 2016.

2. Howard Bryant, "The Fix Is In: Does Tennis Have a PED Problem?" *ESPN the Magazine*, February 18, 2013, 8.

3. Katie Thomas, "Doping Scandals in Tennis Are Few, but Concerns Persist," *New York Times*, September 10, 2009.

4. Bryant, "Fix Is In," 8.

5. Thomas, "Doping Scandals."

6. Bryant, "Fix Is In," 8.

7. Lynn Zinser, "Tennis Strengthens Testing for Drugs," *New York Times*, March 8, 2013.

8. Zinser, "Tennis Strengthens Testing."

9. Amanda Coletta, "Speedskater Poised to Upend Rule of Sports' Highest Court," *New York Times*, February 11, 2016.

10. Greg Garber, "Recent Drug News Depressing," ESPN.com, August 1, 2013, http://espn.go.com.

11. Courtney Nguyen, "What's the Secret to Rafael Nadal's Rapid Recovery from His Knee Injury?" SI.com, October 8, 2013.

12. Nguyen, "What's the Secret?" See also A. S. Wasterlain et al., "Systemic Effects of Platelet-Rich Plasma Injection," *American Journal of Sports Medicine*, January 2013, 186–93.

13. Garber, "Recent Drug News."

14. Garber, "Recent Drug News."

15. Associated Press, "Rafael Nadal Sues French Official for Defamation over Doping Allegation," *New York Times*, April 25, 2016.

16. Christopher Clarey, "I.T.F.'s Antidoping Policy Poses Test for New Leader," *New York Times*, December 6, 2015.

17. Clarey, "I.T.F.'s Antidoping Policy."

18. Greg Beacham, "Failed Drug Test Has Sharapova, 28, Facing Lengthy Ban from Competition," *Washington Post*, March 8, 2016.

19. Patrick Reevell, "New Ban on a Drug Hits Russian Athletes Hard," *New York Times*, March 10, 2016.

20. Andrew Pollack, "Effects of Meldonium on Athletes Are Hazy," *New York Times*, March 10, 2016.

21. Rebecca R. Ruiz and Ben Rothenberg, "Russian Hackers Draw Attention to Drug-Use Exemptions for Athletes," *New York Times*, September 14, 2016.

22. Associated Press, "Manufacturer: 4–6 Weeks Normal Treatment for Drug in Maria Sharapova Case," ESPN.com, March 8, 2016 (last visited March 9, 2016), www.espn.go.com.

23. Christopher Clarey, "Erasing the Bitter Taste without Absolving Sharapova," *New York Times*, June 12, 2016.

## 10. THE IOC, WADA, IAAF, AND STATE-SPONSORED DOPING IN RUSSIA

1. "Doping in Sport: A Cold-War Chill," *Economist*, November 14, 2015, 51.

2. Simon Austin, "WADA Act on Doping Report, Revoking Accreditation of Russian Lab," *International New York Times*, November 10, 2015, www.nytimes.com.

3. Will Hobson, "Alerted to Doping in '10, Wada Didn't Investigate," *Washington Post*, June 3, 2016.

4. Sally Jenkins, "IOC's Sleight of Hand: Focusing on Doping in Lieu of Human Rights," *Washington Post*, May 19, 2016.

5. Austin, "WADA Act on Doping Report."

6. Rebecca R. Ruiz, "Officials Accused of Extortion to Clear Athletes Who Doped," *New York Times*, January 14, 2016.

7. "Doping in Sport," 51.

8. Michael Powell, "Winter Sports Athletes Ask for the Doping Spotlight," *New York Times*, March 29, 2016.

9. "Doping in Sport," 51.

10. "Doping in Sport," 51.

11. Victor Mather and Christopher Clarey, "Governing Body's Move Could Jar 2016 Olympics," *New York Times*, November 14, 2015.

12. Juliet Macur, "A Second Chance for Sebastian Coe to Clean Up His Sport," *New York Times*, January 14, 2016.

13. Patrick Reevell, "New Drug Guidelines May Overturn Suspensions," *New York Times*, April 14, 2016.

14. Patrick Reevell, "Russia Says Uncertainty about Doping Results Led to Withdrawal of Teams," *New York Times*, April 9, 2016.

15. Reevell, "New Drug Guidelines."

16. Rebecca R. Ruiz and Michael Schwirtz, "Russian Insider Says State-Run Doping Fueled Olympic Gold," *New York Times*, May 12, 2016.

17. Rebecca R. Ruiz, "Mystery in Sochi Doping Case Lies with Tamper-Proof Bottle," *New York Times*, May 13, 2016.

18. Juliet Macur, "Revelations of State-Backed Doping Should Bar Russia from Rio Olympics," *New York Times*, May 12, 2016.

19. Editorial Board, "Can Russia Clean Up in Time for Rio?" *New York Times*, May 13, 2016.

20. Rebecca R. Ruiz, "Russian Sports Doping: Explained," *New York Times*, May 16, 2016.

21. Editorial Board, "Shamelessly 'Ashamed' in Moscow," *New York Times*, May 17, 2016.

22. Tim Layden, "Bear Down," *Sports Illustrated*, June 27, 2016, 17.

23. Will Hobson, "Many Hurdles Must Be Cleared to Ban Russia for Doping," *Washington Post*, May 22, 2016.

24. Michael Powell, "In Russian Doping Scandal, Time for a Punishment to Fit the Crime," *New York Times*, June 16, 2016.

25. Powell, "In Russian Doping Scandal."

26. Will Hobson, "IOC Doping Crackdown Could Lead to Athlete Bans," *Washington Post*, May 17, 2016.

27. Rebecca R. Ruiz, "Justice Department Opens Investigation into Russian Doping Scandal," *New York Times*, May 17, 2016.

28. Jenkins, "IOC's Sleight of Hand."

29. Vanessa Barbara, "An Olympic Catastrophe," *New York Times*, July 3, 2016.

30. Christopher Clarey, "Watchdogs Show Teeth and, Finally Some Spine," *New York Times*, June 18, 2016.

31. Layden, "Bear Down," 17.

32. Rebecca R. Ruiz, "Russia's Track and Field Team Barred from Rio Olympics," *New York Times*, June 17, 2016.

33. Rick Maese, "Track Officials Ban Russia from Games over Doping," *Washington Post*, June 18, 2016.

34. Rebecca R. Ruiz, "After Russian Ban, I.O.C. President Addresses Antidoping Efforts," *New York Times*, June 21, 2016.

35. Will Hobson, "Federations Scramble on How to Handle Russian Athletes," *Washington Post*, June 27, 2016.

36. Rebecca R. Ruiz, "Rio Doping Lab Suspended as Games Near," *New York Times*, June 25, 2016.

37. Richard Sandomir and Andrew Jacobs, "Russian Track Team to Miss Olympics, American Audiences? Not Likely." *New York Times*, June 19, 2016.

38. Rebecca R. Ruiz and Ben Rothenberg, "Russian Hackers Draw Attention to Drug-Use Exemptions for Athletes," *New York Times*, September 14, 2016.

39. Rebecca Ruiz, "Olympics History Rewritten: New Doping Tests Topple the Podium," *New York Times*, November 21, 2016.

## I I. REGULATING PEDS TO PROMOTE ATHLETES' HEALTH

1. American Academy of Pediatrics, Policy Statement, "Use of Performance-Enhancing Substances," *Pediatrics* 115, no. 4 (April 2005): 1103, Reaffirmed and Retired, February 2008 and May 2008, doi:10.1542/peds.2005-0085.

2. Matt Pearce, "Diana Nyad Completes Cuba to U.S. Swim, Reaches a Lifelong Dream," *Los Angeles Times*, September 2, 2013.

3. Katrina Karkazis and Rebecca Jordan-Young, "The Trouble with Too Much T," *New York Times*, April 10, 2014.

## 12. A LITANY OF SPORTS-RELATED IMPAIRMENTS

1. Jordan Heck, "Richard Sherman: 'I See a Concussion Movie Every Sunday,'" December 31, 2015, www.sportingnews.com.

2. Richard Hoffer, "Bittersweet Science," *Sports Illustrated*, December 3, 2012, 15.

3. Hoffer, "Bittersweet Science," 15.

4. Richard O'Brien, "Emile Griffith," *Sports Illustrated*, August 5, 2013, 17.

5. Clyde Haberman, "Boxing Is a Brutal, Fading Sport, Could Football Be Next?" *International New York Times*, November 8, 2015.

6. Erika A. Diehl, "What's All the Headache: Reform Needed to Cope with the Effects of Concussions in Football," *Journal of Law and Health* 23, no. 1 (2010): 88, citing the Center for Injury Research and Policy.

7. Don Brady and Flo Brady, "Research-Based Practice: Sport-Related Concussions," *NASP Communique* 39, no. 8 (June 2011) (last viewed March 27, 2014), www.nasponline.org/publications/cq/39/8/sport-related-concussions .

8. "Schools and Hard Knocks," *Economist*, March 5, 2016, 14.

9. "Schools and Hard Knocks."

10. "Schools and Hard Knocks."

11. "Concussion: Bang to Rights," *Economist*, March 5, 2016, 73–74, Science and Technology section.

12. Brady and Brady, "Research-Based Practice."

13. Ken Belson, "Study Bolsters Link between Routine Hits and Brain Disease," *New York Times*, December 3, 2012.

14. "Concussion: Bang to Rights," 74.

15. Ariana Eunjung Cha, "Brain Damage in Young Athletes Stays Long after Concussions, Scientists Find," *Washington Post*, July 12, 2016.

16. Rick Maese, "Chastain Will Donate Brain for Research," *Washington Post*, March 4, 2016.

17. Brady and Brady, "Research-Based Practice."

18. Diehl, "What's All the Headache," 89.

19. Brady and Brady, "Research-Based Practice."

20. Diehl, "What's All the Headache," 88.

21. Cynthia W. Majerske et al., "Concussion in Sports: Postconcussive Activity Levels, Symptoms, and Neurocognitive Performance," *Journal of Athletic Training* 43, no. 3 (May–June 2008): 265.

22. Zack Schonbrun, "'You Can't Put Ice over a Migraine,' a Lurking Malady in the N.F.L.," *New York Times*, December 13, 2015.

23. P. McCrory et al., "Can We Manage Sport Related Concussions in Children the Same as in Adults?" *British Journal of Sports Medicine* 38, no. 5 (2004): 516.

24. "Concussion: Bang to Rights," 74.

25. Rick Maese, "Navy Running Back McKamey, 19, Dies after Days in Coma," *Washington Post*, March 26, 2014.

26. Rick Maese, "Navy Player Is in Coma: Family Defends Program," *Washington Post*, March 25, 2014.

27. Bill Pennington, "Hidden Threats to Young Athletes," *New York Times*, May 12, 2013.

28. Frank Bruni, "Safety, Sports and Kids," *New York Times*, December 20, 2015.

29. Pennington, "Hidden Threats."

30. Sandeep Jauhar, "EKG Screening for College Athletes," *New York Times*, January 26, 2016.

31. Lindsey Tanner, "Athletes' Deaths in Workouts Prompt New Guidelines," Associated Press in the *Washington Post*, July 3, 2012.

32. Pennington, "Hidden Threats."

33. Tanner, "Athletes' Deaths."

34. Tanner, "Athletes' Deaths."

35. Pennington, "Hidden Threats."

36. Michael Ollove, "Schools Move to Protect Athletes, but They Don't Provide Trainers," *Washington Post*, October 7, 2014.

37. Pennington, "Hidden Threats."

38. Bruni, "Safety, Sports and Kids."

39. John Branch, "For N.F.L.'s Injury Carts, a History That Expands beyond Tunnel to Field," *New York Times*, November 8, 2015.

40. Branch, "N.F.L.'s Injury Carts."

41. Preston Williams, "Knee Injury a 'National Epidemic' Felt Acutely in Area," *Washington Post*, January 24, 2013.

42. Sally Jenkins, "To Understand Vonn's Greatness, Start at Nexus of Speed and Fear," *Washington Post*, February 9, 2013.

43. Patricia Hart, "Field of Nightmares," *Texas Monthly*, May 2006 (last visited December 15, 2015), www.texasmonthly.com.

44. Nathan Seppa, "Contact Sports and the Risk of Staph Infections," *Washington Post*, October 21, 2014.

45. Johnette Howard, "Why Sports Can Be a Breeding Ground for Dangerous MRSA Infections," ESPN.com, October 16, 2015 (last visited December 15, 2015), espn.go.com.

46. Howard, "Breeding Ground."

47. Tadd Haislop, "Multiple Surgeries Claim 'Parts of' Fells' Foot," *Sporting News*, October 16, 2015 (last visited December 15, 2015), www.sportingnews.com.

## 13. CONCUSSIONS IN THE NFL

1. Steve Rushin, "Brain Traumatic," *Sports Illustrated*, October 21, 2013, 64.

2. Ken Belson, "Frank Gifford Had Brain Disease, His Family Announces," *New York Times*, December 1, 2015.

3. Special to the *New York Times*, "Staubach Retirement Expected; Concussions a Concern," *New York Times*, March 15, 1980.

4. Mark Fainaru-Wada and Steve Fainaru, "League of Denial," *Sports Illustrated*, October 7, 2013, 64.

5. Fainaru-Wada and Fainaru, "League of Denial," 64.

6. Duff Wilson, "Medical Adviser for Baseball Lists Exaggerated Credentials," *New York Times*, March 30, 2005.

7. Fainaru-Wada and Fainaru, "League of Denial," 65.

8. Tom Friend, "Pro Football; Looking at Concussions, and the Repercussions," *New York Times*, February 18, 1995.

9. Dave Anderson, "N.F.L. Concussions Are Not Really Funny," *New York Times*, November 4, 1996.

10. Fainaru-Wada and Fainaru, "League of Denial," 65; Mark Fainaru-Wada and Steve Fainaru, "Head-on Collision," *ESPN the Magazine*, October 14, 2013, 33, 35, 36.

11. Fainaru-Wada and Fainaru, "League of Denial," 65–66.

12. Fainaru-Wada and Fainaru, "Head-on Collision," 35.

13. Fainaru-Wada and Fainaru, "Head-on Collision," 35.

14. Alan Schwarz, Walt Bogdanich, and Jacqueline Williams, "N.F.L. Concussion Studies Found to Have Deep Flaws," *New York Times*, March 25, 2016.

15. Fainaru-Wada and Fainaru, "Head-on Collision," 35–36.

16. Fainaru-Wada and Fainaru, "League of Denial," 66; Fainaru-Wada and Fainaru, "Head-on Collision," 38.

17. Federal Trade Commission, Staff Letter to John E. Villafranco, Esquire, April 24, 2013.

18. Fainaru-Wada and Fainaru, "League of Denial," 66.

19. Greg Garber, "A Tormented Soul," ESPN.com, January 28, 2005 (last visited April 11, 2014), http://sports.espn.go.com/nfl/news/story?id=1972285 .

20. Garber, "Tormented Soul."

21. Garber, "Tormented Soul."

22. Garber, "Tormented Soul."

23. Fainaru-Wada and Fainaru, "League of Denial," 67.

24. "Concussion: Bang to Rights," *Economist*, March 5, 2016, 73, Science and Technology section.

25. Fainaru-Wada and Fainaru, "League of Denial," 67.

26. Garber, "Tormented Soul."

27. Jani (Estate of Mike Webster) v. NFL Bell/Rozelle Pension Fund, 209 Fed. Appx. 305 (4th Cir. 2006).

28. Jim Corbett, "Tagliabue Hands Off to Goodell as NFL's Next Commissioner," *USA Today*, August 9, 2006.

29. Fainaru-Wada and Fainaru, "Head-on Collision," 36, 40.

30. Fainaru-Wada and Fainaru, "Head-on Collision," 41.

31. Fainaru-Wada and Fainaru, "Head-on Collision," 41.

32. Fainaru-Wada and Fainaru, "League of Denial," 68.

33. Fainaru-Wada and Fainairu, "League of Denial," 68.

34. Benedict Carey, "On C.T.E. and Athletes, Science Remains in Its Infancy," *New York Times*, March 27, 2016.

35. Fainaru-Wada and Fainaru, "League of Denial," 68.

36. Alan Schwarz, "Dementia Risk Seen in Players in N.F.L. Study," *New York Times*, September 30, 2009.

37. Schwarz, "Dementia Risk Seen in Players."

38. Schwarz, "Dementia Risk Seen in Players."

39. Alan Schwarz, "N.F.L.'s Dementia Study Has Flaws, Experts Say," *New York Times*, October 27, 2009.

40. Alan Schwarz, "Dementia Debate Could Intensify," *New York Times*, October 1, 2009. See also Mark Maske, "Study: Increased Dementia in Ex-players," *Washington Post*, October 1, 2009.

41. Maske, "Study."

42. See Judy Battista, "N.F.L. Players Live Longer Than Other Men, Study Says," *New York Times*, May 8, 2012.

43. Schwarz, "Dementia Debate."

44. Alan Schwarz, "N.F.L. Acknowledges Long-Term Concussion Effects," *New York Times*, December 21, 2009.

45. Schwarz, "Long-Term Concussion Effects."

46. Deborah Blum, "Will Science Take the Field?" *New York Times*, February 5, 2010.

47. Blum, "Will Science Take the Field?"

48. Blum, "Will Science Take the Field?"

49. Blum, "Will Science Take the Field?"

50. Alan Schwarz, "House Panel Criticizes New N.F.L. Doctors," *New York Times*, May 24, 2010.

51. Schwarz, "House Panel Criticizes."

52. Alan Schwarz, "On Linking Brain Damage and Behavior," *New York Times*, June 25, 2010.

53. Schwarz, "Linking Brain Damage and Behavior."

54. Alan Schwarz, "Suicide Reveals Signs of a Disease Seen in N.F.L.," *New York Times*, September 13, 2010.

55. Schwarz, "Suicide Reveals Signs."

56. Associated Press, "Penn Backup RB Ambrogi Commits Suicide," October 12, 2005.

57. Associated Press, "Concussions Reported in NFL Up 21 Percent from Last Season," December 13, 2010 (updated July 26, 2012).

58. Associated Press, "Concussions Reported."

59. Gary Mihoces, "Kickoff Returns, Concussions Drop in 2011 after Rule Change," *USA Today*, February 2, 2012.

60. Steve Fainaru and Mark Fainaru-Wada, "NFL's Progress on Concussions Blurred by Inconsistencies," December 13, 2012, www.pbs.org .

61. Fainaru and Fainaru-Wada, "Progress on Concussions Blurred."

62. Jason Reid, "Seau's Death Forces Uncomfortable Questions for Football Fans," *Washington Post*, May 13, 2012.

63. Mary Pilon and Ken Belson, "Seau Suffered from Brain Disease," *New York Times*, January 10, 2013.

64. Reid, "Seau's Death."

65. Alan Schwarz, "A Suicide, a Last Request, a Family's Questions," *New York Times*, February 22, 2011.

66. Pilon and Belson, "Seau Suffered."

67. Fainaru-Wada and Fainaru, "League of Denial," 68.

68. Ken Belson, "Bubba Smith, N.F.L. Star and Actor, Had C.T.E.," *New York Times*, May 24, 2016.

69. Pilon and Belson, "Seau Suffered."

70. David Epstein, "Conclusions? Too Early," *Sports Illustrated*, January 21, 2013, http://www.si.com/vault/2013/01/21/106273507/conclusions-too-early.

## 14. CONCUSSION-RELATED LAWSUITS FILED AGAINST THE NFL

1. Rummana Hussain, "Hoge Wins Lawsuit against Doctor," *Chicago Tribune*, July 22, 2000.

2. Alan Schwarz, "Lawsuit Cites Mishandling of Football Concussions," *New York Times*, March 18, 2010.

3. Rick Maese, "Players Come Together to Take on NFL," *Washington Post*, June 7, 2008.

4. Gene M. Wang, "SN Concussion Report: NFL Could Lose Billions in Player Lawsuits," *Sporting News*, August 22, 2012 (last visited April 21, 2014), http://sportingnews.com/nfl/story/2012-08-22/nfl-concussion- . . .

5. Associated Press, "Seau's Family Sues NFL over Concealing Evidence of Brain Injury Risks," *Washington Post*, January 24, 2013.

6. Nathan Fenno, "Many Ex-Redskins among Those Suing NFL over Effects of Brain Injuries," *Washington Times*, June 20, 2012.

7. Associated Press, "N.F.L. Retirees' Suit Is Dismissed," *New York Times*, May 29, 2012.

8. Associated Press, "N.F.L. Retirees' Suit."

9. Associated Press, "Seau's Family Sues."

10. Mike Wise, "Mixed Messages Are Causing Headaches," *Washington Post*, January 29, 2013.

11. Ken Belson and Jon Hurdle, "Crowded Courtroom for N.F.L. Lawsuit," *New York Times*, April 9, 2013.

12. Paul M. Barrett, "Will Brain Injury Lawsuits Doom or Save the NFL?" *Bloomberg Businessweek*, January 31, 2013.

13. Ken Belson, "Concussion Case Nears Key Phase for N.F.L.," *New York Times*, August 28, 2013.

14. James Andrew Miller, "N.F.L. Pressure Said to Lead ESPN to Quit Film Project," *New York Times*, August 23, 2013.

15. Rick Maese and Cindy Boren, "NFL and Retired Players Settle Concussion Lawsuits," *Washington Post*, August 30, 2013.

16. Maese and Boren, "NFL and Retired Players Settle."

17. Mike Wise, "Real Chance to Make an Impact Lost with Settlement," *Washington Post*, August 30, 2013.

18. Kent Babb and Mark Maske, "Goodell Says NFL Is Safer Than Ever," *Washington Post*, October 4, 2013.

19. Cindy Boren, "Dorsett Reveals He Has CTE," *Washington Post*, November 7, 2013.

20. Mark Maske, "Not on the Sidelines," *Washington Post*, June 8, 2016.

21. Mark Fainaru-Wada and Steve Fainaru, "Concerns over Lawyer Pay in NFL Deal," ESPN.com, December 16, 2013 (last viewed April 23, 2014), http://espn.go.com/espn/print?id=101462287&type=HeadlineNews&i . . .

22. Fainaru-Wada and Fainaru, "Concerns over Lawyer Pay."

23. Fainaru-Wada and Fainaru, "Concerns over Lawyer Pay."

24. Ken Belson, "Payouts May Reach a Wider Pool of Retirees," *New York Times*, December 20, 2013.

25. Alan Schwarz, "Uncertainty over Whether N.F.L. Settlement's Money Will Last," *New York Times*, January 29, 2014.

26. Ken Belson, "No Quick or Clear Solution in N.F.L. Settlement," *New York Times*, March 9, 2014.

27. Rick Maese, "Ex-players: NFL Pushed Risky Drug Use," *Washington Post*, May 21, 2014.

28. Associated Press, "Ex-players: NFL Illegally Used Drugs," ESPN.com, May 20, 2014 (last visited May 27, 2014), www.espn.com.

29. Joe Nocera, "N.F.L.'s Bogus Settlement for Brain-Damaged Former Players," *New York Times*, August 11, 2015.

30. Nocera, "N.F.L.'s Bogus Settlement."

31. Michael McCann, "Shield Law," *Sports Illustrated*, April 4, 2016, 12.

32. Ken Belson, "No Suicide Talk at N.F.L. Function," *New York Times*, July 25, 2015; Nocera, "N.F.L.'s Bogus Settlement."

33. Belson, "No Suicide Talk"; Ken Belson, "Hall Presents a Compromise to Let Seau's Daughter Speak," *New York Times*, August 1, 2015.

34. Ken Belson, "Sony Altered 'Concussion' Film to Prevent N.F.L. Protests, Emails Show," *New York Times*, September 1, 2015.

35. Manohla Dargis, "An Autopsy Sets Off an Epic Clash of Doctors and N.F.L.," *New York Times*, December 25, 2015.

36. Sarah Latimer, "NFL Disputes ESPN Report on Funding of Brain Study," *Washington Post*, December 23, 2015.

37. NFL Notebook, "NFL VP Concedes CTE, Sport Are Linked," *Washington Post*, March 15, 2016. See also Mark Maske, "NFL Stands by CTE Admission," *Washington Post*, March 16, 2016.

38. Ken Belson and Alan Schwarz, "N.F.L. Shifts on Concussions, and Game May Never Be the Same," *New York Times*, March 15, 2016.

39. Steven M. Rothman, "America's Concussion Obsession," *New York Times*, December 22, 2015.

40. Rick Maese, "$1 Billion Concussion Settlement Is Upheld," *Washington Post*, April 19, 2016.

41. ESPN.com News Services. "Appeals Court Upholds $1 Billion Concussion Settlement," April 18, 2016, http://espn.go.com.

42. Ken Belson, "Appeals Court Affirms Landmark N.F.L. Concussion Settlement," *New York Times*, April 18, 2016.

43. Rick Maese, "Report: NFL Tried Influencing NIH Study," *Washington Post*, May 24, 2016.

44. Maese, "NFL Tried Influencing Study."

45. Maese, "NFL Tried Influencing Study."

46. Sally Jenkins, "The NFL Acts as If It's above Science and the Law—and That's Unacceptable," *Washington Post*, May 25, 2016.

47. Maese, "NFL Tried Influencing Study."

48. Mark Maske, "Goodell Defends NFL Report," *Washington Post*, May 25, 2016.

49. Ken Belson, "Bubba Smith, N.F.L. Star and Actor, Had C.T.E.," *New York Times*, May 24, 2016.

50. Ken Belson, "Judge Tells N.F.L. to Reveal Some Secrets about Concussions," *New York Times*, October 31, 2016.

## 15. FOOTBALL'S UNHOLY TRINITY

1. Dan Steinberg, "Norman: I'm Like a Rogue Savage," *Washington Post*, June 10, 2016.

2. Arthur Kretchmer, "Butkus: One Season and One Injury with the Meanest Man Alive," *Playboy*, October 1971 (last viewed April 30, 2014), http://thestacks.deadspin.com/butkus-one-season-and-one-injury-with-the-meanest-man-1245969242.

3. David Fleming, "Knee-Jerk Reaction," *ESPN the Magazine*, November 26, 2012, 21.

4. Kevin Seifert, "Chop Blocks Eliminated, PAT Snaps from 15 Permanent," ESPN.com, March 22, 2016.

5. Fleming, "Knee-Jerk Reaction," 21.

6. Jason Reid, "NFL's Message to Meriweather Contains No Ambiguity," *Washington Post*, October 22, 2013.

7. Gene Wang and Mark Maske, "Meriweather: 'You've Got to Tear People's ACLs and Mess Up Knees' on Hits," *Washington Post*, October 29, 2013.

8. Bill Pennington, "Odell Beckham Jr. Suspended for One Game," *New York Times*, December 21, 2015.

9. Katherine Terrell, "New Orleans Saints Bounty Scandal Timeline," *New Orleans Times-Picayune*, December 12, 2012 (last visited April 29, 2014), NOLA.com.

10. Terrell, "New Orleans Saints Bounty."

11. Terrell, "New Orleans Saints Bounty."

12. Pat Yasinskas, "Report: Gregg Williams Leaving Saints," ESPN.com, January 15, 2012 (last visited April 29, 2014), http://espn.go.com.

13. Mike Wise, "Gregg Williams's True Nature Exposed," *Washington Post*, March 2, 2012.

14. Terrell, "New Orleans Saints Bounty."

15. Steve Coll, "The N.F.L.'s Bounty Game," *New Yorker*, March 3, 2012 (last visited March 26, 2014), www.newyorker.com.

16. Coll, "N.F.L.'s Bounty Game."

17. Coll, "N.F.L.'s Bounty Game."

18. Wise, "Gregg Williams's True Nature."

19. Wise, "Gregg Williams's True Nature."

20. Judy Battista, "Ruling on Bounty Appeals Will Be Signal to the Public," *New York Times*, April 5, 2012.

21. Mike Wise, "Gregg Williams, Redskins Played an Ugly Game with Bounties," *Washington Post*, March 3, 2012.

22. Coll, "N.F.L.'s Bounty Game."

23. Wise, "Ugly Game."

24. Battista, "Ruling on Bounty Appeals."

25. Battista, "Ruling on Bounty Appeals."

26. Terrell, "New Orleans Saints Bounty."

27. Mark Maske, "Discipline Dropped in Saints Bounty Case," *Washington Post*, December 12, 2012.

28. Judy Battista, "Tagliabue Lifts Suspensions but Not Blame in Bounty Case," *New York Times*, December 12, 2012.

29. Maske, "Discipline Dropped."

30. Battista, "Tagliabue Lifts Suspensions."

31. Harvey Araton, "Cuban the Firebrand, and the Futurist," *New York Times*, March 30, 2014.

32. Jon Wertheim, "Trying Times," *Sports Illustrated*, December 10, 2012, 30.

33. Wertheim, "Trying Times," 30.

34. David DiSalvo, "Is Malcolm Gladwell Right, Should College Football Be Banned to Save Brains?" *Forbes*, July 21, 2013 (last viewed April 5, 2014), http://www.forbes.com/sites/daviddisalvo/2013/07/21/is-malcolm-gladwell-right-should-college-football-be-banned.

35. Mike Wise, "NFL Is Losing Concussion Battle—and without a Cultural Shift, It Will Lose War," *Washington Post*, November 14, 2012.

36. "Schools and Hard Knocks," *Economist*, March 5, 2016, 14.

37. Chuck Culpepper, "Ivy League Dummy Could Help Save Football," *Washington Post*, April 23, 2016.

38. Wise, "NFL Is Losing Concussion Battle."

39. George F. Will, "Out of Bounds," *Washington Post*, September 19, 2013.

40. Will, "Out of Bounds."

41. Araton, "Cuban the Firebrand."

42. Jay Mathews, "At Many Leading Schools Football Fails to Make the Cut," *Washington Post*, April 7, 2013.

43. Steve Rushin, "Brain Traumatic," *Sports Illustrated*, October 21, 2013, 64.

## 16. CHILDREN PLAYING FOOTBALL

1. Gary Belsky and Neil Fine, "One Way to Make Football Safer," *Washington Post*, April 24, 2016.

2. Alan Schwarz, Walt Bogdanich, and Jacqueline Williams, "N.F.L. Concussion Studies Found to Have Deep Flaws," *New York Times*, March 25, 2016.

3. Sally Jenkins, "On Head Trauma, Goodell Couches Neglect in Nonsense," *Washington Post*, January 6, 2016.

4. Jenkins, "On Head Trauma."

5. George D. Lundberg, "The N.F.L.'s Collision with the Future," *New York Times*, January 5, 2016.

6. Cindy Boren, "Another NFL Owner Questions Link to CTE," *Washington Post*, March 24, 2016. See also Mark Maske, "NFL Still Has Lack of Clarity on CTE Link," *Washington Post*, March 24, 2015.

7. Boren, "Another NFL Owner."

8. Maske, "NFL Still Has Lack of Clarity."

9. Kevin Seifert, "Roger Goodell Says CTE Link Consistent with NFL's Position," ESPN.com, March 23, 2016.

10. Ken Belson, "Football's Risks Sink In, Even in the Heart of Texas," *New York Times*, May 11, 2014.

11. Alan Schwarz, "N.F.L.'s Influence on Safety at Youth Levels Is Cited," *New York Times*, October 30, 2009.

12. Schwarz, "N.F.L.'s Influence on Safety."

13. Schwarz, "N.F.L.'s Influence on Safety."

14. Alan Schwarz, "Learning from Sadness," *New York Times*, November 7, 2010.

15. Editorial, "Clarity about Concussions," *Washington Post*, June 22, 2016.

16. Editorial, "Clarity about Concussions."

17. Sean Gregory, "Can Roger Goodell Save Football?" *Time*, December 17, 2012, 39.

18. Gregory, "Can Roger Goodell Save Football?," 39.

19. Gregory, "Can Roger Goodell Save Football?"

20. Sally Jenkins and Rick Maese, "Football Is the (Dangerous) Family Business," *Washington Post*, July 22, 2013.

21. Mark Maske, "NFL's New Rules Aim to Curb Injury," *Washington Post*, April 17, 2012.

22. Mark Maske, "NFL Changes, for Safety's Sake," *Washington Post*, March 25, 2013.

23. Anahad O'Connor, "Trying to Reduce Head Injuries, Youth Football Limits Practices," *New York Times*, June 13, 2012.

24. Ken Belson, "Concussion Study Makes Case to Curb Practice Hits," *New York Times*, July 26, 2013.

25. Chelsea Janes, "MPSSAA to Implement Safe Tackling Program," *Washington Post*, May 6, 2014.

26. Rick Maese, "Trying to Protect Players from the Ground Up," *Washington Post*, October 25, 2013.

27. Mike Dougherty, "A Sport at a Crossroad," *Journal News* (A Gannett Company), October 20, 2013.

28. Belson, "Concussion Study."

29. Belson, "Concussion Study."

30. Steven M. Rothman, "America's Concussion Obsession," *New York Times*, December 22, 2015.

31. Maese, "Trying to Protect Players."

32. Maese, "Trying to Protect Players."

33. Janes, "Safe Tackling Program."

34. Dougherty, "Sport at a Crossroad."

35. Sally Jenkins, "Tackling the Problem of Kids' Football," *Washington Post*, October 3, 2013.

36. Maese, "Trying to Protect Players."

37. Ben Shpigel, "Football Faces 'Turning Point' on Safety Risk," *New York Times*, June 20, 2012.

38. Jenkins and Maese, "Family Business."

39. Jenkins, "On Head Trauma."

40. Judy Battista, "N.F.L. Joins with G.E. in Effort to Detect Concussions," *New York Times*, February 3, 2013.

41. Battista, "N.F.L. Joins with G.E."

42. Battista, "N.F.L. Joins with G.E."

43. Battista, "N.F.L. Joins with G.E."

44. Ken Belson, "New Tests for Brain Trauma Create Hope, and Skepticism," *New York Times*, December 25, 2013.

45. Belson, "New Tests."

46. Belson, "New Tests."

47. Ken Belson, "New Concussion Guidelines Stress Individual Treatment," *New York Times*, March 18, 2013.

48. Battista, "N.F.L. Joins with G.E."

49. Belson, "New Concussion Guidelines."

50. Rick Maese, "NFL, Military Partner on Concussions," *Washington Post*, June 13, 2013.

51. Belson, "Football's Risks Sink In."

52. Belson, "Football's Risks Sink In."

53. M. D. Shear and Ken Belson, "Obama's Conference on Concussions Highlights a Paradox for the N.F.L.," *New York Times*, May 30, 2014.

54. Shear and Belson, "Obama's Conference."

55. Adam Kilgore, "Truth about Player Safety, and Consequences," *Washington Post*, November 24, 2015.

56. Sally Jenkins, "For NFL, Protocol Reveals a Disconnect," *Washington Post*, December 5, 2015.

57. Rick Maese, "Study Stresses Impact of Subconcussive Trauma," *Washington Post*, April 1, 2016.

58. See "Walk Off," *Sports Illustrated*, March 18, 2018, 18; Mark Maske, "Not on the Sidelines," *Washington Post*, June 8, 2016.

59. Bennet Omalu, "Don't Let Kids Play Football," *New York Times*, December 7, 2015.

60. Editorial Sunday Review, "Head Trauma Haunts the Gridiron," *New York Times*, October 15, 2016.

## 17. FOLLOWING SUIT

1. Jeff Z. Klein, "Boogaard Lawsuit May Shake Up Hockey," *New York Times*, September 26, 2012.

2. John Branch, "In Suit over Death, Boogaard's Family Blames the N.H.L.," *New York Times*, May 12, 2013.

3. John Branch, "Derek Boogaard: A Brain 'Going Bad,'" *New York Times*, December 5, 2011.

4. Klein, "Boogaard Lawsuit."

5. John Branch, "After a Life of Punches, Ex-N.H.L. Enforcer Is a Threat to Himself," *New York Times*, June 1, 2016.

6. Jeff Z. Klein, "Wave of Concussions Hits the N.H.L.," *New York Times*, February 26, 2013.

7. See Jason Diamos, "Injured Lindros Ponders the Future," *New York Times*, March 19, 2006.

8. Klein, "Wave of Concussions."

9. Brian Cazeneuve, "Chris Pronger Has a Headache," *Sports Illustrated*, April 22, 2013, http://www.si.com/vault/2013/04/22/106312919/chris-pronger-has-a-headache.

10. Cazeneuve, "Chris Pronger."

11. Adam Kilgore, "Ex-players Fight the NHL Yet Try to Remain Loyal to Game," *Washington Post*, May 26, 2016.

12. Jeff Z. Klein, "The Science behind a Call for Safer Hockey," *New York Times*, October 2, 2013.

13. Jeff Z. Klein, "Who Is Susceptible to Concussions?" *New York Times*, March 9, 2014.

14. Kilgore, "Ex-players Fight the NHL."

15. Ken Belson and Jeff Z. Klein, "Ten Former N.H.L. Players Sue League over Head Injuries," *New York Times*, November 25, 2013.

16. Jeff Z. Klein and Stu Hackel, "A Stricter Standard for Safety's Sake," *New York Times*, December 29, 2013.

17. Klein and Hackel, "Stricter Standard."

18. Jeff Z. Klein and Ken Belson, "N.H.L. Promoted Violence for Profit Regardless of Health Risk, Players' Suit Says," *New York Times*, April 11, 2014.

19. Allan Muir, "NHL Hit by New Concussion Lawsuit Filed by 29 Players," *Sports Illustrated*, February 10, 2015, www.si.com.

20. Gary Mihoces, "Judge Denies NHL Bid to Halt Concussion Lawsuit," *USA Today*, March 25, 2015, www.usatoday.com.

21. Adam Kilgore, "NHL's Motion to Dismiss Suit Denied," *Washington Post*, May 19, 2016.

22. Klein and Belson, "N.H.L. Promoted Violence."

23. John Branch, "In Emails, N.H.L. Officials Conceded Concussion Risks of Fights," *New York Times*, March 29, 2016.

24. John Branch, "Members of Congress Ask N.H.L. for More Concussion Information," *New York Times*, October 16, 2016.

25. See Adrian Arrington v. NCAA, No. 11-cv-06356 (N.D. Ill Sept. 12, 2012).

26. NCAA Press Release, "NCAA Reaches Proposed Settlement in Concussion Lawsuit," July 29, 2014.

27. NCAA Press Release, "NCAA Reaches Proposed Settlement."

28. Associated Press, "Archie Griffin's Brother, Others File Suits over Concussions," *New York Times*, June 9, 2016.

29. Ben Strauss, "Six Concussion Suits Are Filed against Colleges and N.C.A.A.," *New York Times*, May 17, 2016.

30. Associated Press, "Archie Griffin's Brother."

31. Associated Press, "Archie Griffin's Brother."

32. Roger Groves, "Coming to a College near You: More Concussion Litigation," *Forbes*, May 25, 2016 (last visited June 10, 2016), www.forbes.com.

## 18. CONCUSSION CONCERNS FOR
## FEMALE ATHLETES

1. Chelsea Janes, "Addressing a Problem Head-On," *Washington Post*, April 24, 2014.

2. Chelsea Janes, "Fears of Concussions Lead to Heading Bans," *Washington Post*, June 1, 2014.

3. Amie Just, "Scurry's Next Big Save: Women's Brain Health," *Washington Post*, June 20, 2016.

4. Rick Maese, "Chastain Will Donate Brain for Research," *Washington Post*, March 4, 2016.

5. Just, "Scurry's Next Big Save."

6. Janes, "Fears of Concussions."

7. Just, "Scurry's Next Big Save."

8. Janes, "Addressing a Problem."

9. Caitlin Dewey, "Tending to a New Goal," *Washington Post*, November 3, 2013.

10. Chelsea Janes, "Reducing the Number of Concussions in High School Girls' Soccer Is a Daunting Task," *Washington Post*, April 24, 2014.

11. Dewey, "Tending to a New Goal."

12. Maese, "Chastain Will Donate."

13. Just, "Scurry's Next Big Save."

14. Just, "Scurry's Next Big Save."

15. Seth Berkman, "Women's Hockey Grows Bigger, Faster and Dire," *International New York Times*, December 18, 2015.

16. Berkman, "Women's Hockey."

17. Pat Borzi, "Amanda Kessel, Top College Player out of Action since Sochi, Returns," *New York Times*, February 6, 2016.

18. Berkman, "Women's Hockey."

## 19. BRAIN AND OTHER SEVERE INJURIES IN BASEBALL

1. Chelsea Janes, "Fears of Concussions Lead to Heading Bans," *Washington Post*, June 1, 2014.

2. ESPN.com News Services, "Ryan Freel Had CTE, Parents Say," December 15, 2013 (last visited April 28, 2014), http://espn.go.com/espn/print?id=10142581&type-HeadlineNews&i . . .

3. Associated Press, "Ryan Freel, Concussion-Plagued Baseball Player, Dies at 36," *New York Times*, December 24, 2012.

4. Associated Press, "MLB Rule Will Limit Collisions at Home Plate," *Washington Post*, February 25, 2014.

5. Tyler Kepner, "The Play at the Plate: Safer," *New York Times*, December 11, 2013.

6. Mark Saxon, "Chase Utley Suspended 2 Games for Slide into Reuben Tejada, Will Appeal," ESPN.com, October 12, 2015 (last visited December 29, 2015), www.espn.go.com; Tyler Kepner, "It's Unsafe at Second, and Some Want New Rules for Slides," *New York Times*, October 11, 2015.

7. Saxon, "Chase Utley Suspended."

8. Stuart Miller, "Safety Sometimes Prevails over Accuracy in Calling the First Out of a Double Play," *New York Times*, May 4, 2014.

9. Benjamin Hoffman, "Rule Revisions on Slide Seem to Muddy Issue," *New York Times*, February 26, 2016. See also MLBPA/MLB News Release, "MLB, MLBPA Adopt Slide Rule on Double Plays, Pace of Game Changes," February 26, 2016.

10. Joe Nocera, "A Fan Injured by a Hard Foul Challenges Assumption That Teams Can Avoid Liability," *New York Times*, November 21, 2015.

11. Nocera, "Fan Injured."

12. Rawlings v. Cleveland Indians Baseball Co., Inc., 2015-Ohio-4587 (November 5, 2015) as reported by Dan Trevas, Court News Ohio, November 5, 2015 (last visited January 7, 2016), www.courtnewsohio.gov/cases.

13. David Glovin, "Baseball Caught Looking as Fouls Injure 1,750 Fans a Year," *Bloomberg Business*, September 9, 2014 (last visited December 30, 2015), www.bloomberg.com.

14. Glovin, "Baseball Caught Looking."

15. Nocera, "Fan Injured."

16. David Waldstein, "Fan Injuries Spur M.L.B. to Call for Netting at Stadiums," *New York Times*, December 10, 2015.

17. Joe Nocera, "Baseball's New Policy Encourages Adding Only a Little New Protection," *New York Times*, December 19, 2015.

18. Joe Nocera, "A Fine Line Separates Ball and Fan," *New York Times*, April 16, 2016.

19. Nocera, "Fine Line."

20. Nocera, "Fine Line."

21. Joe Nocera, "Senseless Injury," *New York Times*, Nov. 4, 2016.

## 20. PERFORMANCE-RISK REWARDS UNDERMINE HEALTH

1. All quotations in this chapter are from P. David Howe, *Sport, Professionalism, and Pain: Ethnographies of Injury and Risk* (New York: Routledge, 2004).

## 21. ARM INJURIES TO ELITE YOUNG PITCHERS IN BASEBALL

1. See David Sheinin, "Arms Torn to Shreds," *Washington Post*, May 4, 2014; Tom Verducci, "As Fernandez Goes Down, Here's a Solution to Arm

Injury Epidemic," *Sports Illustrated*, May 13, 2014, http://sportsillustrated.cnn.com/mlb/news/20140513/jose-fernandez-miami-marlins-injury/.

2. Verducci, "Fernandez Goes Down."

3. Verducci, "Fernandez Goes Down."

4. Johnnie Whitehead and Dick Patrick, "How Much Is Too Much for Young Arms," *USA Today*, August 17, 2006.

5. Sheinin, "Arms Torn to Shreds."

6. Sheinin, "Arms Torn to Shreds."

7. Verducci, "Fernandez Goes Down."

8. Sheinin, "Arms Torn to Shreds."

9. Verducci, "Fernandez Goes Down."

10. Chris Jones, "Magic Mark," *ESPN the Magazine*, June 9, 2014, 136.

11. Jeff Passan, "Book Excerpt: Are High School Pitchers Throwing Too Hard Too Soon," *Sports Illustrated*, April 4, 2016, 59. From *The Arm: Inside the Billion-Dollar Mystery of the Most Valuable Commodity in Sports* (New York: HarperCollins, 2016).

12. David Epstein, " Sports Should Be Child's Play," *New York Times*, June 10, 2014.

13. "Youth Baseball Throwing Arm Injuries Are Rising Dramatically," *Science Daily*, March 11, 2010 (last visited May 20, 2014), www.sciencedaily.com/releases/2010/03/100310083443.htm.

14. Passan, "High School Pitchers," 59.

## 22. FOOTBALL INJURIES IN THE NFL AND COLLEGE

1. NCAA, "Football Injuries," PDF (last visited June 15, 2016), www.ncaa.org.

2. *Wall Street Journal*, "In the NFL, Which Body Part Gets Hurt the Most?" January 27, 2014, wsj.com.

3. Nathaniel Vinton, "Concussions Are on the Rise in the NFL: League Releases Data That Shows 58% Increase in Regular Season Concussions," *Daily News*, January 30, 2016 (last visited June 15, 2016), www.dailynews.com.

4. Carl Prine, "Bloody Sundays," *IRE Journal* 28, no. 4 (July–August 2005) (last visited May 16, 2014), http://www.questia.com/read/1P3-897062681/bloody-sundays.

5. Prine, "Bloody Sundays."

6. Prine, "Bloody Sundays."

7. Prine, "Bloody Sundays."

8. Prine, "Bloody Sundays."

9. Prine, "Bloody Sundays."

## 23. THE NCAA PROVIDES SHAMEFULLY INADEQUATE HEALTH CARE FOR ITS STUDENT-ATHLETES

1. See Juliet Macur, "Gaining Rights amid Guarded Words," *New York Times*, March 28, 2014.

2. Mike Wise, "Lesson of This Health Union Talk: This Isn't Really about Money," *Washington Post*, April 13, 2014.

3. Liz Clarke, "Emmert: Unionization 'Inappropriate,'" *Washington Post*, April 7, 2014.

4. Steve Eder, "Labor Case Filed by Injured Player in '70s Has Echoes Today," *New York Times*, April 22, 2014.

5. Eder, "Labor Case Filed."

6. Eder, "Labor Case Filed."

7. Eder, "Labor Case Filed."

8. Eder, "Labor Case Filed."

9. Kevin B. Blackistone, "Why College Needs Divorce from Football, Basketball," *Diverse Issues in Higher Education* 30, no. 25 (January 16, 2014).

10. Ben Strauss, "A Fight to Save College Athletes from the Ordeal of Injury Costs," *New York Times*, April 25, 2014.

11. Strauss, "Fight to Save College Athletes."

12. Bill Pennington, "In a Moment It Can All Be Gone," *New York Times*, April 5, 2013.

13. Pennington, "In a Moment."

14. Strauss, "Fight to Save College Athletes."

15. Jeff Greer, "Kevin Ware to Transfer from Louisville," *New York Times*, March 29, 2014.

## 24. STIGMA, STEREOTYPES, AND SECRECY UNDERMINE ATHLETES' MENTAL HEALTH

1. Rick Maese, "Concussions, Mental Health Are Linked," *Washington Post*, December 7, 2014.

2. Jon Wertheim, "McKinley's Apparent Suicide Casts Light on Athletes' Risk of Depression," *Sports Illustrated*, September 21, 2010, http://sportsillustrated.cnn.com.

3. Jon Wertheim, "Prisoners of Depression," *Sports Illustrated*, September 8, 2003, http://sportsillustrated.cnn.com/vault.

4. Robert Lipsyte, "Backtalk; Harnisch a Reluctant Role Model," *New York Times*, November 22, 1998.

5. Wertheim, "Prisoners of Depression."

6. Wertheim, "McKinley's Apparent Suicide."

7. Lipsyte, "Backtalk."

8. Wertheim, "Prisoners of Depression."

9. Kostya Kennedy, "Brotherly Love," *Sports Illustrated*, October 22, 2001.

10. Wertheim, "Prisoners of Depression."

11. William C. Rhoden, "On the Court, Finding an Outlet, and a Voice," *New York Times*, February 26, 2012.

12. Sally Jenkins, "Chamique Holdsclaw Confronts Her 'Little Secret' of Depression," *Washington Post*, May 17, 2012.

13. Joseph White, "Holdsclaw Looking for Fresh Start, Traded to Los Angeles," *USA Today*, March 21, 2005.

14. Rhoden, "On the Court."

15. Mame M. Kwayie, "Chamique Holdsclaw Speaks on Her Depression," *Ebony*, August 14, 2014 (last visited December 30, 2014), www.ebony.com.

16. Sally Jenkins, "Holdsclaw's Rocky Road to a Clear Head," *Washington Post*, May 28, 2012.

17. Filip Bondy, "Chamique Holdsclaw's Star Fades as Arrest Is Another Sad Chapter for Former Queens Basketball Star," *New York Daily News*, November 17, 2012.

18. Rachel George, "Holdsclaw Indicted for Shooting Incident with Girlfriend," *USA Today*, February 27, 2013.

19. Rachel Axon, "Chamique Holdsclaw Pleads Guilty to Assault," *USA Today*, June 14, 2013.

20. See John W. Parry, *Mental Disability, Violence, Future Dangerousness: Myths behind the Presumption of Guilt* (Lanham, Md.: Rowman & Littlefield, 2013).

21. Pablo S. Torre, "The Mystery Pick Is Royce White," *Sports Illustrated*, July 2, 2012, 44.

22. William C. Rhoden, "Civility Need Not Be Excluded from the Culture of the N.F.L.," *New York Times*, November 10, 2013.

23. Phil Taylor, "The Influence of Anxiety," *Sports Illustrated*, January 21, 2013, 70.

24. Taylor, "Influence of Anxiety," 70.

25. See John W. Parry, *Disability Discrimination Law, Evidence and Testimony* (Chicago: American Bar Association, 2008), 171–80.

26. Taylor, "Influence of Anxiety," 70.

27. Taylor, "Influence of Anxiety."

28. Rhoden, "Civility."

29. Jeff Zillgitt, "Rookie on a Mission," *USA Today*, February 8, 2013.

30. Sarah Lyall, "White Is a Player with a Cause, but without a Team," *New York Times*, December 9, 2013.

31. Dan Favale, "Sacramento Kings Reportedly 'Likely' to Sign Royce White to 10-Day Contract," Bleacher Report, February 26, 2014, www.bleacherreport. com.

32. George Dohrmann, "A Coach Unbalanced," *Sports Illustrated*, December 1, 2014, 54–60.

33. Dohrmann, "Coach Unbalanced."

34. Rich Cimini, "Ainge: 'I Had to Go Get Help before I Died,'" ESPN.com, March 31, 2011 (last visited January 20, 2015).

35. Associated Press, "Jets Rookie Ainge Suspended Four Games for Violating Steroids Policy," November 22, 2008 (last visited January 21, 2015), www. espn.go.com .

36. Cimini, "Ainge."

37. Cimini, "Ainge."

38. Cimini, "Ainge."

39. Associated Press, "Jets' Ainge Announces Retirement; Cites Injuries," June 23, 2011 (last visited January 21, 2015), www.espn.go.com.

40. Local8Now.com, "Crimetracker: Former Vol QB Arrested for DUI," July 28, 2013 (last visited January 21, 2015), www.local8now.com.

41. Jeff Olson, "A Victory That Means Much More," *Sports Illustrated*, December 17, 2012.

42. Olson, "Victory."

43. ESPN.com News Services, "'Fail Mary' Official Fighting Depression," January 13, 2015 (last visited January 13, 2015), http://www.espn.go.com.

44. ESPN.com News Services, "'Fail Mary' Official."

45. ESPN.com News Services, "'Fail Mary' Official."

46. Adam Kilgore, "Nats Bullish on Barrett after Bout with 'the Yips,'" *Washington Post*, February 24, 2014.

47. Kilgore, "Nats Bullish on Barrett."

48. Michael Bamberger, "Emotional Rescue," *Sports Illustrated*, November 26, 2012, 15.

49. Karen Crouse and Bill Pennington, "Panic Attack Leads to Hospital on Way to Golfer's First Victory," *New York Times*, November 13, 2012.

50. Karen Crouse, "Carefree Spirit Becomes the Face of Anxiety," *New York Times*, January 4, 2013.

51. Bill Pennington, "To Calm Jittery Nerves, Keegan Bradley Embraces Them," *New York Times*, July 15, 2016.

52. Crouse, "Carefree Spirit."

53. Chris Jones, "Status Update," *ESPN the Magazine*, March 18, 2013, 24.

54. Jones, "Status Update," 24.

## CONCLUSION

1. Rick Maese, "In U.S., Drug Testing Is Quite a Serious Business," *Washington Post*, July 18, 2016.

2. Bill Pennington, "The Trusted Grown-Ups Who Steal Millions from Youth Sports," *New York Times*, July 7, 2016.

3. Norman Chad, "It's College Football Season. What's Wrong with College Football? Everything," *Washington Post*, September 19, 2016.

4. Rebecca R. Ruiz, "WADA Tells Lawmakers It Lacked 'Clear Authority' to Investigate Russian Sports," *New York Times*, July 9, 2016.

5. Rebecca R. Ruiz, "Rio Doping Lab Suspended as Games Near," *New York Times*, June 25, 2016.

6. Maese, "Quite a Serious Business."

# BIBLIOGRAPHY

Abshir, Idil. "Kenya's Gold Medal for Corruption." *New York Times*, August 23, 2016, Opinion Pages.

Adrian Arrington v. NCAA. No. 11-cv-06356 (N.D. Ill Sept. 12, 2012).

American Academy of Neurology Press Release. "AAN Issues Sports-Related Concussion Guideline." March 13, 2013.

American Academy of Pediatrics, Policy Statement. "Use of Performance-Enhancing Substances." *Pediatrics* 115, no. 4 (April 2005): 1103. Reaffirmed and Retired, February 2008 and May 2008. doi:10.1542/peds.2005-0085.

Anderson, Dave. "N.F.L. Concussions Are Not Really Funny." *New York Times*, November 4, 1996.

Araton, Harvey. "Cuban the Firebrand, and the Futurist." *New York Times*, March 30, 2014.

———. "It's Time to Reconsider Barry Bonds for the Hall of Fame." *New York Times*, July 24, 2015.

———. "Oden Has a Fragile Body but a Strengthened Spirit." *New York Times*, November 2, 2013.

Associated Press. "Archie Griffin's Brother, Others File Suits over Concussions." *New York Times*, June 9, 2016.

———. "Concussions Reported in NFL Up 21 Percent from Last Season." December 13, 2010. Updated July 26, 2012.

———. "Ex-players: NFL Illegally Used Drugs." ESPN.com. May 20, 2014. Last visited May 27, 2014.www.espn.com.

———. "Inside The Report: Doping Scheme Had Magicians, Cocktails." July 18, 2016.

———. "Jets' Ainge Announces Retirement; Cites Injuries." June 23, 2011. Last visited January 21, 2015. espn.go.com.

———. "Jets Rookie Ainge Suspended Four Games For Violating Steroids Policy." November 22, 2008. Last visited January 21, 2015. espn.go.com.

———. "Manufacturer: 4–6 Weeks Normal Treatment for Drug in Maria Sharapova Case." ESPN.com. March 8, 2016. Last visited March 9, 2016. www.espn.go.com .

———. "Mets' Mejia Banned for Life." February 12, 2016. Last visited February 19, 2016. www.timesunion.com.

———. "MLB Rule Will Limit Collisions at Home Plate." *Washington Post*, February 25, 2014.

———. "N.F.L. Retirees' Suit Is Dismissed." *New York Times*, May 29, 2012.

———. "Penn Backup RB Ambrogi Commits Suicide." ESPN.com. October 12, 2005. http://www.espn.com/college-football/news/story?id=2188851.

———. "Rafael Nadal Sues French Official for Defamation over Doping Allegation." *New York Times*, April 25, 2016.

———. "Ryan Freel, Concussion-Plagued Baseball Player, Dies at 36." *New York Times*, December 24, 2012.

———. "Seau's Family Sues NFL over Concealing Evidence of Brain Injury Risks." *Washington Post*, January 24, 2013.

———. "Study Claims Imaging Tests Show Larger Rubber Core." January 3, 2007. http://sports.espn.go.com/mlb/news/story?id=2719191.

———. "Tiger Woods Doctor in Doping Probe." *Richmond Times-Dispatch*, December 15, 2009.

———. "Urlacher Would Hide Injury." *New York Times*, November 16, 2012.

Austen, Ian. "British Cyclist Releases Test Results but Does Little to Silence His Critics." *New York Times*, December 4, 2015.

———. "Report Describes How Armstrong Mastered Undermining Antidoping Tests." *New York Times*, October 12, 2012.

Austin, Simon. "WADA Act on Doping Report, Revoking Accreditation of Russian Lab." *International New York Times*, November 10, 2015. www.nytimes.com.

Axon, Rachel. "Chamique Holdsclaw Pleads Guilty to Assault." *USA Today*, June 14, 2013.

Babb, Kent. "Threat of Head Injuries Constant." *Washington Post*, October 10, 2012.

Babb, Kent, and Mark Maske. "Goodell Says NFL Is Safer Than Ever." *Washington Post*, October 4, 2013.

Bamberger, Michael. "Emotional Rescue." *Sports Illustrated*, November 26, 2012, 15.

Barbara, Vanessa. "An Olympic Catastrophe." *New York Times*, July 3, 2016.

Barrett, Paul M. "Will Brain Injury Lawsuits Doom or Save the NFL?" *Bloomberg Businessweek*, January 31, 2013.

Battista, Judy. "Drug of Focus Is at Center of Suspensions." *New York Times*, December 2, 2012.

———. "N.F.L. Joins with G.E. in Effort to Detect Concussions." *New York Times*, February 3, 2013.

———. "N.F.L. Players Live Longer Than Other Men, Study Says." *New York Times*, May 8, 2012.

———. "Ruling on Bounty Appeals Will Be Signal to the Public." *New York Times*, April 5, 2012.

———. "Tagliabue Lifts Suspensions but Not Blame in Bounty Case." *New York Times*, December 12, 2012.

Beacham, Greg. "Failed Drug Test Has Sharapova, 28, Facing Lengthy Ban from Competition." *Washington Post*, March 8, 2016.

Belsky, Gary, and Neil Fine. "One Way to Make Football Safer." *Washington Post*, April 24, 2016.

Belson, Ken. "Appeals Court Affirms Landmark N.F.L. Concussion Settlement." *New York Times*, April 18, 2016.

———. "Bubba Smith, N.F.L. Star and Actor, Had C.T.E." *New York Times*, May 24, 2016.

———. "Concussion Case Nears Key Phase for N.F.L." *New York Times*, August 28, 2013.

———. "Concussion Study Makes Case to Curb Practice Hits." *New York Times*, July 26, 2013.

———. "Football's Risks Sink In, Even in the Heart of Texas." *New York Times*, May 11, 2014.

———. "Frank Gifford Had Brain Disease, His Family Announces." *New York Times*, December 1, 2015.

———. "Hall Presents a Compromise to Let Seau's Daughter Speak." *New York Times*, August 1, 2015.

———. "Judge Tells N.F.L. to Reveal Some Secrets about Concussions." *New York Times*, October 31, 2016.

———. "Judges Skeptical of Retirees' Settlement Appeal." *New York Times*, November 20, 2015.

———. "New Concussion Guidelines Stress Individual Treatment." *New York Times*, March 18, 2013.

———. "New Tests for Brain Trauma Create Hope, and Skepticism." *New York Times*, December 25, 2013.

———. "N.F.L. Concussion Settlement Payments Can Begin after Supreme Court Defers." *New York Times*, December 12, 2016.

———. "Nicklas Backstrom Misses Final after Failed Drug Test." *New York Times*, February 23, 2014.

———. "No Quick or Clear Solution in N.F.L. Settlement." *New York Times*, March 9, 2014.

———. "No Suicide Talk at N.F.L. Function." *New York Times*, July 25, 2015.

———. "Payouts May Reach a Wider Pool of Retirees." *New York Times*, December 20, 2013.

———. "A Player Concussed, and a Policy Questioned." *New York Times*, November 23, 2013.

———. "Retired N.F.L. Players Appeal Ruling on Concussion Settlement." *New York Times*, April 28, 2016.

———. "Sony Altered 'Concussion' Film to Prevent N.F.L. Protests, Emails Show." *New York Times*, September 1, 2015.

———. "Study Bolsters Link between Routine Hits and Brain Disease." *New York Times*, December 3, 2012.

———. "To the N.F.L., 40 Winks Is as Vital as the 40-Yard Dash." *New York Times*, October 1, 2016.

Belson, Ken, and Jon Hurdle. "Crowded Courtroom for N.F.L. Lawsuit." *New York Times*, April 9, 2013.

Belson, Ken, and Jeff Z. Klein. "Ten Former N.H.L. Players Sue League over Head Injuries." *New York Times*, November 25, 2013.

Belson, Ken, and Jere Longman. "Baseball Dopers' New Drug Is an Old One Used by East Germany." *International New York Times*, May 6, 2016.

Belson, Ken, and Mary Pilon. "Concern Raised over Athletes' Use of Painkiller before Games." *New York Times*, April 12, 2012.

Belson, Ken, and Alan Schwarz. "N.F.L. Shifts on Concussions, and Game May Never Be the Same." *New York Times*, March 15, 2016.

Bennett, Dashiell. "The Jay Cutler Criticism Is the Reason Why the NFL's Concussion Problem Is Not Going Away." *Business Insider*, January 24, 2011. Last visited May 27, 2014. www.businessinder.com.

Berkman, Seth. "Women's Hockey Grows Bigger, Faster and Dire." *International New York Times*, December 18, 2015.

Blackistone, Kevin B. "Why College Needs Divorce from Football, Basketball." *Diverse Issues in Higher Education* 30, no. 25 (January 16, 2014).

*Bloomberg Businessweek.* "Testing Makes Perfect." April 4, 2016, 20.

Blum, Deborah. "Will Science Take the Field?" *New York Times*, February 5, 2010.

Bondy, Filip. "Chamique Holdsclaw's Star Fades as Arrest Is Another Sad Chapter for Former Queens Basketball Star." *New York Daily News*, November 17, 2012.

Boren, Cindy. "Another NFL Owner Questions Link to CTE." *Washington Post*, March 24, 2016.

———. "Dorsett Reveals He Has CTE." *Washington Post*, November 7, 2013.

Borzi, Pat. "Amanda Kessel, Top College Player out of Action since Sochi, Returns." *New York Times*, February 6, 2016.

Boswell, Thomas. "Ali: An Appreciation." *Washington Post*, June 5, 2016.

Boyle, Robert H. *Sport: Mirror of American Life.* Boston: Little, Brown, 1963.

Brady, Don, and Flo Brady. "Research-Based Practice: Sport-Related Concussions." *NASP Communique* 39, no. 8 (June 2011). Last viewed March 27, 2014. www.nasponline.org/publications/cq/39/8/sport-related-concussions.

Branch, John. "After a Life of Punches, Ex-N.H.L. Enforcer Is a Threat to Himself." *New York Times*, June 1, 2016.

———. "Derek Boogaard: A Brain 'Going Bad.'" *New York Times*, December 5, 2011.

————. "For N.F.L.'s Injury Carts, a History That Expands beyond Tunnel to Field." *New York Times*, November 8, 2015.

————. "In Emails, N.H.L. Officials Conceded Concussion Risks of Fights." *New York Times*, March 29, 2016.

————. "In Suit over Death, Boogaard's Family Blames the N.H.L." *New York Times*, May 12, 2013.

————. "Members of Congress Ask N.H.L. for More Concussion Information." *New York Times*, October 16, 2016.

Brokaw, Tom. *The Greatest Generation* . New York: Random House, 1998.

Bruni, Frank. "Safety, Sports and Kids." *New York Times*, December 20, 2015.

Bryant, Howard. "The Fix Is In: Does Tennis Have a PED Problem?" *ESPN the Magazine*, February 18, 2013, 8.

————. "The Not-So-Fine Line." *ESPN the Magazine*, September 17, 2012, 10.

————. "Spring Thaw." *ESPN the Magazine*, March 31, 2014, 8.

Burnside, Scott. "Backstrom Victim of Testing Debacle." ESPN.com. February 23, 2014.

Carey, Benedict. "On C.T.E. and Athletes, Science Remains in Its Infancy." *New York Times*, March 27, 2016.

Carrera, Katie. "Backstrom Will Get Silver Medal; IOC Says Ban 'Fully Justified.'" *Washington Post*, March 15, 2014.

Carrera, Katie, and Dave Sheinin. "Caps' Backstrom Fails IOC Drug Test." *Washington Post*, February 24, 2014.

Cazeneuve, Brian. "Chris Pronger Has a Headache." *Sports Illustrated*, April 22, 2013. http://www.si.com/vault/2013/04/22/106312919/chris-pronger-has-a-headache.

————. "You Gotta Play Hurt." *Sports Illustrated*, May 3, 2014, 53–59.

Cha, Ariana Eunjung. "Brain Damage in Young Athletes Stays Long after Concussions, Scientists Find." *Washington Post*, July 12, 2016.

Chad, Norman. "It's College Football Season. What's Wrong with College Football? Everything." *Washington Post*, September 19, 2016.

————. "Lance, Oprah and the Search for Truth." *Washington Post*, January 21, 2013.

Cimini, Rich. "Ainge: 'I Had To Go Get Help before I Died." ESPN.com. March 31, 2011. Last visited January 20, 2015.

Clarey, Christopher. "Erasing the Bitter Taste without Absolving Sharapova." *New York Times*, June 12, 2016.

————. "I.T.F.'s Antidoping Policy Poses Test for New Leader." *New York Times*, December 6, 2015.

————. "Tennis's Watchdog Seems to Operate in the Dark." *New York Times*, January 18, 2016.

————. "Watchdogs Show Teeth and, Finally Some Spine." *New York Times*, June 18, 2016.

Clarke, Liz. "Emmert: Unionization 'Inappropriate.'" *Washington Post*, April 7, 2014.

Coletta, Amanda. "Speedskater Poised to Upend Rule of Sports' Highest Court." *New York Times*, February 11, 2016.

Coll, Steve. "The N.F.L.'s Bounty Game." *New Yorker*, March 3, 2012. Last visited March 26, 2014. www.newyorker.com.

Corbett, Jim. "Tagliabue Hands Off to Goodell as NFL's Next Commissioner." *USA Today*, August 9, 2006.

Crouse, Karen. "Carefree Spirit Becomes the Face of Anxiety." *New York Times*, January 4, 2013.

————. "Shadow of Doping Is Never Far from Pool." *New York Times*, August 2, 2015.

Crouse, Karen, and Bill Pennington. "Panic Attack Leads to Hospital on Way to Golfer's First Victory." *New York Times*, November 13, 2012.

Culpepper, Chuck. "Ivy League Dummy Could Help Save Football." *Washington Post*, April 23, 2016.

Dargis, Manohla. "An Autopsy Sets Off an Epic Clash of Doctors and N.F.L." *New York Times*, December 25, 2015.

Das, Andrew. "Chelsea Manager May Allow Doctor Back on the Bench." *New York Times*, August 15, 2015.

Davis, Seth. "The Demons of Rex Chapman." *Sports Illustrated*, July 27, 2015, 47.
Dewey, Caitlin. "Tending to a New Goal." *Washington Post*, November 3, 2013.
Diamos, Jason. "Injured Lindros Ponders the Future." *New York Times*, March 19, 2006.
Diehl, Erika A. "What's All the Headache: Reform Needed to Cope with the Effects of Concussions in Football." *Journal of Law and Health* 23, no. 1 (2010): 83–124.
DiSalvo, David. "Is Malcolm Gladwell Right, Should College Football Be Banned to Save Brains?" *Forbes*, July 21, 2013. Last viewed April 5, 2014. http://www.forbes.com/sites/daviddisalvo/2013/07/21/is-malcolm-gladwell-right-should-college-football-be-banned.
Dohrmann, George. "A Coach Unbalanced." *Sports Illustrated*, December 1, 2014, 54–60.
Dolnick, Sam. "Russian Biathlon Coach Had Suspicions, Too." *New York Times*, February 7, 2014.
Dougherty, Mike. "A Sport at a Crossroad." *Journal News* (A Gannett Company), October 20, 2013.
*Economist.* "Athlete's Dilemma." July 20, 2013, 71.
———. "Concussion: Bang to Rights." March 5, 2016, 73–74, Science and Technology section.
———. "Doping in Sport: A Cold-War Chill." November 14, 2015, 51.
———. "Schools and Hard Knocks." March 5, 2016, 14.
———. "Testing Times." July 20, 2013, 12.
Eder, Steve. "Labor Case Filed by Injured Player in '70s Has Echoes Today." *New York Times*, April 22, 2014.
———. "Lawyer Says the Yankees Misled Rodriguez about His Injuries." *New York Times*, August 18, 2013.
———. "M.L.B. Seeks Records on Rodriguez Doctor." *New York Times*, October 15, 2013.
———. "Rodriguez Sues, Targeting Baseball and Medical Treatment." *New York Times*, October 5, 2013.
Editorial Board. "Can Russia Clean Up in Time for Rio?" *New York Times*, May 13, 2016.
———. "Shamelessly 'Ashamed' in Moscow." *New York Times*, May 17, 2016.
Editorial Sunday Review. "Head Trauma Haunts the Gridiron." *New York Times*, October 15, 2016.
Epstein, David. "Conclusions? Too Early." *Sports Illustrated*, January 21, 2013. http://www.si.com/vault/2013/01/21/106273507/conclusions-too-early.
———. "Moving the Needle." *Sports Illustrated*, October 29, 2012, 17–18.
———. "Sports Should Be Child's Play." *New York Times*, June 10, 2014.
Epstein, David, and George Dohrmann. "The Zany Story of Two Self Ordained Sports Science Entrepreneurs." *Sports Illustrated*, February 4, 2013, 58–66.
ESPN.com News Services. "Appeals Court Upholds $1 Billion Concussion Settlement." April 18, 2016. http://espn.go.com.
———. "'Fail Mary' Official Fighting Depression." January 13, 2015. Last visited January 13, 2015. www.espn.go.com.
———. "Russia Won't Be Fully Banned from Olympics." July 24, 2016. Last visited July 24, 2016. http://www.espn.go.com.
———. "Ryan Freel Had CTE, Parents Say." December 15, 2013. Last visited April 28, 2014. http://espn.go.com/espn/print?id=10142581&type-HeadlineNews&I. . .
Fainaru, Steve, and Mark Fainaru-Wada. "NFL's Progress on Concussions Blurred by Inconsistencies." December 13, 2012. www.pbs.org.
Fainaru-Wada, Mark, and Steve Fainaru. "Concerns over Lawyer Pay in NFL Deal." ESPN.com. December 16, 2013. Last viewed April 23, 2014. http://espn.go.com/espn/print?id=101462287&type=HeadlineNews&i. . .
———. "Head-on Collision." *ESPN the Magazine*, October 14, 2013, 33–40.
———. *League of Denial*. New York: Three Rivers Press, 2013.
———. "League of Denial." *Sports Illustrated*, October 7, 2013, 64–68.
Favale, Dan. "Sacramento Kings Reportedly 'Likely' to Sign Royce White to 10-Day Contract." Bleacher Report. February 26, 2014. www.bleacherreport.com.
Federal Trade Commission. Staff Letter to John E. Villafranco, Esquire. April 24, 2013.
Feinstein, John. "Strasburg Decision Is Still Haunting." *Washington Post*, September 24, 2013.

Fenno, Nathan. "Former UCLA Football Captain Sues NCAA and Pac-12 over Concussions."
  *Los Angeles Times*, October 5, 2016.
———. "Many Ex-Redskins among Those Suing NFL over Effects of Brain Injuries." *Washington Times*, June 20, 2012.
Fleming, David. "Knee-Jerk Reaction." *ESPN the Magazine*, November 26, 2012, 21.
Friend, Tom. "Pro Football; Looking at Concussions, and the Repercussions." *New York Times*,
  February 18, 1995.
Garber, Greg. "Recent Drug News Depressing." ESPN.com. August 1, 2013. http://espn.go.
  com.
———. "A Tormented Soul." ESPN.com. January 28, 2005. Last visited April 11, 2014. http://
  sports.espn.go.com/nfl/news/story?id=1972285.
George, Rachel. "Holdsclaw Indicted for Shooting Incident with Girlfriend." *USA Today*,
  February 27, 2013.
Glovin, David. "Baseball Caught Looking as Fouls Injure 1,750 Fans a Year." *Bloomberg
  Business*, September 9, 2014. Last visited December 30, 2015. www.bloomberg.com.
Graham, Pat. "Track Stars Tyson Gay, Asafa Powell, Sherone Simpson All Fail Drug Tests."
  Associated Press, July 14, 2013.
Greer, Jeff. "Kevin Ware to Transfer from Louisville." *New York Times*, March 29, 2014.
Gregory, Sean. "Can Roger Goodell Save Football?" *Time*, December 17, 2012, 36–43.
Groves, Roger. "Coming to a College Near You: More Concussion Litigation." *Forbes*, May
  25, 2016. Last visited June 10, 2016. www.forbes.com.
Haberman, Clyde. "Boxing Is a Brutal, Fading Sport, Could Football Be Next?" *International
  New York Times*, November 8, 2015.
Haislop, Tadd. "Multiple Surgeries Claim 'Parts of' Fells' Foot." *Sporting News*, October 16,
  2015. Last visited December 15, 2015. www.sportingnews.com.
Halberstam, David. *The Best and the Brightest.* New York: Random House, 1969.
Hall-Flavin, D. K. "Borderline Personality Disorder: A Clinical Perspective." BPDFamily.com.
  March 8, 2012. www.bpdfamily.com.
Hamilton, Tracee. "Athletes Continue to Prove That They Need a Boost in Supplementary
  Education." *Washington Post*, July 30, 2013.
———. "If RGIII Gets the Green Light, Fans Should Buckle Up." *Washington Post*, December
  12, 2012.
———. "Redskins Fail to Learn from RGIII Injury." *Washington Post*, March 22, 2013.
———. "We Can Handle the Truth—Really." *Washington Post*, July 19, 2013.
Hart, Patricia. "Field of Nightmares." *Texas Monthly*, May 2006. Last visited December 15,
  2015. www.texasmonthly.com.
Harvard University Football Players Study. "Protecting and Promoting the Health of NFL
  Players: Legal and Ethical Analysis and Recommendations." November 17, 2016. football-
  playershealth.harvard.edu.
Heflick, Nathan A. "Man Up Roethlisberger, It Was Only a Concussion." *Psychology Today*,
  November 30, 2009.
Hobson, Will. "Alerted to Doping in '10, Wada Didn't Investigate." *Washington Post*, June 3,
  2016.
———. "Federations Scramble on How to Handle Russian Athletes." *Washington Post*, June
  27, 2016.
———. "IOC Doping Crackdown Could Lead to Athlete Bans." *Washington Post*, May 17,
  2016.
———. "Many Hurdles Must Be Cleared to Ban Russia for Doping." *Washington Post*, May
  22, 2016.
Hoffer, Richard. "Bittersweet Science." *Sports Illustrated*, December 3, 2012, 15.
Hoffman, Benjamin. "Rule Revisions on Slide Seem to Muddy Issue." *New York Times*, February 26, 2016.
Howard, Johnette. "Why Sports Can Be a Breeding Ground for Dangerous MRSA Infections."
  ESPN.com. October 16, 2015. Last visited December 15, 2015. espn.go.com.
Howe, P. David. *Sport, Professionalism, and Pain: Ethnographies of Injury and Risk.* New
  York: Routledge, 2004.

Hussain, Rummana. "Hoge Wins Lawsuit against Doctor." *Chicago Tribune*, July 22, 2000.

Janes, Chelsea. "Addressing a Problem Head-On." *Washington Post*, April 24, 2014.

———. "Fears of Concussions Lead to Heading Bans." *Washington Post*, June 1, 2014.

———. "MPSSAA to Implement Safe Tackling Program." *Washington Post*, May 6, 2014.

———. "Reducing the Number of Concussions in High School Girls' Soccer Is a Daunting Task." *Washington Post*, April 24, 2014.

Jani (Estate of Mike Webster) v. NFL Bell/Rozelle Pension Fund, 209 Fed. Appx. 305 (4th Cir. 2006).

Jauhar, Sandeep. "EKG Screening for College Athletes." *New York Times*, January 26, 2016.

Jenkins, Sally. "Chamique Holdsclaw Confronts Her 'Little Secret' of Depression." *Washington Post*, May 17, 2012.

———. "For NFL, Protocol Reveals a Disconnect." *Washington Post*, December 5, 2015.

———. "Holdsclaw's Rocky Road to a Clear Head." *Washington Post*, May 28, 2012.

———. "IOC's Sleight of Hand: Focusing on Doping in Lieu of Human Rights." *Washington Post*, May 19, 2016.

———. "The NFL Acts as If It's above Science and the Law—and That's Unacceptable." *Washington Post*, May 25, 2016.

———. "The NFL Players Will Want to Keep an Eye on the Huff Case." *Washington Post*, September 15, 2016.

———. "On Head Trauma, Goodell Couches Neglect in Nonsense." *Washington Post*, January 6, 2016.

———. "Tackling the Problem of Kids' Football." *Washington Post*, October 3, 2013.

———. "To Understand Vonn's Greatness, Start at Nexus of Speed and Fear." *Washington Post*, February 9, 2013.

———. "USADA's Campaign Is Far from Fair." *Washington Post*, August 25, 2012.

———. "WADA Report Misses the Mark by Focusing on Wrong Targets." *Washington Post*, December 10, 2016.

Jenkins, Sally, and Rick Maese. "Do No Harm: Medical Care in the NFL Plays to a Different Standard, Often Yielding Troubling Results." *Washington Post*, March 17, 2013.

———. "Football Is the (Dangerous) Family Business." *Washington Post*, July 22, 2013.

———. "In the NFL Culture, Pain and Drugs Are the Norm." *Washington Post*, April 14, 2013.

Jones, Chris. "Crime and Punishment." *ESPN the Magazine*, June 10, 2013, 124.

———. "Magic Mark." *ESPN the Magazine*, June 9, 2014, 136.

———. "Status Update." *ESPN the Magazine*, March 18, 2013, 24.

Jones, Mike. "As Griffin Recovers, Who's Responsible Going Forward?" *Washington Post*, March 29, 2013.

———. "Old School Player, New Reality." *Washington Post*, August 23, 2013.

———. "Shanahan: Robert Griffin III Has 'Mild LCL' Sprain." *Washington Post*, December 10, 2012. http://www.washingtonpost.com/blogs/football-insider/wp/2012/12/10/shanahan-robert-griffin-iii-has-mild-lcl-sprain/.

Just, Amie. "Scurry's Next Big Save: Women's Brain Health." *Washington Post*, June 20, 2016.

Karkazis, Katrina, and Rebecca Jordan-Young. "The Trouble with Too Much T." *New York Times*, April 10, 2014.

Keating, Peter. "Who's Cheating Who?" *ESPN the Magazine*, September 2, 2013, 14.

Kennedy, Kostya. "Brotherly Love." *Sports Illustrated*, October 22, 2001.

Kepner, Tyler. "As Baseball Playoffs Begin, an Issue That Has Not Left the Park." *New York Times*, October 4, 2016.

———. "It's Unsafe at Second, and Some Want New Rules for Slides." *New York Times*, October 11, 2015.

———. "The Play at the Plate: Safer." *New York Times*, December 11, 2013.

———. "A Slugger Fights for the Yankees, but Mostly against Them." *New York Times*, August 18, 2013.

Khurshudyan, Isabelle. "Capitals' Diet Now Includes More Than Just Winning." *Washington Post*, December 10, 2015.

Kilgore, Adam. "Ex-players Fight the NHL Yet Try to Remain Loyal to Game." *Washington Post*, May 26, 2016.

———. "Huff Set to Return Home as Dispute over His Care is Mediated." *Washington Post*, September 17, 2016.

———. "Medical Marijuana and the NFL." *Washington Post*, June 6, 2016.

———. "Nats Bullish on Barrett after Bout with 'the Yips.'" *Washington Post*, February 24, 2014.

———. "NHL's Motion To Dismiss Suit Denied." *Washington Post*, May 19, 2016.

———. "Truth about Player Safety, and Consequences." *Washington Post*, November 24, 2015.

———. "Wilson's Dangerous Concussion Claim." *Washington Post*, August 28, 2015.

Kilgore, Adam, and James Wagner. "Gio Gonzalez Will Not Be Suspended in Biogenesis Investigation (Updated)." *Washington Post*, August 5, 2013. Last visited February 20, 2014. www.washingtonpost.com.

Kindred, David. "Fantasy League." *Washington Post*, January 20, 2013.

Klein, Jeff Z. "Boogaard Lawsuit May Shake Up Hockey." *New York Times*, September 26, 2012.

———. "Coaches Defy Doctors after Players' Concussions, Study Finds." *New York Times*, November 20, 2012.

———. "The Science behind a Call for Safer Hockey." *New York Times*, October 2, 2013.

———. "Wave of Concussions Hits the N.H.L." *New York Times*, February 26, 2013.

———. "Who Is Susceptible to Concussions?" *New York Times*, March 9, 2014.

Klein, Jeff Z., and Ken Belson. "N.H.L. Promoted Violence for Profit Regardless of Health Risk, Players' Suit Says." *New York Times*, April 11, 2014.

Klein, Jeff Z., and Stu Hackel. "A Stricter Standard for Safety's Sake." *New York Times*, December 29, 2013.

Kretchmer, Arthur. "Butkus: One Season and One Injury with the Meanest Man Alive." *Playboy*, October 1971. Last viewed April 30, 2014. http://thestacks.deadspin.com/butkus-one-season-and-one-injury-with-the-meanest-man-1245969242.

Kwayie, Mame M. "Chamique Holdsclaw Speaks on Her Depression." *Ebony*, August 14, 2014. Last visited December 30, 2014. www.ebony.com.

Latimer, Sarah. "NFL Disputes ESPN Report on Funding of Brain Study." *Washington Post*, December 23, 2015.

Lattman, Peter, and Natasha Singer. "Learning the Hard Way about a Banned Ingredient." *New York Times*, March 17, 2013.

Layden, Tim. "Bear Down." *Sports Illustrated*, June 27, 2016, 17.

Lipsyte, Robert. "Backtalk; Harnisch a Reluctant Role Model." *New York Times*, November 22, 1998.

Local8Now.com. "Crimetracker: Former Vol QB Arrested for DUI." July 28, 2013. Last visited January 21, 2015. www.local8now.com.

Lundberg, George D. "The N.F.L.'s Collision with the Future." *New York Times*, January 5, 2016.

Lyall, Sarah. "White Is a Player with a Cause, but without a Team." *New York Times*, December 9, 2013.

Macur, Juliet. "Anti-doping Agency Exposed Armstrong, but What about the Others?" *New York Times*, October 21, 2013.

———. "Anti-doping Lab's Flaws Put Olympics in Bind." *New York Times*, November 16, 2013.

———. "Armstrong Faces New Doping Charges." *New York Times*, June 13, 2012.

———. "Cycling May Turn Armstrong into a Sympathetic Figure Yet." *New York Times*, July 17, 2015.

———. "Doping Rules Are Tougher Only If Applied." *New York Times*, November 12, 2013.

———. "Gaining Rights amid Guarded Words." *New York Times*, March 28, 2014.

———. "Revelations of State-Backed Doping Should Bar Russia from Rio Olympics." *New York Times*, May 12, 2016.

———. "A Second Chance for Sebastian Coe to Clean Up His Sport." *New York Times*, January 14, 2016.

———. "Six Concussions Later, Jordan Reed Fears Heartache of Losing Football." *New York Times*, October 31, 2016.

———. "There's a Dark Cloud over Our Sport." *New York Times*, February 7, 2014.

Maese, Rick. "Chastain Will Donate Brain for Research." *Washington Post*, March 4, 2016.

———. "Concussions, Mental Health Are Linked." *Washington Post*, December 7, 2014.

———. "Ex-players: NFL Pushed Risky Drug Use." *Washington Post*, May 21, 2014.

———. "In U.S., Drug Testing Is Quite a Serious Business." *Washington Post*, July 18, 2016.

———. "Navy Player Is in Coma: Family Defends Program." *Washington Post*, March 25, 2014.

———. "Navy Running Back McKamey, 19, Dies after Days in Coma." *Washington Post*, March 26, 2014.

———. "NFL, Military Partner on Concussions." *Washington Post*, June 13, 2013.

———. "$1 Billion Concussion Settlement Is Upheld." *Washington Post*, April 19, 2016.

———. "Players Come Together to Take on NFL." *Washington Post*, June 7, 2008.

———. "Report: NFL Should Overhaul Player Care." *Washington Post*, November 17, 2016.

———. "Report: NFL Tried Influencing NIH Study." *Washington Post*, May 24, 2016.

———. "Study Stresses Impact of Subconcussive Trauma." *Washington Post*, April 1, 2016.

———. "Survey: Players Distrust Team Medical Staff." *Washington Post*, February 1, 2013.

———. "Track Officials Ban Russia from Games over Doping." *Washington Post*, June 18, 2016.

———. "Trying to Protect Players from the Ground Up." *Washington Post*, October 25, 2013.

Maese, Rick, and Matt Bonesteel. "Investigation Exposes Full Scope of Russian Doping." *Washington Post*, December 10, 2016.

Maese, Rick, and Cindy Boren. "NFL and Retired Players Settle Concussion Lawsuits." *Washington Post*, August 30, 2013.

Majerske, Cynthia W., Jason P. Mihalik, Dianxu Ren, Michael W. Collins, Cara Camiolo Reddy, Mark R. Lovell, and Amy K. Wagner. "Concussion in Sports: Postconcussive Activity Levels, Symptoms, and Neurocognitive Performance." *Journal of Athletic Training* 43, no. 3 (May–June 2008): 265–74.

Mangan, J. A., ed. *Militarism, Sport, Europe: War without Weapons.* New York: Routledge, 2003.

Maske, Mark. "Congress Might Bypass NFLPA on HGH Issues." *Washington Post*, January 29, 2013.

———. "Discipline Dropped in Saints Bounty Case." *Washington Post*, December 12, 2012.

———. "Goodell Defends NFL Report." *Washington Post*, May 25, 2016.

———. "NFL Changes, for Safety's Sake." *Washington Post*, March 25, 2013.

———. "NFL Stands by CTE Admission." *Washington Post*, March 16, 2016.

———. "NFL Still Has Lack of Clarity on CTE Link." *Washington Post*, March 24, 2015.

———. "NFL's New Rules Aim to Curb Injury." *Washington Post*, April 17, 2012.

———. "Not a Healthy Way to Make a Living." *Washington Post*, November 10, 2013.

———. "Not on the Sidelines." *Washington Post*, June 8, 2016.

———. "Redskins Fined $20,000 for Robert Griffin Concussion Announcement." *Washington Post*, October 19, 2012.

———. "Study: Increased Dementia in Ex-players." *Washington Post*, October 1, 2009.

Maske, Mark, and Mike Jones. "Adderall Use Said to Be behind the Suspension of C. Griffin." *Washington Post*, December 6, 2012.

Mather, Victor, and Christopher Clarey. "Governing Body's Move Could Jar 2016 Olympics." *New York Times*, November 14, 2015.

Mathews, Jay. "At Many Leading Schools Football Fails to Make the Cut." *Washington Post*, April 7, 2013.

McCann, Michael. "Shield Law." *Sports Illustrated*, April 4, 2016, 12.

McCrory, P., A. Collie, V. Anderson, and G. Davis. "Can We Manage Sport Related Concussions in Children the Same as in Adults?" *British Journal of Sports Medicine* 38, no. 5 (2004): 516–19.

McDonnell, Terry. "As Time Goes By." *Sports Illustrated*, July 9, 2012.

McMurphy, Brett. "McMurphy's Law: Inconsistency Epitomizes Drug Policies." CBS Sports, November 1, 2011. www.cbssports.com.

Mehlman, Maxwell J. *The Price of Perfection: Individualism and Society in the Era of Biomedical Enhancement.* Baltimore: Johns Hopkins University Press, 2009.

Miah, Andy. *Genetically Modified Athletes.* New York: Routledge, 2004.

Mihoces, Gary. "Judge Denies NHL Bid to Halt Concussion Lawsuit." *USA Today*, March 25, 2015. www.usatoday.com.

———. "Kickoff Returns, Concussions Drop in 2011 after Rule Change." *USA Today*, February 2, 2012.

Miller, James Andrew. "N.F.L. Pressure Said to Lead ESPN to Quit Film Project." *New York Times*, August 23, 2013.

Miller, Stuart. "Safety Sometimes Prevails over Accuracy in Calling the First Out of a Double Play." *New York Times*, May 4, 2014.

Mitchell, George. "Drugs in Sports an Ongoing Menace." *Washington Post*, January 10, 2014.

MLBPA/MLB News Release. "MLB, MLBPA Adopt Slide Rule on Double Plays, Pace of Game Changes." February 26, 2016.

Muir, Allan. "NHL Hit by New Concussion Lawsuit Filed by 29 Players." *Sports Illustrated*, February 10, 2015. www.si.com.

Nathan, Alan M., Lloyd V. Smith, Warren L. Faber, and Daniel A. Russell. "Corked Bats, Juiced Balls, and Humidors: The Physics of Cheating in Baseball." *American Journal of Physics* 79, no. 6 (June 2011): 575–80.

NCAA. "Football Injuries." PDF. Last visited June 15, 2016. www.ncaa.org.

———. "Understanding the NCAA's Drug Testing Policies." Last visited February 26, 2014. www.ncas.org/health-and-safety/policy/drug-testing.

NCAA Press Release. "NCAA Reaches Proposed Settlement in Concussion Lawsuit." July 29, 2014.

*New York Times.* Special to the *New York Times.* "Staubach Retirement Expected; Concussions a Concern." March 15, 1980.

NFL. "Report: Adderall Remains Drug of Choice for Many NFL Players." Last visited February 24, 2014. www.nfl.com/news/story/Oap1000000242017/article/report-adderall-remains-drug-of-choice-for-many-nfl-players.

Nguyen, Courtney. "What's the Secret to Rafael Nadal's Rapid Recovery from His Need Surgery." SI.com, October 8, 2013.

Nocera, Joe. "Baseball's New Policy Encourages Adding Only a Little New Protection." *New York Times*, December 19, 2015.

———. "A Fan Injured by a Hard Foul Challenges Assumption That Teams Can Avoid Liability." *New York Times*, November 21, 2015.

———. "A Fine Line Separates Ball and Fan." *New York Times*, April 16, 2016.

———. "N.F.L.'s Bogus Settlement for Brain-Damaged Former Players." *New York Times*, August 11, 2015.

———. "Senseless Injury." *New York Times*, November 4, 2016.

Nutt, Amy Ellis. "Heading a Soccer Ball Can Cause Brain Damage." *Washington Post*, October 26, 2016.

O'Brien, Richard. "Emile Griffith." *Sports Illustrated*, August 5, 2013, 17.

O'Connor, Anahad. "Trying to Reduce Head Injuries, Youth Football Limits Practices." *New York Times*, June 13, 2012.

Ollove, Michael. "Schools Move to Protect Athletes, but They Don't Provide Trainers." *Washington Post*, October 7, 2014.

Olney, Buster. "Just Say Yes." *ESPN the Magazine*, December 24, 2012, 60–61.

Olson, Jeff. "A Victory That Means Much More." *Sports Illustrated*, December 17, 2012.

Omalu, Bennet. "Don't Let Kids Play Football." *New York Times*, December 7, 2015.

Padawer, Ruth. "Too Fast to Be Female." *New York Times Magazine*, July 3, 2016, MM32.

Palmer, Brian. "Armstrong Case Illustrates Doping's Enduring Appeal to Cyclists." *Washington Post*, January 1, 2013.

Parry, John W. *Disability Discrimination Law, Evidence and Testimony.* Chicago: American Bar Association, 2008.
———. *Mental Disability, Violence, Future Dangerousness: Myths behind the Presumption of Guilt.* Lanham, Md.: Rowman & Littlefield, 2013.
Passan, Jeff. "Book Excerpt: Are High School Pitchers Throwing Too Hard Too Soon." *Sports Illustrated*, April 4, 2016, 59. From *The Arm: Inside the Billion-Dollar Mystery of the Most Valuable Commodity in Sports.* New York: HarperCollins, 2016.
Pearce, Matt. "Diana Nyad Completes Cuba to U.S. Swim, Reaches a Lifelong Dream." *Los Angeles Times*, September 2, 2013.
Pelissero, Tom. "Players to Be Blood-Tested in Camp for HGH Study." *USA Today*, July 22, 2013.
Pells, Eddie, and Pat Graham. "Tyson Gay Tests Positive for Banned Substances: 2 Other Track Stars Fail Drug Tests." Associated Press, July 14, 2013.
Pennington, Bill. "Hidden Threats to Young Athletes." *New York Times*, May 12, 2013.
———. "In a Moment It Can All Be Gone." *New York Times*, April 5, 2013.
———. "Odell Beckham Jr. Suspended for One Game." *New York Times*, December 21, 2015.
———. "The Trusted Grown-Ups Who Steal Millions from Youth Sports." *New York Times*, July 7, 2016.
———. "To Calm Jittery Nerves, Keegan Bradley Embraces Them." *New York Times*, July 15, 2016.
Persky, Anna Stolley. "Playing It Safe: Are Concussions Ruining Sports?" *Washington Lawyer*, April 2013, 22–28.
Pilon, Mary, and Ken Belson. "Seau Suffered from Brain Disease." *New York Times*, January 10, 2013.
Pilon, Mary, and Gina Kolata. "New to Most Fans, IGF-1 Has Long Been Banned as a Performance Enhancer." *New York Times*, January 29, 2013.
Pollack, Andrew. "Effects of Meldonium on Athletes Are Hazy." *New York Times*, March 10, 2016.
Powell, Michael. "After Spree of Doping, a Time to Reform." *New York Times*, December 10, 2016.
———. "In Russian Doping Scandal, Time for a Punishment to Fit the Crime." *New York Times*, June 16, 2016.
———. "Jake Arrieta Shows He's Human, despite Accusations to the Contrary." *New York Times*, April 29, 2016.
———. "Rose's Ban, a Product of His Flaws, Highlights Others' Faults." *New York Times*, December 20, 2015.
———. "Winter Sports Athletes Ask for the Doping Spotlight." *New York Times*, March 29, 2016.
Price, S. L. "It Would Hurt More Not to Play." *Sports Illustrated*, December 7, 2015, 58.
———. "Judge Ye Not." *Sports Illustrated*, August 13, 2012, 76.
Prine, Carl. "Bloody Sundays." *IRE Journal* 28, no. 4 (July–August 2005). Last visited May 16, 2014. http://www.questia.com/read/1P3-897062681/bloody-sundays.
Prunty, Brendan. "Anyone Have a Lozenge?" *New York Times*, November 22, 2015.
Rapp, Geoffrey. "Blue Sky Steroids." *Journal of Criminal Law & Criminology* 99, no. 3 (2009): 599.
Rawlings v. Cleveland Indians Baseball Co., Inc., 2015-Ohio-4587 (November 5, 2015) as reported by Dan Trevas, Court News Ohio, November 5, 2015. Last visited January 7, 2016. www.courtnewsohio.gov/cases.
Reevell, Patrick. "New Ban on a Drug Hits Russian Athletes Hard." *New York Times*, March 10, 2016.
———. "New Drug Guidelines May Overturn Suspensions." *New York Times*, April 14, 2016.
———. "Russia Says Uncertainty about Doping Results Led to Withdrawal of Teams." *New York Times*, April 9, 2016.
Reid, Jason. "NFL's Message to Meriweather Contains No Ambiguity." *Washington Post*, October 22, 2013.

———. "Seau's Death Forces Uncomfortable Questions for Football Fans." *Washington Post*, May 13, 2012.

Rhoden, William C. "Civility Need Not Be Excluded from the Culture of the N.F.L." *New York Times*, November 10, 2013.

———. "On the Court, Finding an Outlet, and a Voice." *New York Times*, February 26, 2012.

———. "Sports of the Times—George Atkinson's Old-School Values." *New York Times*, December 8, 2009. Accessed December 8, 2012. www.nytimes.com/2009/12/08/sports/football/08rhoden.html ?r=1&ref=sports.

———. "When Players Put Team First, They Put Themselves at Risk." *New York Times*, October 25, 2015.

Ritholtz, Barry. "Congratulations, You Were Drafted! Prepare to Go Broke." *Big Picture* (blog), June 1, 2014. http://ritholtz.com/2014/06/congratulations-you-were-drafted-prepare-to-go-broke-2/.

Rohan, Tim. "Antidoping Agency Delays Publication of Research." *New York Times*, August 22, 2013.

Rosenberg, Michael. "Knees and Wants." *Sports Illustrated*, December 9, 2013, 70.

Rothman, Steven M. "America's Concussion Obsession." *New York Times*, December 22, 2015.

Ruiz, Rebecca R. "After Russian Ban, I.O.C. President Addresses Antidoping Efforts." *New York Times*, June 21, 2016.

———. "Drugs Pervade Sport in Russia, World Anti-Doping Agency Report Finds." *New York Times*, November 9, 2015.

———. "Justice Department Opens Investigation into Russian Doping Scandal." *New York Times*, May 17, 2016.

———. "Mystery in Sochi Doping Case Lies with Tamper-Proof Bottle." *New York Times*, May 13, 2016.

———. "Officials Accused of Extortion to Clear Athletes Who Doped." *New York Times*, January 14, 2016.

———. "Olympics History Rewritten: New Doping Tests Topple the Podium." *New York Times*, November 21, 2016.

———. "Rio Doping Lab Suspended as Games Near." *New York Times*, June 25, 2016.

———. "Russian Sports Doping: Explained." *New York Times*, May 16, 2016.

———. "Russia's Track and Field Team Barred from Rio Olympics." *New York Times*, June 17, 2016.

———. "Sports Arbitration Court Ruling against German Speedskater Claudia Pechstein Is Upheld." *New York Times*, June 7, 2016.

———. "U.S. Athletes Weigh a Boycott over Russian Doping." *New York Times*, December 4, 2016.

———. "WADA Tells Lawmakers It Lacked 'Clear Authority' to Investigate Russian Sports." *New York Times*, July 9, 2016.

Ruiz, Rebecca R., and Ben Rothenberg. "Russian Hackers Draw Attention to Drug-Use Exemptions for Athletes." *New York Times*, September 14, 2016.

Ruiz, Rebecca R., and Michael Schwirtz. "Russian Insider Says State-Run Doping Fueled Olympic Gold." *New York Times*, May 12, 2016.

Rushin, Steve. "Brain Traumatic." *Sports Illustrated*, October 21, 2013, 64.

Sandomir, Richard, and Andrew Jacobs. "Russian Track Team to Miss Olympics, American Audiences? Not Likely." *New York Times*, June 19, 2016.

Sands, Robert R. *Anthropology, Sport and Culture.* New York: Praeger, 1999.

Saxon, Mark. "Chase Utley Suspended 2 Games for Slide into Reuben Tejada, Will Appeal." ESPN.com. October 12, 2015. Last visited December 29, 2015. www.espn.go.com.

Schmidt, Michael S. "Ripples of H.G.H. Test in England Are Being Felt across the U.S." *New York Times*, February 28, 2010.

Schonbrun, Zack. "'You Can't Put Ice over a Migraine,' a Lurking Malady in the N.F.L." *New York Times*, December 13, 2015.

Schrotenboer, Brent. "First Year of HGH Testing in NFL Catches No One." *USA Today*, February 2, 2015. Last visited December 17, 2015. www.usatoday.com.

Schwarz, Alan. "Dementia Debate Could Intensify." *New York Times*, October 1, 2009.

———. "Dementia Risk Seen in Players in N.F.L. Study." *New York Times*, September 30, 2009.

———. "House Panel Criticizes New N.F.L. Doctors." *New York Times*, May 24, 2010.

———. "Lawsuit Cites Mishandling of Football Concussions." *New York Times*, March 18, 2010.

———. "Learning from Sadness." *New York Times*, November 7, 2010.

———. "N.F.L. Acknowledges Long-Term Concussion Effects." *New York Times*, December 21, 2009.

———. "N.F.L.'s Dementia Study Has Flaws, Experts Say." *New York Times*, October 27, 2009.

———. "N.F.L.'s Influence on Safety at Youth Levels Is Cited." *New York Times*, October 30, 2009.

———. "On Linking Brain Damage and Behavior." *New York Times*, June 25, 2010.

———. "Rules Trickle Down; Cash Won't." *New York Times*, August 30, 2013.

———. "A Suicide, a Last Request, a Family's Questions." *New York Times*, February 22, 2011.

———. "Suicide Reveals Signs of a Disease Seen in N.F.L." *New York Times*, September 13, 2010.

———. "Uncertainty over Whether N.F.L. Settlement's Money Will Last." *New York Times*, January 29, 2014.

Schwarz, Alan, Walt Bogdanich, and Jacqueline Williams. "N.F.L. Concussion Studies Found to Have Deep Flaws." *New York Times*, March 25, 2016.

*Science Daily.* "Youth Baseball Throwing Arm Injuries Are Rising Dramatically." March 11, 2010. Last visited May 20, 2014. www.sciencedaily.com/releases/2010/03/100310083443.htm.

Scorecard. "The Race Goes On." *Sports Illustrated*, August 31, 2015, 16.

Seifert, Kevin. "Chop Blocks Eliminated, PAT Snaps from 15 Permanent." ESPN.com. March 22, 2016.

———. "Roger Goodell Says CTE Link Consistent with NFL's Position." ESPN.com. March 23, 2016.

Seppa, Nathan. "Contact Sports and the Risk of Staph Infections." *Washington Post*, October 21, 2014.

Shear, M. D., and Ken Belson. "Obama's Conference on Concussions Highlights a Paradox for the N.F.L." *New York Times*, May 30, 2014.

Sheinin, David. "Arms Torn to Shreds." *Washington Post*, May 4, 2014.

———. "IAAF Bans Russian Track Team." *Washington Post*, November 14, 2014.

Shipley, Amy. "Growing Old Gracefully." *Washington Post*, May 20, 2012.

———. "A Shadow of Doubt." *Washington Post*, July 5, 2012.

Shpigel, Ben. "Football Faces 'Turning Point' on Safety Risk." *New York Times*, June 20, 2012.

Smith, Adrian, and Dilwyn Porter. *Sport and National Identity in the Post-War World.* New York: Psychology Press, 2004.

*Sports Illustrated.* "Go Figure." March 3, 2014, 16.

———. Special Report. "10 Years After." June 4, 2012.

———. "They Said It." July 22, 1968.

———. "Walk Off." March 18, 2018, 18.

Steinberg, Dan. "Norman: I'm Like a Rogue Savage." *Washington Post*, June 10, 2016.

Strauss, Ben. "A Fight to Save College Athletes from the Ordeal of Injury Costs." *New York Times*, April 25, 2014.

———. "Six Concussion Suits Are Filed against Colleges and N.C.A.A." *New York Times*, May 17, 2016.

Suttie, Ian Dishart. *The Origins of Love and Hate.* London: Kegan Paul, Trench, Trubner, 1935.

Svrluga, Barry. "Gordon's Suspension Alters Marlins' Plans." *Washington Post*, April 30, 2016.

Svrluga, Barry, and Mark Maske. "NFL, MLB to Probe Allegations in Report." *Washington Post*, December 28, 2015.

Tanner, Lindsey. "Athletes' Deaths in Workouts Prompt New Guidelines." Associated Press in the *Washington Post*, July 3, 2012.

Taylor, Phil. "The Influence of Anxiety." *Sports Illustrated*, January 21, 2013, 70.

Terrell, Katherine. "New Orleans Saints Bounty Scandal Timeline." *New Orleans Times-Picayune*, December 12, 2012. Last visited April 29, 2014. NOLA.com.

Thomas, Katie. "Doping Scandals in Tennis Are Few, but Concerns Persist." *New York Times*, September 10, 2009.

Torre, Pablo S. "The Mystery Pick Is Royce White." *Sports Illustrated*, July 2, 2012, 44.

Tracy, Marc. "Concussions Ended His Football Dreams. Now He Helps Others Achieve Theirs." *New York Times*, November 20, 2015.

Tucker, Ross, and Jonathan Dugas. "How to Fight Doping in Sports." *New York Times*, August 1, 2015.

Turner, Dan. "Armstrong: Nobody's Buying the Witch-Hunt Line, Lance." *Los Angeles Times*, August 24, 2012.

Verducci, Tom. "As Fernandez Goes Down, Here's a Solution to Arm Injury Epidemic." *Sports Illustrated*, May 13, 2014. http://sportsillustrated.cnn.com/mlb/news/20140513/jose-fernandez-miami-marlins-injury/.

———. "Here We Go Again." *Sports Illustrated*, November 19, 2012, 22.

———. "Swampland Chronicles." *Sports Illustrated*, February 11, 2013, 16–17.

Vinton, Nathaniel. "Concussions Are on the Rise in the NFL: League Releases Data That Shows 58% Increase in Regular Season Concussions." *Daily News*, January 30, 2016. Last visited June 15, 2016. www.dailynews.com.

Wagner, James. "Nats' Gonzalez Quiet over Report." *Washington Post*, February 3, 2013.

Waldstein, David. "Fan Injuries Spur M.L.B. to Call For Netting at Stadiums." *New York Times*, December 10, 2015.

*Wall Street Journal*. "In the NFL, Which Body Part Gets Hurt the Most?" January 27, 2014. wsj.com.

Wang, Gene M. "SN Concussion Report: NFL Could Lose Billions in Player Lawsuits." *Sporting News*, August 22, 2012. Last visited April 21, 2014. http://sportingnews.com/nfl/story/2012-08-22/nfl-concussion-. . .

———. "Terps' Mincy Out for Year with ACL." *Washington Post*, December 1, 2013.

Wang, Gene, and Mark Maske. "Meriweather: 'You've Got to Tear People's ACLs and Mess Up Knees' on Hits." *Washington Post*, October 29, 2013.

Washington Nationals. "Aaron Barrett Stats Summary." Last visited January 22, 2015. http://washington.nationals.mlb.com/team/player.jsp?player_id=502578#gameType=%27R%27.

*Washington Post*. Editorial. "Clarity about Concussions." June 22, 2016.

———. NFL Notebook. "NFL VP Concedes CTE, Sport Are Linked." March 15, 2016.

Wasterlain, A. S., et al. "The Systemic Effects of Platelet-Rich Plasma Injection." *American Journal of Sports Medicine*, January 2013.

Wendel, Tim. "In 1968, Sports Helped Temper a Year of Rage and Upheaval." *New York Times*, February 18, 2012.

Wertheim, Jon. "McKinley's Apparent Suicide Casts Light on Athletes' Risk of Depression." *Sports Illustrated*, September 21, 2010. http://sportsillustrated.cnn.com.

———. "Prisoners of Depression." *Sports Illustrated*, September 8, 2003. http://sportsillustrated.cnn.com/vault.

———. "Trying Times." *Sports Illustrated*, December 10, 2012, 30.

———. "Why Men Cheat." *Sports Illustrated*, August 19, 2013, 17–18.

White, Joseph. "Holdsclaw Looking for Fresh Start, Traded to Los Angeles." *USA Today*, March 21, 2005.

Whitehead, Johnnie, and Dick Patrick. "How Much Is Too Much for Young Arms." *USA Today*, August 17, 2006.

Wieners, Brad. "Liestrong." *Bloomberg Businessweek*, October 17, 2012, 86.

*Wikipedia.* S.v. "List of Suspensions in the National Football League." Last visited February 24, 2014. http://en.wikipedia.org/wiki/List_of_players_and_coaches_suspended_by_the_ NFL.

Will, George F. "Out of Bounds." *Washington Post*, September 19, 2013.

Williams, Preston. "Knee Injury a 'National Epidemic' Felt Acutely in Area." *Washington Post*, January 24, 2013.

Wilson, Duff. "Medical Adviser for Baseball Lists Exaggerated Credentials." *New York Times*, March 30, 2005.

Wise, Mike. "Gregg Williams, Redskins Played an Ugly Game with Bounties." *Washington Post*, March 3, 2012.

———. "Gregg Williams's True Nature Exposed." *Washington Post*, March 2, 2012.

———. "Lance, Manti and Modern Mythmaking." *Washington Post*, January 19, 2013.

———. "Lesson of This Health Union Talk: This Isn't Really about Money." *Washington Post*, April 13, 2014.

———. "Mixed Messages Are Causing Headaches." *Washington Post*, January 29, 2013.

———. "NFL Is Losing Concussion Battle—and without a Cultural Shift, It Will Lose War." *Washington Post*, November 14, 2012.

———. "Real Chance to Make an Impact Lost with Settlement." *Washington Post*, August 30, 2013.

———. "Rose's Call to Sit Out Is Right One." *Washington Post*, May 8, 2013.

Wolff, Alexander. "The Powers That Be." *Sports Illustrated*, May 20, 2016, 14.

———. "United We Sit." *Sports Illustrated*, October 20, 2014, 64.

Yasinskas, Pat. "Report: Gregg Williams Leaving Saints." ESPN.com. January 15, 2012. Last visited April 29, 2014. http://espn.go.com.

Zillgitt, Jeff. "Rookie on a Mission." *USA Today*, February 8, 2013.

Zinser, Lynn. "Tennis Strengthens Testing for Drugs." *New York Times*, March 8, 2013.

———. "To Baseball's Chagrin, Steroid Era Goes On." *New York Times*, August 24, 2012.

# INDEX

# ABOUT THE AUTHOR

**John Weston Parry** is a lawyer, writer, and host of a website (sportpatholgies.com) that identifies and discusses health and other pathologies in America's most popular sports. He is the former director of the American Bar Association's Commission on Disability Rights (1982–2012) and editor/editor-in-chief of the *Mental and Physical Disability Law Reporter* (1979–2011). He has published numerous articles and books on mental disability and health law, diversity, and the rights of persons with disabilities, including *Mental Disability, Violence, Future Dangerousness: Myths behind the Presumption of Guilt* (Rowman & Littlefield, 2013). He is a recipient of the Manfred Guttmacher Award from the American Psychiatric Association and the American Academy of Psychiatry and Law.